# Acaricides Resistance in Ticks

Sachin Kumar
Raquel Cossío-Bayúgar
Estefan Miranda-Miranda
Anil Kumar Sharma
Ashok Kumar Chaubey
Editors

# Acaricides Resistance in Ticks

## A Global Problem

Springer

*Editors*
Sachin Kumar
Entomology Laboratory
Division of Parasitology
ICAR-Indian Veterinary Research
Institute, Izatnagar
Bareilly, Uttar Pradesh, India

Constituent Government College
Meerapur Banger
Bijnor, Uttar Pradesh, India

Estefan Miranda-Miranda
Instituto Nacional de Investigaciones
Agrícolas y Pecuarias
Mexico City, Mexico

Raquel Cossío-Bayúgar
Instituto Nacional de Investigaciones
Agrícolas y Pecuarias
Mexico City, Mexico

Anil Kumar Sharma
Uttaranchal University
Dehradun, Uttarakhand, India

Ashok Kumar Chaubey
Ch. Charan Singh University
Meerut, Uttar Pradesh, India

ISBN 978-981-97-7410-4 ISBN 978-981-97-7411-1 (eBook)
https://doi.org/10.1007/978-981-97-7411-1



This Springer imprint is published by the registered company Springer Nature Singapore Pte Ltd.
The registered company address is: 152 Beach Road, #21-01/04 Gateway East, Singapore 189721, Singapore

# Preface

Ticks are haematophagous ectoparasite of mammals, birds and reptiles, distributed worldwide and have significant medical and veterinary importance due to the direct damage they cause to their hosts and as vectors of human and animal pathogens. They are among the most competent and versatile vectors of pathogens and are second only to mosquitoes in terms of the number of human pathogens they transit, and the most important vector of pathogens affecting cattle worldwide. Direct injuries to animals can be very serious, especially in tropical climates, and are mainly observed in infestations with ixodid ticks. It is estimated the global costs of ticks and tick-borne diseases (TTBDs) in cattle range between US$ 13.9 and US$ 18.7 billion annually. Among various one-host cattle ticks, *Rhipicephalus microplus* is the most prevalent species found in different parts of the world. Widespread increases in acaricide resistance to most available acaricides threaten both global livestock industries and public health.

Apart from residue in food and environment and acaricide resistance problems in tick species, resistance monitoring tools, biochemical and molecular bioassays and resistance mechanisms, the current status of global resistant tick problem inspired the editors to utilize their vast experience on the subject to publish a book entitled *Acaricide Tick Resistance: A Global Problem*. This book is collectively written by the internationally recognized tick researchers and experts from prestigious organizations and covers in-depth information on different aspects of ticks and resistance, published by Springer Nature. This book is intended for the benefit of students, researchers, teachers, entrepreneurs and policymakers and for the advancement of tick research.


Bareilly, Uttar Pradesh, India — Sachin Kumar
Mexico City, Mexico — Raquel Cossío-Bayúgar
Mexico City, Mexico — Estefan Miranda-Miranda
Dehradun, Uttarakhand, India — Anil Kumar Sharma
Meerut, Uttar Pradesh, India — Ashok Kumar Chaubey

# Contents

# Editors and Contributors

## About the Editors

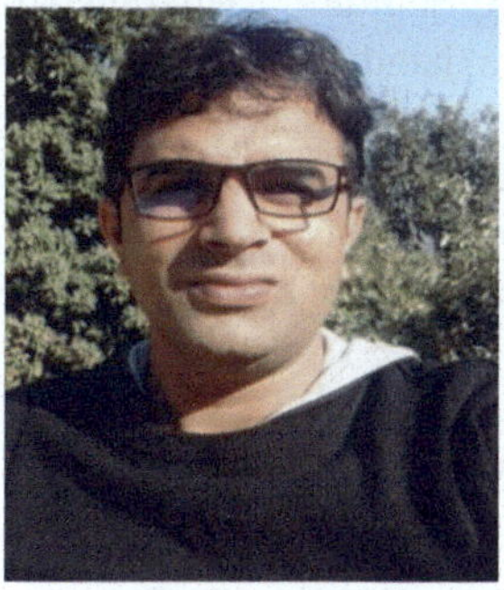

**Sachin Kumar, PhD, NPDF** is a Young Scientist in the Parasitology Division, ICAR-Indian Veterinary Research Institute, Izatnagar 243,122, Bareilly, Uttar Pradesh, India. He is exclusively working on characterization of multi-acaricide resistant tick species, resistance mechanisms, tick-borne pathogen diseases and drug development. He has characterized a number of tick populations from different states of India and has published more than 61 international research papers and holds 03 patents. He has developed an antitick natural formulation and commercialized it. He has been completed 2–3 project on cattle tick funded by the Indian Government.

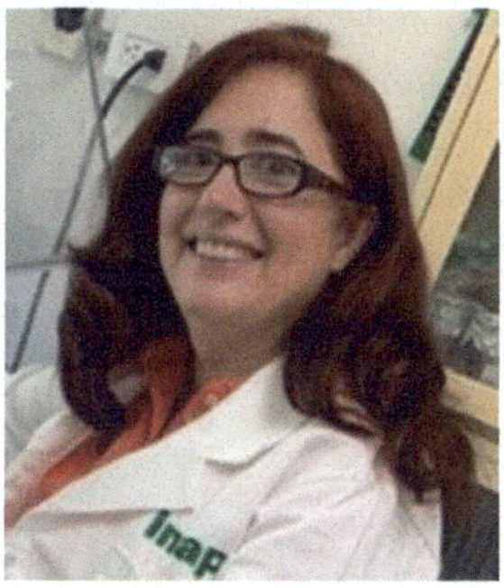


**Raquel Cossío-Bayúgar, PhD, PDF** is a Senior Scientific Researcher at the National Center for Disciplinary Research in Animal Health and Safety (CENID-SAI), Mexico. Her main area of research includes cattle tick, acaricide resistance, in vitro tick cell culture, tick physiology, immunology and tick response to pathogens, with more than 60 international research publications.

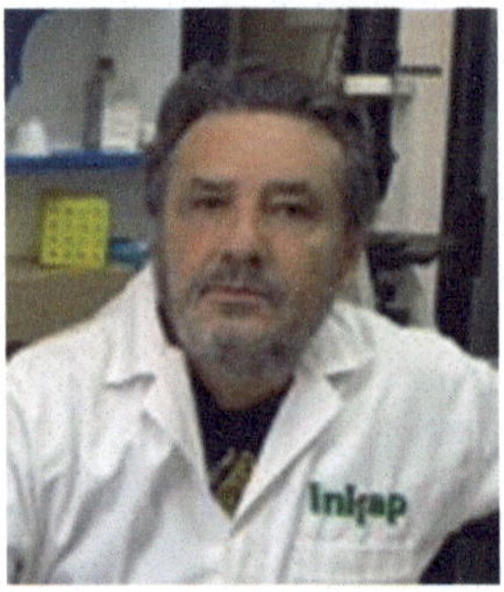

**Estefan Miranda-Miranda, PhD, PDF** has been a Senior Scientific Researcher for 35 years at the National Center for Disciplinary Research in Animal Health and Safety (CENID-SAI), Mexico. Dr. Miranda's work is focused on parasite antiparasitic resistance, molecular biology and parasite physiology. Dr. Miranda has published numerous scientific papers on the subject.

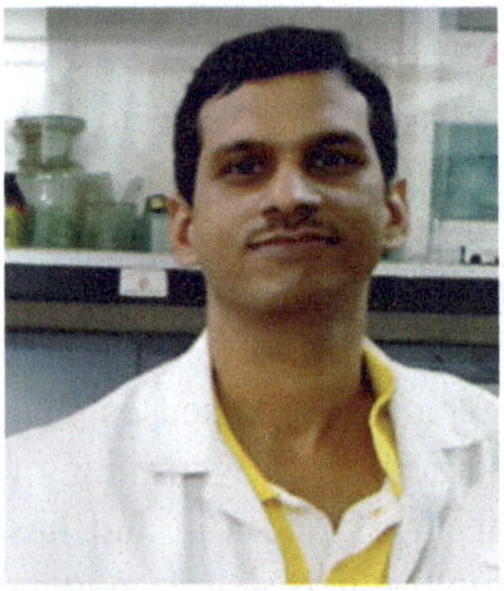

**Anil Kumar Sharma, PhD, PDF** is an Assistant Professor in School of Agriculture, Uttaranchal University, Dehradun, Uttarakhand, India. He has extensively worked on acaricide resistance, herbal drug development, resistant tick management and the development of resistance monitoring tools. He has published more than 60 international and national research articles and holds two patents. He has contributed to the development of four "Antitick Herbal Technologies" and one has been commercialized.

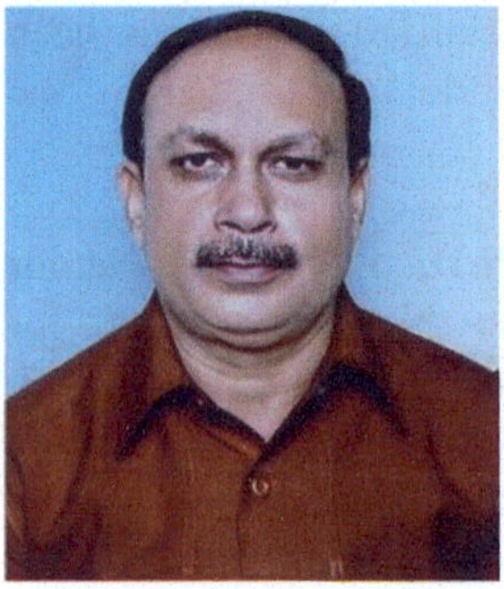

**Ashok Kumar Chaubey, PhD, FSPPS, FAIR** is a Senior Professor and Coordinator in the Department of Zoology and Environmental Science, CCS University, Meerut, Uttar Pradesh, India. He has published more than 104 national and international research papers, edited 04 books, guided 15 PhD and 52 MPhil students and completed 06 research projects. He has worked on nematology, environmental biology, zoology and helminthology.

## Contributors

**Hugo Aguilar-Diaz** National Center for Disciplinary Research in Animal Health and Safety, INIFAP, Carretera Federal Cuernavaca-Cuautla 8534, Jiutepec, Morelos, Mexico

**Imtiaz Ahmad** Department of Botany and Zoology, Bacha Khan University, Charsadda, Pakistan

**Abid Ali** Department of Zoology, Abdul Wali Khan University, Mardan, Pakistan

**Consuelo Almazán** Immunology and Vaccines Laboratory, Faculty of Natural Sciences, Autonomous University of Queretaro, Queretaro, Mexico

**Bader S. Alotaibi** Department of Clinical Laboratory Sciences, College of Applied Medical Sciences, Al-Quwayiyah, Shaqra University, Riyadh, Saudi Arabia

**Itzel Amaro-Estrada** National Center for Disciplinary Research in Animal Health and Safety, INIFAP, Carretera Federal Cuernavaca-Cuautla 8534, Jiutepec, Morelos, Mexico

**Fayaz Asad** Department of Botany and Zoology, Bacha Khan University, Charsadda, Pakistan

**Hanène Belkahia** Laboratory of Microbiology, National School of Veterinary Medicine of Sidi Thabet, University of Manouba, Sidi Thabet, Tunisia

**Edgar Castro-Saines** National Center for Disciplinary Research in Animal Health and Safety, INIFAP, Carretera Federal Cuernavaca-Cuautla 8534, Jiutepec, Morelos, Mexico

**Gajanan M. Chigure** Department of Veterinary Parasitology, College of Veterinary and Animal Sciences, Nagpur, Maharashtra, India

**Iván Corona-Guerrero** Immunology and Vaccines Laboratory, Faculty of Natural Sciences, Autonomous University of Queretaro, Queretaro, Mexico

**Raquel Cossío-Bayúgar** Instituto Nacional de Investigaciones, Agrícolas y Pecuarias, Mexico City, Mexico

**Itabajara da Silva Vaz Junior** Centro de Biotecnologia, Universidade Federal do Rio Grande do Sul, Campus do Vale, Porto Alegre, RS, Brazil

Faculdade de Veterinária, Universidade Federal do Rio Grande do Sul, Campus do Vale, Porto Alegre, RS, Brazil

**Ixchel Guadalupe Díaz-Esquivel** National Center for Disciplinary Research in Animal Health and Safety, INIFAP, Carretera Federal Cuernavaca-Cuautla 8534, Jiutepec, Morelos, Mexico

**Gabriela J. Flota-Burgos** Campus de Ciencias Biológicas y Agropecuarias, Facultad de Medicina Veterinaria y Zootecnia, Universidad Autónoma de Yucatán, Mérida, Yucatán, Mexico

**Diego Josimar Hernández-Silva** Immunology and Vaccines Laboratory, Faculty of Natural Sciences, Autonomous University of Queretaro, Queretaro, Mexico

**Furhan Iqbal** Institute of Zoology, Bahauddin Zakariya University, Multan, Pakistan

**Nitin D. Jadhav** Department of Veterinary Pharmacology and Toxicology, College of Veterinary and Animal Sciences, Parbhani, MAFSU, Nagpur, Maharashtra, India

**Adil Khan** Department of Botany and Zoology, Bacha Khan University, Charsadda, Pakistan

**Afshan Khan** Department of Zoology, Abdul Wali Khan University Mardan, Mardan, Pakistan

**Haseeb Ullah Khan** Department of Botany and Zoology, Bacha Khan University, Charsadda, Pakistan

**Murad Khan** Department of Botany and Zoology, Bacha Khan University, Charsadda, Pakistan

**Saba Kousar** Department of Zoology, The Women University Multan, Multan, Pakistan

**Sachin Kumar** Entomology Laboratory, Division of Parasitology, ICAR-Indian Veterinary Research Institute, Izatnagar, Bareilly, Uttar Pradesh, India

Constituent Government College, Meerapur Banger, Bijnor, Uttar Pradesh, India

**Renato León** Laboratorio de Entomología Médica & Medicina Tropical LEMMT, Colegio de Ciencias Biológicas y Ambientales COCIBA, Universidad San Francisco de Quito USFQ, Quito, Ecuador

**Daniel Gustavo López-Díaz** Immunology and Vaccines Laboratory, Faculty of Natural Sciences, Autonomous University of Queretaro, Queretaro, Mexico

**Nosheen Malak** Department of Zoology, Abdul Wali Khan University Mardan, Mardan, Pakistan

**Naunain Mehmood** Department of Zoology, University of Sargodha, Sargodha, Pakistan

Department of Veterinary Medicine, University of Sassari, Sassari, Italy

**Estefan Miranda-Miranda** Instituto Nacional de Investigaciones, Agrícolas y Pecuarias, Mexico City, Mexico

**Rodrigo Morales-García** Immunology and Vaccines Laboratory, Faculty of Natural Sciences, Autonomous University of Queretaro, Queretaro, Mexico

**Juan Mosqueda** Immunology and Vaccines Laboratory, Faculty of Natural Sciences, Autonomous University of Queretaro, Queretaro, Mexico

**Hira Muqaddas** Department of Zoology, The Women University Multan, Multan, Pakistan

**Sadaf Niaz** Department of Zoology, Abdul Wali Khan University Mardan, Mardan, Pakistan

**Angel Salvador Ortega-Catalán** National Center for Disciplinary Research in Animal Health and Safety, INIFAP, Carretera Federal Cuernavaca-Cuautla 8534, Jiutepec, Morelos, Mexico

**Luís Fernando Parizi** Centro de Biotecnologia, Universidade Federal do Rio Grande do Sul, Campus do Vale, Porto Alegre, RS, Brazil

**Aldo Josué Pavón-Rocha** Immunology and Vaccines Laboratory, Faculty of Natural Sciences, Autonomous University of Queretaro, Queretaro, Mexico

**Ximena Pérez-Otáñez** Instituto de Investigación en Zoonosis (CIZ), Universidad Central del Ecuador, Quito, Ecuador

Centre for Earth and Climate Research, Université Catholique de Louvain, Louvain-la-Neuve, Belgium

**María Martina Esperanza Perez-Soria** Immunology and Vaccines Laboratory, Faculty of Natural Sciences, Autonomous University of Queretaro, Queretaro, Mexico

**Rosa Estela Quiroz-Castañeda** National Center for Disciplinary Research in Animal Health and Safety, INIFAP, Carretera Federal Cuernavaca-Cuautla 8534, Jiutepec, Morelos, Mexico

**Madiha Rasool** Department of Zoology, The Women University Multan, Multan, Pakistan

Institute of Zoology, Bahauddin Zakariya University, Multan, Pakistan

**Richar Rodríguez-Hidalgo** Facultad de Medicina Veterinaria y Zootecnia, Universidad Central del Ecuador, Quito, Ecuador

Instituto de Investigación en Zoonosis (CIZ), Universidad Central del Ecuador, Quito, Ecuador

**Roger I. Rodríguez-Vivas** Campus de Ciencias Biológicas y Agropecuarias, Facultad de Medicina Veterinaria y Zootecnia, Universidad Autónoma de Yucatán, Mérida, Yucatán, Mexico

**José A. Rosado Aguilar** Campus de Ciencias Biológicas y Agropecuarias, Facultad de Medicina Veterinaria y Zootecnia, Universidad Autónoma de Yucatán, Mérida, Yucatán, Mexico

**Mourad Ben Said** Laboratory of Microbiology, National School of Veterinary Medicine of Sidi Thabet, University of Manouba, Sidi Thabet, Tunisia

Department of Basic Sciences, Higher Institute of Biotechnology of Sidi Thabet, University of Manouba, Sidi Thabet, Tunisia

**M. Sankar** Entomology Laboratory, Division of Parasitology, ICAR-Indian Veterinary Research Institute, Izatnagar, Bareilly, Uttar Pradesh, India

**Rachid Selmi** Laboratory of Microbiology, National School of Veterinary Medicine of Sidi Thabet, University of Manouba, Sidi Thabet, Tunisia

**Nimra Shahid** Department of Zoology, University of Sargodha, Sargodha, Pakistan

**Anil Kumar Sharma** School of Agriculture, Uttaranchal University, Dehradun, Uttarakhand, India

**Carlos Termignoni** Centro de Biotecnologia, Universidade Federal do Rio Grande do Sul, Campus do Vale, Porto Alegre, RS, Brazil

Departamento de Bioquímica, Universidade Federal do Rio Grande do Sul, Porto Alegre, RS, Brazil

**Shakir Ullah** Department of Zoology, Abdul Wali Khan University Mardan, Mardan, Pakistan

**Jéssica Waldman** Centro de Biotecnologia, Universidade Federal do Rio Grande do Sul, Campus do Vale, Porto Alegre, RS, Brazil

**Farhana Yousaf** Department of Zoology, The Women University Multan, Multan, Pakistan

# Introduction to Ticks and Their Resistance to Acaricides

1

Richar Rodríguez-Hidalgo, Ximena Pérez-Otáñez, and Renato León

**Abstract**

This chapter describes the significant economic and health challenges posed by ticks of the genus Ixodidae, particularly *Rhipicephalus* species, infesting livestock in tropical and subtropical regions and worldwide. It addresses the limited understanding of tick-borne diseases caused by hemoparasites, bacteria, and protozoa. These pathogens, transmitted through the bite of an infected vector tick, infect animals and occasionally humans, leading to morbidity and mortality and significant economic losses. It elaborates on the available tick control strategies using acaricides and its environmental repercussions. The increasing resistance to chemical treatments, categorized into acquired, cross-, and multiresistance, is discussed. The intricate process of evolution of resistance to acaricides, influenced by intrinsic and extrinsic factors, including tick genetics and environmental issues, is also examined. Moreover, various resistance mechanisms against

R. Rodríguez-Hidalgo
Facultad de Medicina Veterinaria y Zootecnia, Universidad Central del Ecuador, Quito, Ecuador

Instituto de Investigación en Zoonosis (CIZ), Universidad Central del Ecuador, Quito, Ecuador

X. Pérez-Otáñez
Instituto de Investigación en Zoonosis (CIZ), Universidad Central del Ecuador, Quito, Ecuador

Centre for Earth and Climate Research, Université Catholique de Louvain, Louvain-la-Neuve, Belgium

R. León (✉)
Laboratorio de Entomología Médica & Medicina Tropical LEMMT, Colegio de Ciencias Biológicas y Ambientales COCIBA, Universidad San Francisco de Quito USFQ, Quito, Ecuador
e-mail: rleon@usfq.edu.ec



S. Kumar et al. (eds.), *Acaricides Resistance in Ticks*,
https://doi.org/10.1007/978-981-97-7411-1_1

commonly used acaricides are outlined, including organochlorines, organophosphates, carbamates, amidines, pyrethrins/pyrethroids, and macrocyclic lactones. The chapter suggests integrated management strategies encompassing rational acaricide use, vaccination, nutritional management, and the utilization of natural products. It also emphasizes the importance of genetic resistance in livestock breeds, environmental management, and diagnostic resistance tests. Lastly, it highlights the potential of PCR-based assays for rapid and specific resistance detection, aiding in the selection of effective acaricides.

**Keywords**
Ticks · Acaricide resistance · Livestock management · Vaccination

## 1.1 Introduction

Ticks of the genus Ixodidae, hematophagous ectoparasites of veterinary significance, pose substantial economic burdens on the global livestock industry, particularly in tropical and subtropical regions. They present a significant challenge to animal, human, and environmental health (Valencia et al. 2009). Among these, species of the genus *Rhipicephalus*, commonly known as blue or common cattle ticks, infest up to 80% of the world's livestock, primarily in tropical and subtropical areas (Cortés Vecino et al. 2010; De Clercq et al. 2013; Nava et al. 2009; Pérez-Otáñez et al. 2024; Polanco Echeverry and Ríos Osorio 2016). Moreover, these parasites can affect a diverse range of hosts, including buffaloes, donkeys, horses, goats, sheep, deer, wildlife, and humans (Estrada-Peña et al. 2014; Guglielmone et al. 2021).

Despite their significant impact, the study of ticks and the diseases they transmit to production and companion animals, as well as their environmental and public health effects, has been relatively limited (Enríquez et al. 2020; Maya-Delgado et al. 2020). Hemoparasites, causing diseases such as babesiosis, anaplasmosis, ehrlichiosis, and trypanosomiasis, are examples of bacteria and protozoa that affect animals and, in some cases, humans, and are transmitted by ticks (Chávez-Larrea et al. 2023; Csordas et al. 2018; Le Gall et al. 2018; Muhanguzi et al. 2020).

Agricultural practices significantly influence parasite transmission and tick infestation, directly impacting acaricide resistance (Ghosh and Nagar 2014; Guerrero et al. 2012). Concerns about the environmental repercussions of acaricides are substantial, given their effects on terrestrial and aquatic organisms' physiology, reproduction, and population dynamics (Lumaret et al. 2005; Ruiz and Blanco 2009). Additionally, pesticide accumulation can compromise animal or livestock production by negatively impacting pasture productivity if organic matter decomposition is hindered by the reduction in coprophagous insect populations (Bello Velásquez 2015; Lumaret et al. 2005; Tovar et al. 2016).

While chemical acaricides have been the primary method for tick control due to their low cost and accessibility, their high negative impact on animal, human, and environmental health is increasingly evident. In addition, the rapid emergence of acaricide resistance poses a significant challenge, diminishing the efficacy and efficiency of these products (Bianchi et al. 2003; Le Gall et al. 2018). Efficacy issues with chemicals have been identified since the mid-twentieth century, exacerbating the management challenge of *Rhipicephalus microplus* (Busch et al. 2014; Stone et al. 2014).

## 1.2 Resistance

Resistance manifests as a decrease in the effectiveness of products utilized to control bacteria, parasites, and fungi. Specifically, it is defined as "the ability of a strain or species of bacteria, parasite, or fungus to survive and/or multiply despite the administration and absorption of a drug in doses equal to or greater than those usually recommended, within the host's tolerance limits" (Chapman 1997; Meyer et al. 2012). Three main categories of resistance are identified:

*Acquired resistance:* Arising from a heritable reduction in sensitivity to a drug over time, acquired resistance directly correlates with the drug concentration. Underdosing can lead to the selection of resistant species, allowing the survival of those with specific genetic mutations (Faza et al. 2013; Lees et al. 2014; Lin et al. 2009; Mitchell 1996).

*Cross-resistance:* Shared resistance between different acaricides with similar modes of action characterizes cross-resistance. Notably documented between organophosphates (OP) and carbamates in various *R. microplus* strains, cross-resistance arises due to their common inhibition of acetylcholinesterase (AChE), vital for the invertebrate nervous system (Botello et al. 2011; Li et al. 2005; Madder et al. 2011; Pérez-González et al. 2014). AChE insensitivity is a pivotal mechanism of resistance (Dawkar et al. 2013; Fournier and Mutero 1994). Alternating or rotating acaricides from different groups can reduce selection pressure toward resistance to a specific group.

*Multiresistance:* Resistance to multiple drugs with distinct modes of action characterizes multiresistance. *Rhipicephalus microplus* populations in Mexico exhibit significant multiresistance against several classes of acaricides, including chlorinated hydrocarbons, pyrethroids, organophosphates, and formamidines (Amitraz) (Foil et al. 2004). Mutations at the site of action constitute the most observed resistance mechanism, while metabolic factors may also be involved (Bielza et al. 2007; Sammataro et al. 2005).

Considering the escalating resistance evident in ticks, it becomes crucial to devise inventive strategies aimed at upholding the efficacy of existing treatments. Moreover, there is a pressing need to curtail their usage by adopting sustainable control alternatives that are less harmful to animals and pose minimal risk to human safety, all within the overarching framework of a One Health approach. This underscores the importance of implementing integrated and comprehensive management practices for tick populations, prioritizing the well-being of both animals and public and environmental health (Estrada-Peña et al. 2022).

## 1.3 Evolution of Resistance

The evolution of resistance to acaricides is a multifaceted process influenced by various intrinsic and extrinsic factors (Pérez-Otáñez et al. 2023; Rodríguez-Hidalgo et al. 2017).

Intrinsic factors include genetic determinants affecting parasites, such as the prevalence of resistance alleles, the number of involved genes, initial frequencies of resistance genes, genetic diversity within populations, relative fitness of resistant organisms, potential linkage disequilibrium, and opportunities for genetic recombination (Georghiou and Taylor 1977; Mulchandani et al. 1998).

Sutherst and Comins (1979) delineated a three-dimensional process for resistance genesis, involving its establishment, development, and eventual emergence. It is often the case that genes responsible for resistance onset exist at low levels within tick populations before new acaricides are introduced, paving the way for continued selection under acaricidal pressure (Alonso-Díaz et al. 2013; Roulston et al. 1981). The rate at which resistant alleles become fixed in the population and their impact on tick control efficacy hinge on factors like the original mutation frequency, mode of inheritance of resistant alleles, acaricidal treatment frequency and concentration, and the proportion of the population in refugee status (Sangster 2001).

While the prevalence of resistant genes may initially rise gradually, by the time a decline in treatment efficacy is evident, these genes often become widespread (Stutzer et al. 2013). Selection pressure can act on single or multiple resistance genes, potentially in a sequential manner. However, genetic factors are beyond human control, complicating management efforts (Chevillon et al. 2007, 2013).

Extrinsic factors, from an operational and management perspective, encompass elements like the chemical properties of the drug, potential cross-resistance, drug persistence in hosts, and drug elimination kinetics. Factors such as application thresholds, frequency, and selection, targeted parasite life stages, application methods, treatment timing, spatial distribution, and integration with other control measures are crucial. Suboptimal dosing, drug quality issues, and combinations of multiple products (Mendes et al. 2013a; Paucar-Quishpe et al. 2023) can favor the selection of mutants initially resistant to low acaricide levels (Bianchi et al. 2003; Rezende et al. 2013; Shyma et al. 2012). Resistance is favored when parasite populations are exposed to subtherapeutic drug concentrations due to lack of regulation on the use of drugs, inappropriate treatment protocols, and use of drugs with extended half-lives (Buczek et al. 2015; Paucar-Quishpe et al. 2023).

An important aspect of operational management is the frequent and prolonged use of the same acaricide. For instance, in Queensland, Australia, more than five treatments per season increase resistance risk in livestock ticks (Jonsson et al. 2000b; Paucar-Quishpe et al. 2023), highlighting how high-treatment frequencies facilitate resistance selection. Acaricide effectiveness can significantly vary across regions due to differing practices and tick species (Enayati et al. 2009, 2010; Paucar-Quishpe et al. 2023; Pérez-Otáñez et al. 2023; Rodríguez-Hidalgo et al. 2017; Soberanes Céspedes et al. 2005).

Unlike genetic factors, operational and management aspects are modifiable through appropriate interventions, including educating producers on acaricide rational use, to mitigate resistance progression and preserve intervention efficacy.

Biological factors are critical in resistance evolution and can be categorized into biotic and behavioral aspects. Biotic factors encompass adult tick generation time, offspring count, and reproductive patterns, while behavioral factors influence gene flow and selection probabilities, including isolation, mobility, migration, and feeding habits of ectoparasites (monophagous or polyphagous), as well as the presence of refuges allowing some individuals' survival (Dzemo et al. 2022).

In the context of host–ectoparasite dynamics, these biological factors significantly influence resistance selection mechanisms. Ectoparasites inducing effective host immune responses face reduced resistance pressure as host immunity affects susceptible and resistant ectoparasites equally, decreasing the chances of survival and reproduction of resistant ectoparasites. Additionally, ectoparasite pathogenicity determines the infestation load required to impact production negatively, thus influencing the frequency of acaricidal treatments. Recognizing that a higher proportion of parasites in refuge slows resistance selection underscores the need for effective management of these populations to control the spread of resistance (Rajput et al. 2006; Sangster 2001).

Understanding these biological factors underscores the complexity of resistance management and emphasizes the need for integrated approaches considering both biotic and behavioral elements to effectively mitigate the advancement of acaricide resistance.

## 1.4 Resistance Mechanisms

Understanding the mechanisms behind the development of acaricide resistance in cattle ticks is crucial and urges a basic comprehension of these compounds' mode of action.

### 1.4.1 Resistance to Organochlorines

Organochlorines, introduced in 1946 as synthetic insecticides targeting livestock ticks, are believed to bind to the picrotoxin site on the γ-aminobutyric acid (GABA) chloride ionophore complex. This binding inhibits chloride ion flow into nerves, disrupting inhibitory GABAergic neuron function, leading to hyperexcitation and eventual ectoparasite death (Obaid et al. 2022). Research indicates these compounds also bind to the same site as t-butylbicyclophosphorothionate (TBPS), suggesting mechanisms of resistance involving enhanced metabolism and reduced chemical absorption (Bloomquist and Soderlund 1985; Corley et al. 2012; Kunz and Kemp 1994; Lawrence and Casida 1983; Tanaka et al. 1984; Zheng et al. 2003).

### 1.4.2 Resistance to Organophosphates and Carbamates

Organophosphates and carbamates function by inhibiting AChE, a crucial enzyme for nervous system function. Inhibition of AChE prevents acetylcholine degradation, leading to nervous system overstimulation and tick death (Lovis et al. 2011). Resistance to these compounds, documented worldwide, is primarily attributed to site insensitivity. Point mutations identified in AChE have advanced understanding of the molecular mechanisms underlying this resistance (Faza et al. 2013; Foil et al. 2004; Jamroz et al. 2000; Mendes et al. 2011; Roulston et al. 1981; Temeyer et al. 2013a, b; Van Leeuwen et al. 2009).

### 1.4.3 Resistance to Amidines (Amitraz)

Amitraz, utilized for almost four decades, has displayed resistance in various tick populations. Its speculated mode of action involves interaction with the octopamine receptor. Mutations in the octopamine receptor found in resistant strains suggest alterations in the site of action as a resistance mechanism, though the overall mechanism of resistance to Amitraz remains partly unexplored (Chevillon et al. 2007; Corley et al. 2013; Ducornez et al. 2005; Gong et al. 2013; Li et al. 2007; Mendes et al. 2013b; Rodríguez-Vivas et al. 2012; Soberanes et al. 2002).

### 1.4.4 Resistance to Pyrethrins/Pyrethroids

Pyrethrins and their synthetic derivatives, pyrethroids, act on sodium ion channels, inducing nervous system excitement. Resistance to these compounds is associated with esterase, cytochrome P450 monooxygenase, and glutathione S-transferase activity. Mutations in the $Na^+$ channel have been identified as a site-specific resistance mechanism, revealing the complexity of tick resistance mechanisms (Baffi et al. 2007; Gong et al. 2013; Jamroz et al. 2000; Rodríguez-Vivas et al. 2012; Rosario-Cruz et al. 2009; Stone et al. 2014; Lopes et al. 2013; Weston et al. 2013).

### 1.4.5 Resistance to Macrocyclic Lactones

Macrocyclic lactones, such as avermectins and milbemycins, block electrical activity transmission by stimulating GABA release and binding, resulting in hyperpolarization and paralysis. Despite their efficacy, extensive use has led to partial resistance, with mechanisms still under investigation. Insensitivity of chloride channels regulated by GABA or glutamate is suggested as a possible pathway for resistance (Blackhall et al. 1998; Bloomquist and Soderlund 1985; Campbell et al. 1983; Klafke et al. 2006; Lopes et al. 2013; Lovis et al. 2013; Ono et al. 1983; Perez-Cogollo et al. 2010; Rodríguez-Vivas et al. 2014; Shoop et al. 1995).

## 1.5 Resistance Management

This analysis underscores the intricate and varied mechanisms through which ticks acquire resistance to acaricides, emphasizing the need for integrated and comprehensive approaches. Managing acaricide resistance is pivotal in combating ticks, requiring strategies that span from rationale acaricide use to vaccination.

### 1.5.1 Rational Use of Acaricides

The strategic use of acaricides, coupled with insights into their cycling and the right combination of active ingredients, plays a crucial role in preserving the efficacy of existing compounds.

#### 1.5.1.1 Regular Monitoring

Routine monitoring stands as a cornerstone strategy in prolonging resistance development, emphasizing the application of acaricide every three weeks during peak tick seasons in regions with heightened resistance prevalence. However, it is critical to limit treatments at a maximum of five per season to mitigate the emergence of resistant strains. This underscores the significance of confirming resistance cases in laboratories and adjusting management protocols accordingly (Jonsson et al. 2000b; Sugimoto and Osakabe 2014; Sun et al. 2011; Thullner et al. 2007).

#### 1.5.1.2 Acaricide Rotation

Implementing alternating acaricides with diverse modes of action can alleviate selective pressure on any specific group, potentially slowing significant resistance development. Although data is limited, studies suggest this practice could be effective. Further research is necessary to ascertain optimal rotation strategies, considering its feasibility and economic viability across different scenarios (Adakal et al. 2013; Adehan et al. 2016; Maggi et al. 2011; Rodriguez-Vivas et al. 2011, 2021; Thullner et al. 2007).

## 1.6 Vaccination

The immunization of livestock through vaccines presents a valuable tool in tick control. Vaccines like Gavac®, TickGARD, and TickGARDPLUS, which are based on the Bm86 antigen, have demonstrated effectiveness against various tick species. However, the variability in vaccine efficacy, influenced by the genetic diversity of ticks in different regions, underscores the importance of assessing vaccine effectiveness prior to their introduction into new geographic areas. The synergistic use of vaccines alongside acaricides holds promise in reducing reliance on the latter and, consequently, slowing the development of resistance (Ben Said et al. 2012; Beugnet et al. 1998; de la Fuente et al. 1998; Freeman et al. 2010; Jonsson et al. 2000a; Pereira et al. 2008; Rodriguez-Valle et al. 2013; Tinoco et al. 2023).

## 1.7 Nutritional Management

Adequate nutrition plays a crucial role in maintaining the functionality of the immune system, particularly T cells, whose efficiency can be compromised by protein and energy deficiencies (Lichtman 2013; Rodriguez-Vivas et al. 2018). Research indicates that T cells are vital for acquired resistance against ticks, with evidence suggesting that a protein-rich diet can enhance the host's ability to resist tick infestation (Maharana et al. 2011; Wikel 2013). Experimental studies have confirmed that animals fed low-protein diets exhibit increased susceptibility to ticks compared to those on high-protein diets, which not only resist tick infestation better but also maintain their weight and overall health (Rechav and Hay 1992).

The use of sulfur as a dietary supplement in livestock tick control holds significant importance in integrated management strategies for these ectoparasites. Beyond its known metabolic functions, sulfur has been found to effectively reduce the incidence of tick infestations. Administering sulfur in livestock diets has proven to be an effective adjunct measure in tick control, potentially due to its impact on reducing blood palatability or altering skin conditions, thereby deterring tick infestations or interrupting tick life cycles on treated hosts (repellent effect). This effect could lead to a decrease in tick reproduction and survival rates, positively influencing ectoparasite population management (Avila and Calderón 2021; Egas and López 2023; Herrera et al. 2024; Paternina Durango et al. 2015).

Livestock breeds naturally resistant to ticks, such as *Bos indicus* and its crosses, demonstrate that the host immune system is a significant regulator of resistance. The quality of food directly impacts this resistance capacity, underscoring the importance of nutritional management within integrated tick control programs (Carvalho et al. 2011; Maryam et al. 2012; Mattioli et al. 2000; Otto et al. 2018).

## 1.8 Use of Natural Products

Given the high cost of developing new drugs and vaccines, along with concerns regarding drug resistance and chemical residues, there has been a resurgence of interest in plant products as safe, effective, and economical alternatives for tick control (Abbas et al. 2014; Alotaibi et al. 2023; Obaid et al. 2022). The tradition of using plants to combat ectoparasites is particularly strong in developing countries, where numerous species with acaricidal properties have been identified. Studies have documented a wide range of plant species effective against ticks, highlighting their potential in integrated pest management (de Souza Chagas et al. 2011; George et al. 2014; Godara et al. 2014; Quadros et al. 2020; Rodriguez-Vivas et al. 2018; Showler and Saelao 2022).

Species such as *Commiphora erythraea*, *Artocarpus altilis*, and many others have been recognized for their acaricidal activity, paving the way for the development of commercial formulations based on plant extracts, such as MyggA® Natural and Citriodiol®, which are already in use in some countries for tick control (Freitag and Kells 2013; Gardulf et al. 2004; Medlock et al. 2013). These advancements underscore the importance of continuing research into the effects of plant extracts and the potential value of their combination with conventional methods for more effective and sustainable tick management.

Another appealing measure is the cultivation of grasses that repel or prevent the development of ticks. Species such as *Stylosanthes* spp., *Melinis minutiflora*, and *Andropogon gayanus* have been recognized for inhibiting tick development (Jonsson and Piper 2007; Soares et al. 2010). However, the main drawback of these grasses is their lack of appropriate nutritional value for livestock.

Furthermore, implementing agricultural practices such as cultivating grasses that naturally repel ticks or do not favor their development presents a valuable complementary strategy, although the nutritional adequacy of these grass species for livestock must be considered (Jonsson and Piper 2007; Soares et al. 2010).

The integration of ethnoveterinary products with synthetic acaricides could produce better effects in terms of tick control and delaying tick resistance compared to the use of acaricides alone.

In summary, nutritional management and the use of plants emerge as innovative strategies that, when combined with other management practices, can significantly contribute to tick control and the management of resistance to acaricides, promoting a more comprehensive and sustainable approach to animal health.

## 1.9 Improving Genetic Resistance in Livestock

Historically, certain livestock breeds have exhibited inherent resistance to tick infestations compared to others under similar environmental conditions. This natural resistance is attributed to the animal's immunological response to tick infestation. The utilization of cattle with inherent resistance, notably prevalent in breeds such as zebu and their crosses, has demonstrated more effective tick infestation management. Consequently, in regions grappling with significant tick infestation issues, there is a push for replacing *B. taurus* cattle with more resilient zebu breeds, as well as for the development of *B. indicus* lines with enhanced resistance. In areas where livestock farming faces constraints, the crossbreeding of taurine animals with zebu lines has proven to be a viable alternative (Ayres et al. 2013; O'kelly and Seifert 1969; Frisch et al. 2000; Riek 1962; Roberts 1968; Rodriguez-Valle et al. 2012, 2013; Solomon and Kaaya 1996; Wagland 1975).

## 1.10 Environmental Management

The practice of burning grasslands to stimulate green regrowth during the dry season has been widely embraced as a tick control strategy in various countries. This method, implemented in government-led tick management programs as seen in countries like Cuba, demands meticulous monitoring to effectively target all ectoparasite stages. However, it poses significant challenges for farmers with limited resources and often conflicts with public policies favoring nature and environmental conservation (Baars 1999; Cordoves et al. 1986; Cully 1999; Davidson et al. 1994; Jonsson et al. 1998; Spickett et al. 1992).

In contrast, the alternation and/or rotation of pastures, integrated into animal production management on farms alongside the application of chemical acaricides on the animals, has proven to be a practical measure for tick control. This strategy, more accessible to resource-constrained farmers compared to grassland burning, has been validated by various studies as one of the most economically viable approaches to reduce ectoparasite load (Barnard et al. 1994; Stachurski and Adakal 2010).

A proper design and management of facilities, particularly in feedlots, can help mitigate the risk of tick infestations by creating unfavorable conditions for their free-living stages. Essential factors include adequate ventilation, regular cleaning, and optimal water and food management. Additionally, eliminating or excluding alternative hosts is recommended to minimize infestation pressure (Soberanes Céspedes et al. 2005; Young et al. 1988).

## 1.11 Diagnostic Resistance Tests

The most employed in vitro bioassays include the larval packet test (LPT) (FAO 1984), the larval immersion test (LIT) (Shaw 1966), and the adult immersion test (AIT) (Drummond et al. 1973). In LPT, tick larvae are exposed to chemical-impregnated filter papers, and their subsequent mortality is assessed after 24 h (Githaka et al. 2022; Nogueira Domingues et al. 2012). In LIT, 7- to 10-day-old tick larvae are submerged in various dilutions of acaricide, and their viability is evaluated 24 h post-treatment by counting live and dead larvae (Castro-Janer et al. 2011). The AIT involves determining dose-mortality responses of ticks to acaricides by treating engorged female ticks with a range of dilutions of an acaricide and comparing treated and untreated ticks to assess the treatment's impact on fecundity and fertility (Andreotti et al. 2011; Brito et al. 2011).

These bioassays are valued for their portability and cost-effectiveness. However, they lack direct insights into the genetic mechanisms of resistance, insufficient sensitivity to detect early-stage resistance emergence, and are time-consuming to yield results.

A rapid and sensitive test would be beneficial for determining the resistance status of tick samples, guiding the selection of an appropriate and effective acaricide in resistance management programs. PCR-based assays, designed to be completed within a day, offer the potential to identify specific resistance mechanisms and can be conducted on individual ticks using whole tick larvae or adult hemolymph or cuticular material. Progress in this area includes PCR assays developed to detect site-of-action resistance to pyrethroids and organophosphates (Baffi et al. 2007; Jamroz et al. 2000). Besides providing insights into the molecular basis of acaricide resistance, these assays are intended to furnish valuable information for resistance management programs. With a full range of molecular tests available, initial resistance detection can be performed through PCR assays, followed by larval packet testing if desired, to allow a rapid selection of the best choice of acaricide for eradication of the outbreak (Maya-Delgado et al. 2020; Mendes et al. 2013a).

**Acknowledgments** We thank Dr. Michael J. Turell, retired senior scientist from USAMRIID, Ft. Detrick, MD, USA, for the edition of the text and his valuable comments.

## References

Abbas RZ, Zaman MA, Colwell DD, Gilleard J, Iqbal Z (2014) Acaricide resistance in cattle ticks and approaches to its management: the state of play. Vet Parasitol 203(1-2):6–20. https://doi.org/10.1016/j.vetpar.2014.03.006

Adakal H, Stachurski F, Chevillon C (2013) Tick control practices in Burkina Faso and acaricide resistance survey in *Rhipicephalus* (*Boophilus*) *geigyi* (Acari: Ixodidae). Exp Appl Acarol 59:483–491. https://doi.org/10.1007/s10493-012-9610-5

Adehan SB, Biguezoton A, Adakal H, Assogba MN, Zoungrana S, Gbaguidi AM, Tonouhewa A, Kandé S, Achi L, Kagone H, Adehan R, Mensah GA, De Deken R, Madder M, Farougou S (2016) Acaricide resistance of *Rhipicephalus microplus* ticks in Benin. Afr J Agric Res 11(14):1199–1208

Alonso-Díaz MA, Fernández-Salas A, Martínez-Ibáñez F, Osorio-Miranda J (2013) *Amblyomma cajennense* (Acari: Ixodidae) tick populations susceptible or resistant to acaricides in the Mexican tropics. Vet Parasitol 197(1-2):326–331. https://doi.org/10.1016/j.vetpar.2013.06.004

Alotaibi BS, Malak N, Khan A, Nasreen N, Niaz S, Ahmad I, Khan A, Rodriguez-Vivas RI, Chen CC (2023) Acaricidal assessment of the fungal extract of *Pleurotus ostreatus* against *Rhipicephalus microplus*: role of in vitro and in silico analysis. Heliyon 9(9):e19600. https://doi.org/10.1016/j.heliyon.2023.e19600

Andreotti R, Guerrero FD, Soares MA, Barros JC, Miller RJ, De Léon AP (2011) Acaricide resistance of *Rhipicephalus* (*Boophilus*) *microplus* in State of Mato Grosso do Sul, Brazil. Braz J Vet Parasitol 20(2):127–133

Avila A, Calderón J (2021) Efecto del azufre y Saccharomyces cerevisiae en la dieta de vacas lecheras como repelente de garrapatas en la comunidad El Regadío-Estelí, 2019 Universidad Católica del Trópico Seco “Pbro. https://doi.org/10.25044/25392190.1028

Ayres DR, Pereira RJ, Boligon AA, Silva FF, Schenkel FS, Roso VM, Albuquerque LG (2013) Linear and Poisson models for genetic evaluation of tick resistance in cross-bred Hereford x Nellore cattle. J Anim Breed Genet 130(6):417–424. https://doi.org/10.1111/jbg.12036

Baars RM (1999) The effect of rangeland fires on cattle tick infestation in western Zambia. Trop Anim Health Prod 31(5):275–278. https://doi.org/10.1023/a:1005299605959

Baffi MA, de Souza GRL, Vieira CU, de Sousa CS, Gourlart LR, Bonetti AM (2007) Identification of point mutations in a putative carboxylesterase and their association with acaricide resistance in *Rhipicephalus* (*Boophilus*) *microplus* (Acari: Ixodidae). Vet Parasitol 148(3-4):301–309. https://doi.org/10.1016/j.vetpar.2007.06.016

Barnard DR, Mount GA, Haile DG, Daniels E (1994) Integrated management strategies for *Amblyomma americanum* (acari: ixodidae) on pastured beef cattle. J Med Entomol 31(4):571–585. https://doi.org/10.1093/jmedent/31.4.571

Bello Velásquez AE (2015) Evaluación de lactonas macrocíclicas sobre la población de escarabajos coprofagos. Universidad Veracruzana, Veracruz

Ben Said M, Galai Y, Canales M, Nijhof AM, Mhadhbi M, Jedidi M, de la Fuente J, Darghouth MA (2012) Hd86, the Bm86 tick protein ortholog in *Hyalomma scupense* (syn. *H. detritum*): expression in *Pichia pastoris* and analysis of nucleotides and amino acids sequences variations prior to vaccination trials. Vet Parasitol 183(3):215–223. https://doi.org/10.1016/j.vetpar.2011.07.049

Beugnet F, Chalvet-Monfray K, Sabatier P (1998) Use of a mathematical model to study the control measures of the cattle tick *Boophilus microplus* population in New Caledonia. Vet Parasitol 77(4):277–288. https://doi.org/10.1016/S0304-4017(98)00116-2

Bianchi MW, Barré N, Messad S (2003) Factors related to cattle infestation level and resistance to acaricides in *Boophilus microplus* tick populations in New Caledonia. Vet Parasitol 112(1-2):75–89. https://doi.org/10.1016/S0304-4017(02)00415-6

Bielza P, Espinosa PJ, Quinto V, Abellán J, Contreras J (2007) Synergism studies with binary mixtures of pyrethroid, carbamate and organophosphate insecticides on *Frankliniella occidentalis* (Pergande). Pest Manag Sci 63(1):84–89. https://doi.org/10.1002/ps.1328

Blackhall WJ, Pouliot J-F, Prichard RK, Beech RN (1998) *Haemonchus contortus*: selection at a glutamate-gated chloride channel gene in ivermectin- and moxidectin-selected strains. Exp Parasitol 90(1):42–48. https://doi.org/10.1006/expr.1998.4316

Bloomquist JR, Soderlund DM (1985) Neurotoxic insecticides inhibit GABA-dependent chloride uptake by mouse brain vesicles. Biochem Biophys Res Commun 133(1):37–43. https://doi.org/10.1016/0006-291X(85)91838-8

Botello AR, Botello AL, Borroto CN, Suárez M, Pérez DA, Rodríguez YV, Fajardo H, Pérez KC, González AO, Rodríguez AN, Linares BR, Colicchia MR, Gómez IA, Peraza PS, Gort AM (2011) Control de garrapatas *Riphicephalus* (*Boophilus*) *microplus* en bovinos con el inmunógeno Herber biogar. Rev Electron Vet 12(5):1–10

Brito LG, Barbieri FS, Rocha RB, Oliveira MCS, Ribeiro ES (2011) Evaluation of the efficacy of acaricides used to control the cattle tick, *Rhipicephalus microplus*, in dairy herds raised in the Brazilian Southwestern Amazon. Vet Med Int 2011. https://doi.org/10.4061/2011/806093

Buczek A, Lachowska-Kotowska P, Bartosik K (2015) The effect of synthetic pyrethroids on the attachment and host-feeding behaviour in *Dermacentor reticulatus* females (Ixodida: Amblyommidae). Parasit Vectors 8(1):4–8. https://doi.org/10.1186/s13071-015-0977-0

Busch JD, Stone NE, Nottingham R, Araya-Anchetta A, Lewis J, Hochhalter C, Giles JR, Gruendike J, Freeman J, Buckmeier G, Bodine D, Duhaime R, Miller RJ, Davey RB, Olafson PU, Scoles GA, Wagner DM (2014) Widespread movement of invasive cattle fever ticks (*Rhipicephalus microplus*) in southern Texas leads to shared local infestations on cattle and deer. Parasit Vectors 7(1):188. https://doi.org/10.1186/1756-3305-7-188

Campbell WC, Fisher MH, Stapley EO, Albers-Schönberg G, Jacob TA (1983) Ivermectin: a potent new antiparasitic agent. Science 221(4613):823–828. https://doi.org/10.1126/science.6308762

Carvalho WA, Ianella P, Arnoldi FGC, Caetano AR, Maruyama SR, Ferreira BR, Andreucci Conti LH, Da Silva MRM, Paula JOF, Maia AAM, De Miranda Santos IKF (2011) Haplotypes of the bovine IgG2 heavy gamma chain in tick-resistant and tick-susceptible breeds of cattle. Immunogenetics 63(5):319–324. https://doi.org/10.1007/s00251-011-0515-y

Castro-Janer E, Rifran L, González P, Niell C, Piaggio J, Gil A, Schumaker TTS (2011) Determination of the susceptibility of *Rhipicephalus* (*Boophilus*) *microplus* (Acari: Ixodidae) to ivermectin and fipronil by larval immersion test (LIT) in Uruguay. Vet Parasitol 178(1-2):148–155. https://doi.org/10.1016/j.vetpar.2010.12.035

Chapman HD (1997) Biochemical, genetic and applied aspects of drug resistance in Eimeria parasites of the fowl. Avian Pathol 26(2):221–244. https://doi.org/10.1080/03079459708419208

Chávez-Larrea MA, Cholota-Iza C, Cueva-Villavicencio J, Yugcha-Díaz M, Ron-Román JW, Rodríguez-Cabezas A, Saegerman C, Reyna-Bello A (2023) Molecular identification of

*Trypanosoma theileri* (Laveran, 1902) in cattle from two slaughterhouses in Ecuador and its relation with other haemotropic agents. Front Vet Sci 10:1153069. https://doi.org/10.3389/fvets.2023.1153069

Chevillon C, Ducornez S, de Meeûs T, Koffi B, Gaïa H, Delathière JM, Barré N (2007) Accumulation of acaricide resistance mechanisms in *Rhipicephalus* (*Boophilus*) *microplus* (Acari: Ixodidae) populations from New Caledonia Island. Vet Parasitol 147(3-4):276–288

Chevillon C, de Garine-Wichatitsky M, Barré N, Ducornez S, de Meeûs T (2013) Understanding the genetic, demographical and/or ecological processes at play in invasions: lessons from the southern cattle tick *Rhipicephalus microplus* (Acari: Ixodidae). Exp Appl Acarol 59(1):203–218. https://doi.org/10.1007/s10493-012-9602-5

Cordoves CO, De la Cruz J, Tamayo J, Mesejo J, Fleites R (1986) Experience and perspectives of tick control and eradication in the Republic of Cuba. Rev Cubana Cien Vet 17(1/2):1–13

Corley SW, Piper EK, Jonsson NN (2012) Generation of Full-Length cDNAs for Eight Putative GPCnR from the Cattle Tick, R. microplus using a targeted degenerate PCR and sequencing strategy. PLoS ONE 7(3):1–8. https://doi.org/10.1371/journal.pone.0032480

Corley SW, Jonsson NN, Piper EK, Cutullé C, Stear MJ, Seddon JM (2013) Mutation in the RmβAOR gene is associated with amitraz resistance in the cattle tick *Rhipicephalus microplus*. Proc Natl Acad Sci USA 110(42):16772–16777. https://doi.org/10.1073/pnas.1309072110

Cortés Vecino JA, Betancourt Echeverri JA, Argüelles Cárdenas J, Pulido Herrera LA (2010) Distribution of *Rhipicephalus* (*Boophilus*) *microplus* ticks on cattle and farms from Altiplano Cundiboyacense (Colombia). Rev Corp 11(1):73–84

Csordas BG, Cunha RC, Garcia MV, da Silva SS, Leite FL, Andreotti R (2018) Molecular characterization of the recombinant protein RmLTI-BmCG-LTB: protective immunity against *Rhipicephalus* (*Boophilus*) *microplus*. PLoS ONE 13(2):e0191596. https://doi.org/10.1371/journal.pone.0191596

Cully JF (1999) Lone star tick abundance, fire, and bison grazing in tallgrass prairie. J Range Manag 52(2):139–144. https://doi.org/10.2307/4003507

Davidson WR, Siefken DA, Creekmore LH (1994) Influence of annual and biennial prescribed burning during March on the abundance of *Amblyomma americanum* (Acari: ixodidae) in Central Georgia. J Med Entomol 31(1):72–81. https://doi.org/10.1093/jmedent/31.1.72

Dawkar VV, Chikate YR, Lomate PR, Dholakia BB, Gupta VS, Giri AP (2013) Molecular insights into resistance mechanisms of lepidopteran insect pests against toxicants. J Proteome Res 12(11):4727–4737. https://doi.org/10.1021/pr400642p

De Clercq EM, Estrada-Peña A, Adehan S, Madder M, Vanwambeke SO (2013) An update on distribution models for *Rhipicephalus microplus* in West Africa. Geospat Health 8(1):301–308. https://doi.org/10.4081/gh.2013.75

de la Fuente J, Rodríguez M, Redondo M, Montero C, García-García J, Méndez L, Serrano E, Valdés M, Enriquez A, Canales M, Ramos E, Boué O, Machado H, Lleonart R, de Armas CA, Rey S, Rodríguez JL, Artiles M, García L (1998) Field studies and cost-effectiveness analysis of vaccination with Gavac™ against the cattle tick *Boophilus microplus*. Vaccine 16(4):366–373. https://doi.org/10.1016/S0264-410X(97)00208-9

de Souza Chagas AC, Georgetti CS, de Carvalho CO, de Sena Oliveira MC, Rodrigues RA, Foglio MA, de Magalhãees PM (2011) *In vitro* activity of *Artemisia annua* L (Asteraceae) extracts against *Rhipicephalus* (*Boophilus*) *microplus*. Rev Bras Parasitol Vet 20(1):31–35. https://doi.org/10.1590/s1984-29612011000100007

Drummond R, Ernst S, Trevino JW, Gladney OG (1973) *Boophilus annulatus* and *Boophilus microplus:* laboratory test of insecticides. J Econ Entomol 66:130–133

Ducornez S, Barré N, Miller RJ, de Garine-Wichatitsky M (2005) Diagnosis of amitraz resistance in *Boophilus microplus* in new caledonia with the modified larval packet test. Vet Parasitol 130(3):285–292. https://doi.org/10.1016/j.vetpar.2005.04.018

Dzemo WD, Thekisoe O, Vudriko P (2022) Development of acaricide resistance in tick populations of cattle: a systematic review and meta-analysis. Heliyon 8(1):e08718. https://doi.org/10.1016/j.heliyon.2022.e08718

Egas J, López S (2023) Evaluación del efecto de azufre elemental como alternativa de control de garrapatas y su influencia sobre la producción de leche en ganaderías del noroccidente de Pichincha. Unviersidad Central del Ecuador, Quito

Enayati AA, Asgarian F, Sharif M, Boujhmehrani H, Amouei A, Vahedi N, Boudaghi B, Piazak N, Hemingway J (2009) Propetamphos resistance in *Rhipicephalus bursa* (Acari, Ixodidae). Vet Parasitol 162(1):135–141. https://doi.org/10.1016/j.vetpar.2009.02.005

Enayati AA, Asgarian F, Amouei A, Sharif M, Mortazavi H, Boujhmehrani H, Hemingway J (2010) Pyrethroid insecticide resistance in *Rhipicephalus bursa* (Acari, Ixodidae). Pestic Biochem Physiol 97(3):243–248. https://doi.org/10.1016/j.pestbp.2010.03.003

Enríquez S, Guerrero R, Arrivillaga-Henríquez J, Araujo P, Villacrés E, Enríquez A, Benítez-Ortíz W (2020) New records of ticks of genus Amblyomma Koch, 1844 (Acari: ixodidae) for Ecuador. Acta Parasitol 65(2):430–440. https://doi.org/10.2478/s11686-020-00173-7

Estrada-Peña A, Tarragona EL, Vesco U, de Meneghi D, Mastropaolo M, Mangold AJ, Guglielmone AA, Nava S (2014) Divergent environmental preferences and areas of sympatry of tick species in the *Amblyomma cajennense* complex (Ixodidae). Int J Parasitol 44(14):1081–1089. https://doi.org/10.1016/j.ijpara.2014.08.007

Estrada-Peña A, Mallón AR, Bermúdez S, de la Fuente J, Domingos A, García MPE, Labruna MB, Merino O, Mosqueda J, Nava S, Cruz RL, Szabó M, Tarragona E, Venzal JM (2022) One health approach to identify research needs on *Rhipicephalus microplus* ticks in the Americas. Pathogens 11(10):1180. https://doi.org/10.3390/pathogens11101180

FAO (1984) Ticks and tick borne disease control. A practical field manual. Tick control. Food and Agriculture Organization, Rome, p 299

Faza AP, Pinto ISB, Fonseca I, Antunes GR, de Oliveira Monteiro CM, Daemon E, de Souza Muniz M, Martins MF, Furlong J, de Azevedo Prata MC (2013) A new approach to characterization of the resistance of populations of *Rhipicephalus microplus* (Acari: Ixodidae) to organophosphate and pyrethroid in the state of Minas Gerais, Brazil. Exp Parasitol 134(4):519–523. https://doi.org/10.1016/j.exppara.2013.04.006

Foil LD, Coleman P, Eisler M, Fragoso-Sanchez H, Garcia-Vazquez Z, Guerrero FD, Jonsson NN, Langstaff IG, Li AY, Machila N, Miller RJ, Morton J, Pruett JH, Torr S (2004) Factors that influence the prevalence of acaricide resistance and tick-borne diseases. Vet Parasitol 125(1-2):163–181. https://doi.org/10.1016/j.vetpar.2004.05.012

Fournier D, Mutero A (1994) Modification of acetylcholinesterase as a mechanism of resistance to insecticides. Comp Biochem Physiol C: Pharmacol Toxicol Endocrinol 108(1):19–31. https://doi.org/10.1016/1367-8280(94)90084-1

Freeman JM, Davey RB, Kappmeyer LS, Kammlah DM, Olafson PU (2010) Bm86 midgut protein sequence variation in South Texas cattle fever ticks. Parasit Vectors 3(1):101. https://doi.org/10.1186/1756-3305-3-101

Freitag JA, Kells SA (2013) Efficacy and application considerations of selected residual acaricides against the mold mite *Tyrophagus putrescentiae* (acari: acaridae) in simulated retail habitats. J Econ Entomol 106(4):1920–1926. https://doi.org/10.1603/EC13038

Frisch JE, O'Neill CJ, Kelly MJ (2000) Using genetics to control cattle parasites - the Rockhampton experience. Int J Parasitol 30(3):253–264. https://doi.org/10.1016/S0020-7519(00)00010-2

Gardulf A, Wohlfart I, Gustafson R (2004) A prospective cross-over field trial shows protection of lemon eucalyptus extract against tick bites. J Med Entomol 41(6):1064–1067. https://doi.org/10.1603/0022-2585-41.6.1064

George DR, Finn RD, Graham KM, Sparagano OA (2014) Present and future potential of plant-derived products to control arthropods of veterinary and medical significance. Parasit Vectors 7(1):1–12. https://doi.org/10.1186/1756-3305-7-28

Georghiou GP, Taylor CE (1977) Genetic and biological influences in the evolution of insecticide resistance. J Econ Entomol 70(3):319–323. https://doi.org/10.1093/jee/70.3.319

Ghosh S, Nagar G (2014) Problem of ticks and tick-borne diseases in India with special emphasis on progress in tick control research: a review. J Vector Borne Dis 51:259–270

Githaka NW, Kanduma EG, Wieland B, Darghouth MA, Bishop RP (2022) Acaricide resistance in livestock ticks infesting cattle in Africa: current status and potential mitigation strategies. Curr Res Parasitol Vector-Borne Dis 2(April):100090. https://doi.org/10.1016/j.crpvbd.2022.100090

Godara R, Katoch M, Katoch R, Yadav A, Parveen S, Vij B, Khajuria V, Singh G, Singh NK (2014) *In vitro* acaricidal activity of *Atropa belladonna* and its components, scopolamine and atropine, against *Rhipicephalus* (*Boophilus*) *microplus*. Sci World J 2014:713170. https://doi.org/10.1155/2014/713170

Gong Y, Li T, Zhang L, Gao X, Liu N (2013) Permethrin induction of multiple cytochrome P450 genes in insecticide resistant mosquitoes, *Culex quinquefasciatus*. Int J Biol Sci 9(9):863–871. https://doi.org/10.7150/ijbs.6744

Guerrero FD, Lovis L, Martins JR (2012) Acaricide resistance mechanisms in *Rhipicephalus* (*Boophilus*) *microplus*. Bras J Vet Parasitol 21(1):1–6

Guglielmone AA, Nava S, Robbins RG (2021) Neotropical hard ticks (acari: ixodida: ixodidae). Springer, Cham. https://doi.org/10.1007/978-3-030-72353-8

Herrera Y, Rizo A, Soca M, Iglesias J, Ojeda F, Santana H, Medina R (2024) Evaluación de la actividad acaricida *in vitro* del sulfuro de calcio en *Rhipicephalus* (*Boophilus*) *microplus*. Producción de Rumiantes/Convención AGROPAT 2022 Evaluación, April, 3–7

Jamroz RC, Guerrero FD, Pruett JH, Oehler DD, Miller RJ (2000) Molecular and biochemical survey of acaricide resistance mechanisms in larvae from Mexican strains of the southern cattle tick, *Boophilus microplus*. J Insect Physiol 46(5):685–695. https://doi.org/10.1016/S0022-1910(99)00157-2

Jonsson NN, Piper EK (2007) Integrated control programs for ticks on cattle

Jonsson NN, Mayer DG, Matschoss AL, Green PE, Ansell J (1998) Production effects of cattle tick (*Boophilus microplus*) infestation of high yielding dairy cows. Vet Parasitol 78(1):65–77. https://doi.org/10.1016/S0304-4017(98)00118-6

Jonsson NN, Matschoss AL, Pepper P, Green PE, Albrecht MS, Hungerford J, Ansell J (2000a) Evaluation of TickGARDPLUS, a novel vaccine against *Boophilus microplus*, in lactating Holstein–Friesian cows. Vet Parasitol 88(3-4):275–285. https://doi.org/10.1016/S0304-4017(99)00213-7

Jonsson NN, Mayer DG, Green PE (2000b) Possible risk factors on Queensland dairy farms for acaricide resistance in cattle tick (*Boophilus microplus*). Vet Parasitol 88(1-2):79–92. https://doi.org/10.1016/S0304-4017(99)00189-2

Klafke GM, Sabatini GA, de Albuquerque TA, Martins JR, Kemp DH, Miller RJ, Schumaker TTS (2006) Larval immersion tests with ivermectin in populations of the cattle tick *Rhipicephalus* (*Boophilus*) *microplus* (Acari: Ixodidae) from State of Sao Paulo, Brazil. Vet Parasitol 142(3-4):386–390. https://doi.org/10.1016/j.vetpar.2006.07.001

Kunz SE, Kemp DH (1994) Insecticides and acaricides: resistance and environmental impact. Int Off Epizoot 13(4):1249–1286. https://doi.org/10.20506/rst.13.4.816

Lawrence LJ, Casida JE (1983) Stereospecific action of pyrethroid insecticides on the γ-aminobutyric acid receptor-ionophore complex. Science 221(4618):1399–1401. https://doi.org/10.1126/science.6310756

Le Gall VL, Klafke GM, Torres TT (2018) Detoxification mechanisms involved in ivermectin resistance in the cattle tick, *Rhipicephalus* (*Boophilus*) *microplus*. Sci Rep 8(1):1–10. https://doi.org/10.1177/1094342012440585

Lees K, Jones AK, Matsuda K, Akamatsu M, Sattelle DB, Woods DJ, Bowman AS (2014) Functional characterisation of a nicotinic acetylcholine receptor α subunit from the brown dog tick, *Rhipicephalus sanguineus*. Int J Parasitol 44(1):75–81. https://doi.org/10.1016/j.ijpara.2013.11.002

Li AY, Davey RB, George JE (2005) Carbaryl resistance in Mexican strains of the southern cattle tick (acari: ixodidae). J Econ Entomol 98(2):552–556. https://doi.org/10.1093/jee/98.2.552

Li Y, Chen A, Miller RJ, Davey RB, George J (2007) Acaricide resistance and synergism between permethrin and amitraz against susceptible and resistant strains of *Boophilus microplus* (acari: ixodidae). Pest Manag Sci 63(9):882–889

Lichtman AH (2013) Adaptive immunity and atherosclerosis: mouse tales in the AJP. Am J Pathol 182(1):5–9. https://doi.org/10.1016/j.ajpath.2012.10.006

Lin H, Chuan-hua X, Jin-jun W, Ming L, Wen-cai L, Zhi-mo Z (2009) Resistance selection and biochemical mechanism of resistance to two acaricides in *Tetranychus cinnabarinus* (Boiduval). Pestic Biochem Physiol 93(1):47–52. https://doi.org/10.1016/j.pestbp.2008.11.001

Lopes WDZ, Teixeira WFP, de Matos LVS, Felippelli G, Cruz BC, Maciel WG, Buzzulini C, Fávero FC, Soares VE, de Oliveira GP, da Costa AJ (2013) Effects of macrocyclic lactones on the reproductive parameters of engorged *Rhipicephalus* (*Boophilus*) *microplus* females detached from experimentally infested cattle. Exp Parasitol 135(1):72–78. https://doi.org/10.1016/j.exppara.2013.06.003

Lovis L, Perret JL, Bouvier J, Fellay JM, Kaminsky R, Betschart B, Sager H (2011) A new *in vitro* test to evaluate the resistance level against acaricides of the cattle tick, *Rhipicephalus* (*Boophilus*) *microplus*. Vet Parasitol 182(2–4):269–280. https://doi.org/10.1016/j.vetpar.2011.06.004

Lovis L, Reggi J, Berggoetz M, Betschart B, Sager H (2013) Determination of acaricide resistance in *Rhipicephalus* (*Boophilus*) *microplus* (Acari: Ixodidae) field populations of Argentina, South Africa, and Australia with the larval tarsal test. J Med Entomol 50(2):326–335. https://doi.org/10.1603/ME12127

Lumaret J-P, Martínez M, I. (2005) El impacto de productos veterinarios sobre insectos coprófagos: consecuencias sobre la degradación del estiércol en pastizales. Acta Zool Mex 21(3):137–148

Madder M, Thys E, Achi L, Touré A, De Deken R (2011) *Rhipicephalus* (*Boophilus*) *microplus*: a most successful invasive tick species in West-Africa. Exp Appl Acarol 53(2):139–145. https://doi.org/10.1007/s10493-010-9390-8

Maggi MD, Ruffinengo SR, Mendoza Y et al (2011) Susceptibility of *Varroa destructor* (Acari: Varroidae) to synthetic acaricides in Uruguay: Varroa mites' potential to develop acaricide resistance. Parasitol Res 108:815–821. https://doi.org/10.1007/s00436-010-2122-5

Maharana BR, Baithalu RK, Allaie IM, Mishra C, Samal L (2011) Mechanism of immunity to tick infestation in livestock. Vet World 4(3):131–135. https://doi.org/10.5455/vetworld.2011.131-135

Maryam J, Babar ME, Nadeem A, Hussain T (2012) Genetic variants in interferon gamma (IFN-γ) gene are associated with resistance against ticks in *Bos taurus* and *Bos indicus*. Mol Biol Rep 39(4):4565–4570. https://doi.org/10.1007/S11033-011-1246-8

Mattioli RC, Pandey VS, Murray M, Fitzpatrick JL (2000) Immunogenetic influences on tick resistance in African cattle with particular reference to trypanotolerant N'Dama (*Bos taurs*) and trypanosusceptible Gobra zebu (*Bos indicus*) cattle. Acta Trop 75(3):263–277. https://doi.org/10.1016/S0001-706X(00)00063-2

Maya-Delgado A, Madder M, Benítez-Ortíz W, Saegerman C, Berkvens D, Ron-Garrido L (2020) Molecular screening of cattle ticks, tick-borne pathogens and amitraz resistance in ticks of Santo Domingo de los Tsáchilas province in Ecuador. Ticks Tick-Borne Dis 11(5):101492. https://doi.org/10.1016/j.ttbdis.2020.101492

Medlock JM, Hansford KM, Bormane A, Derdakova M, Estrada-Peña A, George J-C, Golovljova I, Jaenson TGT, Jensen J-K, Jensen PM, Kazimirova M, Oteo JA, Papa A, Pfister K, Plantard O, Randolph SE, Rizzoli A, Santos-Silva MM, Sprong H, Van Bortel W (2013) Driving forces for changes in geographical distribution of *Ixodes ricinus* ticks in Europe. Parasit Vectors 6(1):1–11. https://doi.org/10.1186/1756-3305-6-1

Mendes MC, Lima CKP, Nogueira AHC, Yoshihara E, Chiebao DP, Gabriel FHL, Ueno TEH, Namindome A, Klafke GM (2011) Resistance to cypermethrin, deltamethrin and chlorpyriphos in populations of *Rhipicephalus* (*Boophilus*) *microplus* (Acari: Ixodidae) from small farms of the State of São Paulo, Brazil. Vet Parasitol 178(3–4):383–388. https://doi.org/10.1016/j.vetpar.2011.01.006

Mendes MC, Duarte FC, Martins JR, Klafke GM, Fiorini LC, de Barros ATM (2013a) Characterization of the pyrethroid resistance profile of *Rhipicephalus* (*Boophilus*) *microplus* populations from the states of Rio Grande do Sul and Mato Grosso do Sul, Brazil. Braz J Vet Parasitol 22(3):379–384. https://doi.org/10.1590/S1984-29612013000300010

Mendes EC, Mendes MC, Sato ME (2013b) Diagnosis of amitraz resistance in Brazilian populations of *Rhipicephalus* (*Boophilus*) *microplus* (acari: ixodidae) with larval immersion test. Exp Appl Acarol 61(3):357–369. https://doi.org/10.1007/s10493-013-9697-3

Meyer JM, Ejendal KFK, Avramova LV, Garland-Kuntz EE, Giraldo-Calderón GI, Brust TF, Watts VJ, Hill CA (2012) A "genome-to-lead" approach for insecticide discovery: pharmacological characterization and screening of Aedes aegypti D1-like dopamine receptors. PLoS Negl Trop Dis 6(1):1–15. https://doi.org/10.1371/journal.pntd.0001478

Mitchell GJ (1996) A reflective moment with false cheerfulness. Nurs Sci Q 9(2):53–54. https://doi.org/10.1177/089431849600900204

Muhanguzi D, Byaruhanga J, Amanyire W, Ndekezi C, Ochwo S, Nkamwesiga J, Mwiine FN, Tweyongyere R, Fourie J, Madder M, Schetters T, Horak I, Juleff N, Jongejan F (2020) Invasive cattle ticks in East Africa: morphological and molecular confirmation of the presence of *Rhipicephalus microplus* in south-eastern Uganda. Parasit Vectors 13(1):1–9. https://doi.org/10.1186/s13071-020-04043-z

Mulchandani A, Kaneva I, Chen W (1998) Biosensor for direct determination of organophosphate nerve agents using recombinant *Escherichia coli* with surface-expressed organophosphorus hydrolase. 2. Fiber-optic microbial biosensor. Anal Chem 70(23):5042–5046. https://doi.org/10.1021/ac980643l

Nava S, Guglielmone AA, Mangold AJ (2009) An overview of systematics and evolution of ticks. Front Biosci 14:2857–2877. https://doi.org/10.2741/3418

Nogueira Domingues L, dos Santos Alves Figueiredo B, Passos de Paiva Bello AC, Pinto da Cunha A, Thadeu Medeiros de Barros A, Cerqueira Leite R, Silaghi C, Pfister K, Friche Passos LM (2012) Survey of pyrethroid and organophosphate resistance in Brazilian field populations of *Rhipicephalus* (*Boophilus*) *microplus*: detection of C190A mutation in domain II of the para-type sodium channel gene. Vet Parasitol 189(2-4):327–332. https://doi.org/10.1016/j.vetpar.2012.04.031

O'kelly J, Seifert G (1969) Relationship between resistance to *Boophilus microplus*, nutritional status, and blood composition in shorthorn X hereford cattle. Aust J Biol Sci 22(6):1497. https://doi.org/10.1071/BI9691497

Obaid MK, Islam N, Alouffi A, Khan AZ, da Silva Vaz I, Tanaka T, Ali A (2022) Acaricides resistance in ticks: selection, diagnosis, mechanisms, and mitigation. Front Cell Infect Microbiol 12(July):1–20. https://doi.org/10.3389/fcimb.2022.941831

Ono M, Terao M, Takiguchi Y, Mishima H, Muramatsu S, Ide J (1983) Milbemycins, a new family of macrolide antibiotics fermentation, isolation and physicochemical properties of milbemycins D, E, F, G and H. J Antibiot 36(5):502–508. https://doi.org/10.7164/antibiotics.36.502

Otto PI, Guimarães SEF, Verardo LL, Azevedo ALS, Vandenplas J, Soares ACC, Sevillano CA, Veroneze R, de Fatima A, Pires M, de Freitas C, Prata MCA, Furlong J, Verneque RS, Martins MF, Panetto JCC, Carvalho WA, Gobo DOR, da Silva MVGB, Machado MA (2018) Genome-wide association studies for tick resistance in *Bos taurus* × *Bos indicus* crossbred cattle: a deeper look into this intricate mechanism. J Dairy Sci 101(12):11020–11032. https://doi.org/10.3168/jds.2017-14223

Paternina Durango EM, Maza Angulo LA, Medina Ríos H, Simanca Sotelo JC, Vergara Garay OD (2015) Evaluation of sulfur flower in mineralized salts as repellent of ectoparasites (ticks and flies) in crossbred heifers *Bos taurus* x *Bos indicus* in the valley of the sinu. Livest Res Rural Dev 27:8

Paucar-Quishpe V, Pérez-Otáñez X, Rodríguez-Hidalgo R, Cepeda-Bastidas D, Pérez-Escalante C, Grijalva-Olmedo J, Enríquez S, Arciniegas-Ortega S, Sandoval-Trávez L, Benavides-Erazo B, Vanwambeke SO, Saegerman C, Ron-Garrido L (2023) An economic evaluation of cattle tick acaricide-resistances and the financial losses in subtropical dairy farms of Ecuador: a farm system approach. PLoS ONE 18(6):1–31. https://doi.org/10.1371/journal.pone.0287104

Pereira MC, Labruna MB, Szabó MPJ, Klafke GM (2008) *Rhipicephalus* (*Boophilus*) *microplus*: biologia, controle e resistência. MedVet, São Paulo

Perez-Cogollo LC, Rodriguez-Vivas RI, Ramirez-Cruz GT, Miller RJ (2010) First report of the cattle tick *Rhipicephalus microplus* resistant to ivermectin in Mexico. Vet Parasitol 168(1):165–169. https://doi.org/10.1016/j.vetpar.2009.10.021

Pérez-González IE, Prado-Ochoa MG, Muñoz-Guzmán MA, Vázquez-Valadez VH, Velázquez-Sánchez AM, Avila-Suárez BL, Cuenca-Verde C, Angeles E, Alba-Hurtado F (2014) Effect of new ethyl and methyl carbamates on *Rhipicephalus microplus* larvae and adult ticks resistant to conventional ixodicides. Vet Parasitol 199(3):235–241. https://doi.org/10.1016/j.vetpar.2013.07.042

Pérez-Otáñez X, Vanwambeke SO, Orozco-Alvarez G, Arciniegas-Ortega S, Ron-Garrido L, Rodríguez-Hidalgo R (2023) Widespread acaricide resistance and multi-resistance in *Rhipicephalus microplus* in Ecuador and associated environmental and management risk factors. Ticks Tick-Borne Dis 15(1):102274. https://doi.org/10.1016/j.ttbdis.2023.102274

Pérez-Otáñez X, Rodríguez-Hidalgo R, Enríquez S, Celi-Erazo M, Benítez W, Saegerman C, Vaca-Moyano F, Ron-Garrido L, Vanwambeke SO (2024) High-resolution prediction models for *Rhipicephalus microplus* and *Amblyomma cajennense* s.l. ticks affecting cattle and their spatial distribution in continental Ecuador using bioclimatic factors. Exp Appl Acarol 92:439–462. https://doi.org/10.1007/s10493-023-00883-3

Polanco Echeverry DN, Ríos Osorio LA (2016) Aspectos biológicos y ecológicos de las garrapatas duras. Corpoica Cienc Tecnol 17(1):81–95

Quadros DG, Johnson TL, Whitney TR, Oliver JD, Chávez ASO (2020) Plant-derived natural compounds for tick pest control in livestock and wildlife: pragmatism or Utopia? Insects 11(8):1–25. https://doi.org/10.3390/insects11080490

Rajput ZI, Hu S-H, Chen W-J, Arijo AG, Xiao C-W (2006) Importance of ticks and their chemical and immunological control in livestock. J Zhejiang Univ Sci B 7(11):912–921. https://doi.org/10.1631/jzus.2006.B0912

Rechav Y, Hay L (1992) The effects of nutritional status of rabbits and sheep on their resistance to the ticks *Rhipicephalus evertsi evertsi* and *R. appendiculatus*. Exp Appl Acarol 15(3):171–179. https://doi.org/10.1007/BF01195789

Rezende DDM, Fadini MAM, Oliveira HG, Oliveira CM, Melo JWS, Guedes RNC, Pallini A (2013) Fitness costs associated with low-level dimethoate resistance in *Phytoseiulus macropilis*. Exp Appl Acarol 60(3):367–379. https://doi.org/10.1007/s10493-012-9654-6

Riek R (1962) Studies on the reactions of animals to infestation with ticks. VI. Resistance of cattle to infestation with the tick *Boophilus microplus* (Canestrini). Aust J Agric Res 13(3):532. https://doi.org/10.1071/AR9620532

Roberts JA (1968) Acquisition by the host of resistance to the cattle tick, *Boophilus microplus* (Canestrini). J Parasitol 54(4):657–662

Rodríguez-Hidalgo R, Pérez-Otáñez X, Garcés-Carrera S, Vanwambeke SO, Madder M, Benítez-Ortiz W (2017) The current status of resistance to alpha-cypermethrin, ivermectin, and amitraz of the cattle tick (*Rhipicephalus microplus*) in Ecuador. PLoS ONE 12(4):1–15. https://doi.org/10.1371/journal.pone.0174652

Rodriguez-Valle M, Vance M, Moolhuijzen PM, Tao X, Lew-Tabor AE (2012) Differential recognition by tick-resistant cattle of the recombinantly expressed *Rhipicephalus microplus* serine protease inhibitor-3 (RMS-3). Ticks Tick-Borne Dis 3(3):159–169. https://doi.org/10.1016/j.ttbdis.2012.03.002

Rodriguez-Valle M, Moolhuijzen P, Piper EK, Weiss O, Vance M, Bellgard M, Lew-Tabor A (2013) Rhipicephalus microplus lipocalins (LRMs): genomic identification and analysis of the bovine immune response using in silico predicted B and T cell epitopes. Int J Parasitol 43(9):739–752. https://doi.org/10.1016/j.ijpara.2013.04.005

Rodríguez-Vivas RI, Trees AJ, Rosado-Aguilar JA, Villegas-Perez SL, Hodgkinson JE (2011) Evolution of acaricide resistance: phenotypic and genotypic changes in field populations of *Rhipicephalus* (*Boophilus*) *microplus* in response to pyrethroid selection pressure. Int J Parasitol 4:895–903. https://doi.org/10.1016/j.ijpara.2011.03.012

Rodríguez-Vivas I, Hodgkinson R, Trees JE (2012) Resistencia a los acaricidas en *Rhipicephalus* (*Boophilus*) *microplus*: situación actual y mecanismos de resistencia. Rev Mex Cien Pecuarias 3(1):9–24

Rodríguez-Vivas RI, Pérez-Cogollo LC, Rosado-Aguilar JA, Ojeda-Chi MM, Trinidad-Martinez I, Miller RJ, Li AY, de León AP, Guerrero F, Klafke G (2014) *Rhipicephalus* (*Boophilus*) *microplus* resistant to acaricides and ivermectin in cattle farms of Mexico. Braz J Vet Parasitol 23(2):113–122

Rodriguez-Vivas RI, Jonsson NN, Bhushan C (2018) Strategies for the control of *Rhipicephalus microplus* ticks in a world of conventional acaricide and macrocyclic lactone resistance. Parasitol Res 117(1):3–29. https://doi.org/10.1007/s00436-017-5677-6

Rodriguez-Vivas RI, España ER, Blanco IL, Ojeda-Chi MM, Trinidad-Martinez I, Islas JAT, Bhushan C (2021) 'Monitoring the resistance of *Rhipicephalus microplus* to amitraz, flumethrin, coumaphos, and ivermectin on cattle farms in Mexico'. Vet Parasitol: Reg Stud Rep 26:100644

Rosario-Cruz R, Guerrero FD, Miller RJ, Rodriguez-Vivas RI, Tijerina M, Dominguez-Garcia DI, Hernandez-Ortiz R, Cornel AJ, McAbee RD, Alonso-Diaz MA (2009) Molecular survey of pyrethroid resistance mechanisms in Mexican field populations of *Rhipicephalus* (*Boophilus*) *microplus*. Parasitol Res 105(4):1145–1153. https://doi.org/10.1007/s00436-009-1539-1

Roulston W, Wharton RH, Nolan J, Kerr JD, Wilson JTGTP, Martina S (1981) A survey for resistance in cattle ticks to acaricides. Aust Vet J 57(8):362–371. https://doi.org/10.1111/j.1751-0813.1981.tb00524.x

Ruiz A, Blanco R (2009) Grado de resistencia *Rhipicephalus* (*Boophilus*) *microplus* a productos ixodicidas y su residualidad en lecheen 20 predios de sitema doble proposito de piedemonte llanero

Sammataro D, Untalan P, Guerrero F, Finley J (2005) The resistance of varroa mites (Acari: Varroidae) to acaricides and the presence of esterase. Int J Acarol 31(1):67–74. https://doi.org/10.1080/01647950508684419

Sangster NC (2001) Managing parasiticide resistance. Vet Parasitol 98(1):89–109. https://doi.org/10.1016/S0304-4017(01)00425-3

Shaw RD (1966) Culture of an organophosphorus Resistance, strain of B. microplus and an assessment of its spectrum. Bull Entomol Res 56:389–405

Shoop WL, Mrozik H, Fisher MH (1995) Structure and activity of avermectins and milbemycins in animal health. Vet Parasitol 59(2):139–156. https://doi.org/10.1016/0304-4017(94)00743-V

Showler AT, Saelao P (2022) Integrative alternative tactics for ixodid control. Insects 13(3):302. https://doi.org/10.3390/insects13030302

Shyma KP, Kumar S, Sharma AK, Ray DD, Ghosh S (2012) Acaricide resistance status in Indian isolates of *Hyalomma anatolicum*. Exp Appl Acarol 58(4):471–481. https://doi.org/10.1007/s10493-012-9592-3

Soares SF, Borges LMF, de Sousa Braga R, Ferreira LL, Louly CCB, Tresvenzol LMF, de Paula JR, Ferri PH (2010) Repellent activity of plant-derived compounds against *Amblyomma cajennense* (acari: ixodidae) nymphs. Vet Parasitol 167(1):67–73. https://doi.org/10.1016/j.vetpar.2009.09.047

Soberanes Céspedes N, Rosario Cruz R, Santamaría Vargas M, García Vazquez Z (2005) General esterase activity variation in the cattle tick *Boophilus microplus* and its relationship with organophosphate resistance. Tecn Pecuaria Mexico 43(2):239–246

Soberanes N, Santamaría M, Fragoso H (2002) Primer caso de resistencia al amitraz en la garrapata del ganado Boophilus microplus en México. Técn Pecuaria México 40(1):81–92

Solomon G, Kaaya GP (1996) Comparison of resistance in three breeds of cattle against African ixodid ticks. Exp Appl Acarol 20(4):223–230. https://doi.org/10.1007/BF00054514

Spickett AM, Horak IG, Van Niekerk A, Braack LE (1992) The effect of veld-burning on the seasonal abundance of free-living ixodid ticks as determined by drag-sampling. Onderstepoort J Vet Res 59(4):285–292

Stachurski F, Adakal H (2010) Exploiting the heterogeneous drop-off rhythm of *Amblyomma variegatum* nymphs to reduce pasture infestation by adult ticks. Parasitology 137(7):1129–1137. https://doi.org/10.1017/S0031182009992071

Stone NE, Olafson PU, Davey RB, Buckmeier G, Bodine D, Sidak-Loftis LC, Giles JR, Duhaime R, Miller RJ, Mosqueda J, Scoles G, Wagner DM, Busch JD (2014) Multiple mutations in the para-sodium channel gene are associated with pyrethroid resistance in *Rhipicephalus microplus* from the United States and Mexico. Parasit Vectors 7(1):456. https://doi.org/10.1186/s13071-014-0456-z

Stutzer C, van Zyl WA, Olivier NA, Richards S, Maritz-Olivier C (2013) Gene expression profiling of adult female tissues in feeding *Rhipicephalus microplus* cattle ticks. Int J Parasitol 43(7):541–554. https://doi.org/10.1016/j.ijpara.2013.01.009

Sugimoto N, Osakabe M (2014) Cross-resistance between cyenopyrafen and pyridaben in the twospotted spider mite *Tetranychus urticae* (acari: tetranychidae). Pest Manag Sci 70(7):1090–1096. https://doi.org/10.1002/ps.3652

Sun M, Ren Q, Guan G, Liu Z, Ma M, Gou H, Chen Z, Li Y, Liu A, Niu Q, Yang J, Yin H, Luo J (2011) Virulence of *Beauveria bassiana*, *Metarhizium anisopliae* and *Paecilomyces lilacinus* to the engorged female *Hyalomma anatolicum anatolicum* tick (acari: ixodidae). Vet Parasitol 180(3):389–393. https://doi.org/10.1016/j.vetpar.2011.03.027

Sutherst RW, Comins HN (1979) The management of acaricide resistance in the cattle tick, *Boophilus microplus* (Canestrini) (acari: ixodidae), in Australia. Bull Entomol Res 69(3):519–537. https://doi.org/10.1017/S0007485300019015

Tanaka K, Scott JG, Matsumura F (1984) Picrotoxinin receptor in the central nervous system of the American cockroach: its role in the action of cyclodiene-type insecticides. Pestic Biochem Physiol 22(1):117–127. https://doi.org/10.1016/0048-3575(84)90017-8

Temeyer KB, Olafson PU, Brake DK, Tuckow AP, Li AY, Pérez de León AA (2013a) Acetylcholinesterase of *Rhipicephalus* (*Boophilus*) *microplus* and *Phlebotomus papatasi*: gene identification, expression, and biochemical properties of recombinant proteins. Pestic Biochem Physiol 106(3):118–123. https://doi.org/10.1016/j.pestbp.2013.01.005

Temeyer KB, Tuckow AP, Brake DK, Li AY, Pérez de León AA (2013b) Acetylcholinesterases of blood-feeding flies and ticks. Chem Biol Interact 203(1):319–322. https://doi.org/10.1016/j.cbi.2012.09.010

Thullner F, Willadsen P, Kemp D (2007) Acaricide rotation strategy for managing resistance in the tick *Rhipicephalus* (*Boophilus*) *microplus* (Acarina: Ixodidae): laboratory experiment with a field strain from Costa Rica. J Med Entomol 44(5):817–821. https://doi.org/10.1603/0022-2585(2007)44[817:arsfmr]2.0.co;2

Tinoco T, Ron-garrido L, Perez-otañez X (2023) Preliminary evaluation of the effectiveness of the GAVAC® immunogen and the rational use of acaricides as an alternative for an integrated tick control program in Ecuador Evaluación preliminar de la efectividad del inmunógeno GAVAC® y el uso racional de acaricidas como alternativa de un programa integrado de control de garrapatas en Ecuador. ESPOCH Congr 3(1):793–806. https://doi.org/10.18502/espoch.v3i1.14487

Tovar HL, Noriega JA, Caraballo P (2016) Efecto de la ivermectina sobre la estructura del ensamble de escarabajos coprófagos (Coleoptera: Scarabaeidae: Aphodiinae-Scarabaeinae) en las sabanas colombianas de la región Caribe Ivermectin effect on the structure of the ensembles of dung beetles. Actual Biol 38:157–166. https://doi.org/10.17533/udea.acbi.v38n105a03

Valencia L, Nacimento G, Oquendo G, Agudelo V, Marinilla CIN (2009). Evaluación de una mezcla de cipermetrina + clorpirifós sobre la garrapata Rhipicephalus (Boophilus) microplus en pruebas de campo y de laboratorio en el predio Esteban Jaramillo Román Gómez del Politécnico Colombiano de Marinilla, Antioquia. Revista CES Medicina Veterinaria y Zootecnia, 4(2), 57–65. Retrieved from http://www.redalyc.org/articulo.oa?id=321428102006

Van Leeuwen T, Vontas J, Tsagkarakou A, Tirry L (2009) Mechanisms of acaricide resistance in the two-spotted spider mite *Tetranychus urticae*. In: Ishaaya I, Horowitz AR (eds) Biorational control of arthropod pests: application and resistance management. Springer, Cham, pp 347–393. https://doi.org/10.1007/978-90-481-2316-2_14

Wagland B (1975) Host resistance to cattle tick (*Boophilus microplus*) in Brahman (Bos indicus) cattle. I. Responses of previously unexposed cattle to four infestations with 20,000 larvae. Aust J Agric Res 26(6):1073. https://doi.org/10.1071/AR9751073

Weston DP, Poynton HC, Wellborn GA, Lydy MJ, Blalock BJ, Sepulveda MS, Colbourne JK (2013) Multiple origins of pyrethroid insecticide resistance across the species complex of a nontarget aquatic crustacean, *Hyalella azteca*. Proc Natl Acad Sci 110(41):16532–16537. https://doi.org/10.1073/pnas.1302023110

Wikel S (2013) Ticks and tick-borne pathogens at the cutaneous interface: host defenses, tick countermeasures, and a suitable environment for pathogen establishment. Front Microbiol 4:337. https://doi.org/10.3389/fmicb.2013.00337

Young AS, Groocock CM, Kariuki DP (1988) Integrated control of ticks and tick-borne diseases of cattle in Africa. Parasitology 96(Pt 2):403–432. https://doi.org/10.1017/s0031182000058388

Zheng Y, Priest B, Cully DF, Ludmerer SW (2003) RdlDv, a novel GABA-gated chloride channel gene from the American dog tick *Dermacentor variabilis*. Insect Biochem Mol Biol 33(6):595–599. https://doi.org/10.1016/S0965-1748(03)00038-9

# Basic Biology of Ticks

2

Rachid Selmi, Hanène Belkahia, and Mourad Ben Said

**Abstract**

This chapter thoroughly examines the basic biology of ticks and their significant impact on various ecosystems. It delves into their complex four-stage life cycle, specialized sensory abilities, and capacity to target a wide range of host species, including livestock, pets, and crops. The chapter underscores the crucial role ticks play in transmitting various pathogens, such as those causing Lyme disease and Rocky Mountain spotted fever, highlighting the need for further research and a deeper understanding of tick biology. It discusses the severe consequences of tick infestations, which can lead to the death of livestock, companion animals, and crop plants due to extensive feeding damage, disruption of vital functions, and the introduction of toxins and harmful pathogens. To address the threats posed by ticks, the chapter highlights the need for an integrated approach. This involves improving tick control methods, raising public awareness, and continuing to study the interactions between ticks, their hosts, and the pathogens they carry. By gaining a deeper understanding of the basic biology of ticks, we can create more effective strategies to reduce their impact and preserve the delicate balance of the ecosystems they inhabit. This knowledge can inform policy decisions, guide research priorities, and empower communities to take proactive steps in protecting themselves, their livestock, and their crops from the devastating consequences of tick infestations.

R. Selmi · H. Belkahia
Laboratory of Microbiology, National School of Veterinary Medicine of Sidi Thabet, University of Manouba, Sidi Thabet, Tunisia

M. Ben Said (✉)
Laboratory of Microbiology, National School of Veterinary Medicine of Sidi Thabet, University of Manouba, Sidi Thabet, Tunisia

Department of Basic Sciences, Higher Institute of Biotechnology of Sidi Thabet, University of Manouba, Sidi Thabet, Tunisia


S. Kumar et al. (eds.), *Acaricides Resistance in Ticks*,
https://doi.org/10.1007/978-981-97-7411-1_2

**Keywords**

Ticks · Life cycle · Tick anatomy · Morphology · Physiology · Tick–host interactions · Tick-borne pathogens

## 2.1 Introduction

Ticks belong to the Arthropoda phylum, the Acari subclass, and the Ixodida order. Three tick families have been identified to date: the Ixodidae or hard ticks (694 species), the Argasidae or soft ticks (177 species), and the Nuttalliellidae (a single species) (Fig. 2.1).

Ticks, diminutive parasitic arachnids, thrive on the blood of mammals, birds, and reptiles. Inhabiting a myriad of environments, from forests and grasslands to urban areas (Park et al. 2021), their existence poses both a nuisance and a potential peril, given their capacity to transmit diseases like Lyme disease, Rocky Mountain spotted fever, and ehrlichiosis (Boulanger and Wikel 2021).

Embarking on a four-stage journey (egg, larva, nymph, and adult), the tick's life cycle unfolds intricately. Females deposit thousands of eggs in protected locations, which metamorphose into larvae, diminutive six-legged entities that feed on small hosts like insects or rodents. Post-molt, larvae transition into larger eight-legged nymphs, seeking larger hosts such as birds or mammals for sustenance. Culminating in the adult stage, the apex of their life cycle involves feeding on even larger hosts like humans or livestock, thus perpetuating the species (Hofmeester et al. 2018).

Tick activity undergoes marked fluctuations, with peak activity occurring during the warmer months when temperatures range between 50- and 80-degree Fahrenheit (Hassett et al. 2022; Keesing et al. 2022). Ticks are predominantly found in forests and grasslands, but they also display adaptability and can be found in meadows and even urban areas.

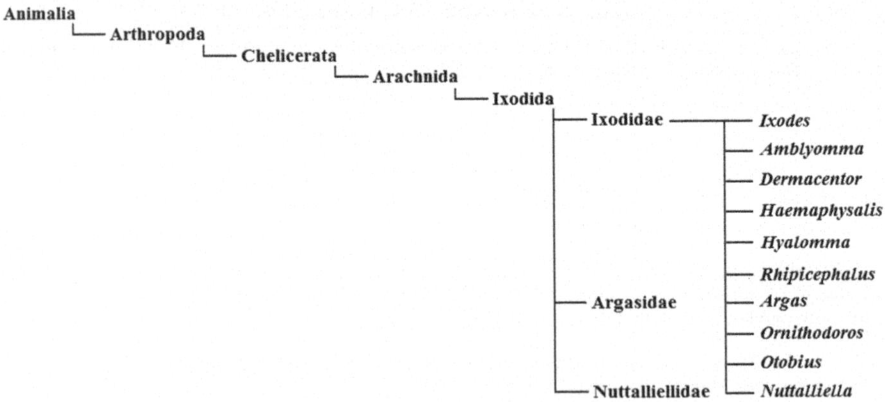


**Fig. 2.1** Classification of ticks. (Modified from Hoogstraal 1956)

Ticks are attracted to heat, carbon dioxide, and movement, which they use to locate potential hosts. They employ crawling to attach themselves to humans and animals (Gherman et al. 2012).

Ticks are known to be vectors for various diseases, including Lyme disease, which is caused by the spirochete bacterium *Borrelia burgdorferi* sensu lato (Keesing et al. 2022). Understanding tick behavior and activity patterns is crucial for assessing the risk of tick exposure and developing effective tick control strategies.

Ticks are arachnids that share anatomical and physiological similarities with spiders, scorpions, and mites (Hoogstraal 1956). They have a robust outer covering called a carapace, which protects them from predators and environmental elements. With eight legs for mobility and a piercing-sucking mouthpart for blood feeding, ticks possess internal systems such as the digestive system, respiratory system, nervous system, and reproductive organs (Deshpande et al. 2023).

Ticks have a significant impact on ecosystems and economies due to their role as vectors of diseases. They can transmit various pathogens to humans and animals, leading to significant health issues and economic consequences (Estrada-Peña et al. 2013). Here, we will explore the diverse dimensions of tick biology and their influence on ecological and economic landscapes.

## 2.2 Overview of Tick Life Cycle and Behavior

### 2.2.1 Life Cycle

The life cycle of ticks is a fascinating and essential aspect of their biology, and a comprehensive understanding of this cycle is crucial for effective control measures and disease prevention. Ticks progress through a four-stage life cycle, encompassing the egg, larva, nymph, and adult stages (Chen et al. 2009; Fourie and Horak 2004). The life cycle initiation involves the female tick laying eggs, a process typically occurring during the spring or fall seasons. These eggs hatch into larvae within a few weeks, with the larvae exhibiting a small size and possessing six legs (Fig. 2.2). Larvae actively seek out their host to feed on during this stage (Sasakawa 2007; Olegário et al. 2011).

Advancing through development, ticks enter the nymph stage, characterized by a larger size and the presence of eight legs. Nymphs transition to larger hosts, including birds or mammals, for their blood meals (Cadenas et al. 2007; Price et al. 2023).

The final stage in the tick life cycle is the adult stage, the largest and most noticeable phase. Adult ticks seek out even larger hosts, such as humans or livestock, to complete their life cycle and obtain necessary blood meals (Espinaze et al. 2015; GarciaGuizzo et al. 2023).

#### 2.2.1.1 Eggs

Ticks are highly fecund, with a single fertilized female capable of producing thousands of eggs. The clutch size and subsequent larval hatch vary among tick species.

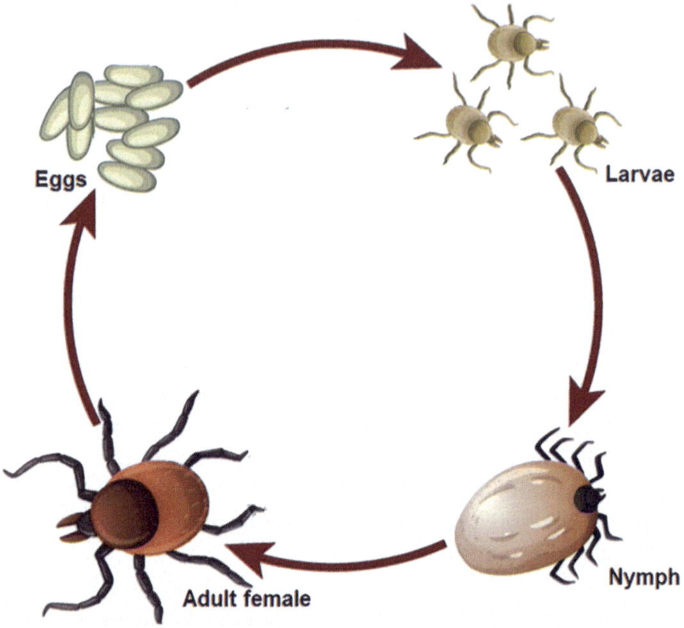


**Fig. 2.2** The main phases of tick life cycle

For example, a *Dermacentor* female can produce a clutch of 3000–4000 eggs, while an *Amblyomma* female can lay as many as 8000 eggs (Brunner et al. 2011).

The mating behavior of ticks differs among species. Metastriate ticks, such as *Amblyomma* spp., *Dermacentor* spp., and *Rhipicephalus sanguineus*, mate on the host animal, with males requiring a blood meal before mating. Male metastriate ticks can mate multiple times and may even change hosts to fertilize additional females. On the other hand, prostriate ticks, like *Ixodes* spp., can mate prior to feeding and often remain in copulation with the female tick throughout her feeding and even after detachment from the host (Kiszewski et al. 2001).

It is important to note that tick populations are not easily controlled as they feed and reproduce largely on wildlife reservoirs. Wildlife hosts in areas frequented by dogs serve as a constant source of new ticks, leading to re-infestations. Effective tick control requires a combination of restricting a dog's exposure to tick-infested environments and monthly application of acaricides year-round (Leschnik et al. 2013).

The oviposition period is the time required by ticks from the moment they start laying eggs until they stop laying (time needed to lay eggs). Table 2.1 shows a summary of the oviposition period as well as the estimated mean of eggs' number laid according to the tick specie.

**Table 2.1** The oviposition period and means of eggs number of different tick species

| Tick specie | Oviposition mean period (days) | Mean eggs' number (eggs) | References |
|---|---|---|---|
| *Rhipicephalus sanguineus* sensu lato | 9–19 | 135–1700 | Hadi and Adventini (2015) |
| *Hyalomma marginatum* | 8–11 | 3500 | Elhachimi et al. (2021) |
| *Hyalomma lusitanicum* | 20–30 | 6320 | Ouhelli and Pandey (1984) |
| *Dermacentor variabilis* | 24–26 | 3850–5209 | Dipeolu (1991) |
| *Amblyomma maculatum* | 28–30 | 4278–5216 | Dipeolu (1991) |
| *Ixodes ricinus* | 15–30 | 613–1927 | Dautel and Knülle (2010) |
| *Ornithodoros rostratus* | 15–20 | 143–413 | Costa et al. (2015) |

#### 2.2.1.2 Larvae

Tick larvae are the first stage of the tick life cycle. They hatch from eggs and are typically six-legged. Tick larvae are very small and usually measure less than 1 mm in length (Benelli 2020). Although tick larvae do not possess the ability to transmit diseases to humans or animals during this stage of their development, they can still attach to a host and feed on its blood. Tick larvae are often found in grassy or wooded areas, where they wait for a potential host to pass by. Once a suitable host is detected, the larvae climb onto it and attach using their mouthparts to begin feeding on the host's blood. While the risk of disease transmission is lower with larvae compared to nymphs or adults, their capacity to latch onto a host and feed on its blood remains an important consideration for ensuring proper protection. The feeding process can take several days to complete (Battur et al. 2009; Benelli 2020). After feeding, the tick larvae detach from the host and drop to the ground. They then molt into the next stage of their life cycle, which is the nymph stage (Benelli 2020).

#### 2.2.1.3 Nymphs

The nymph stage is an important phase in the tick life cycle as it plays a significant role in the transmission of tick-borne diseases (Vechtova et al. 2020). During the nymph stage, ticks must have a blood meal to survive. They can feed on a variety of hosts, including mammals, birds, reptiles, and amphibians. The nymphs need a new host at each stage to continue their development (Benelli 2020). Research has shown that the nymph stage of ticks is associated with the transmission of various pathogens. For example, the nymphs of the blacklegged tick (*Ixodes scapularis*) are known to transmit Lyme disease (Hofmeester et al. 2018). Understanding the biology and behavior of nymph ticks is crucial for the prevention and control of tick-borne diseases. Researchers have conducted studies to investigate the stage-specific transcripts and potential functions during the tick life cycle. These studies aim to identify the genes and molecular mechanisms involved in the nymph stage, which can provide valuable insights into tick biology and the development of control strategies (Battur et al. 2009; Benelli 2020).

#### 2.2.1.4 Adults

The adult stage is an important phase in the tick life cycle as it is during this stage that ticks showed their high potential for transmitting pathogens to humans and animals. At this stage, with the metamorphosis of ticks we can differentiate morphologically, between male and female (Battur et al. 2009; Benelli 2020). During the adult stage, ticks are approximately the size of a sesame seed. They can feed on a variety of hosts, including mammals, birds, reptiles, and amphibians. The adult ticks must have a blood meal at this stage to survive and reproduce (Kiszewski et al. 2001; Brunner et al. 2011). Ticks find their hosts by detecting breath, body odors, body heat, moisture, vibrations, and even shadows. They wait in a position known as "questing," where they hold onto leaves and grass with their third and fourth pair of legs. When a host brushes against the spot where a tick is waiting, it quickly climbs aboard and attaches itself to the host's skin (Vayssier-Taussat 2016).

Ticks transmit pathogens that cause diseases through the process of feeding. Depending on the tick species and its stage of life, preparing to feed can take from 10 min to 2 h. The tick cuts into the skin and inserts its feeding tube, which may have barbs to keep it in place. Ticks also secrete a cement-like substance to stay firmly attached during the meal. They can secrete small amounts of saliva with anesthetic properties, making it difficult for the host to feel their presence. If the tick contains a pathogen, it may be transmitted to the host through the saliva or when the tick ingests the host's blood. After feeding, most ticks drop off and prepare for the next life stage, potentially transmitting any acquired diseases to a new host (Battur et al. 2009; Benelli 2020; Gregory et al. 2022). It is worth noting that ticks, including the adult stage, play a significant role in the transmission of Lyme disease. The bacteria causing Lyme disease, such as *Borrelia burgdorferi*, are primarily spread by infected blacklegged ticks (also known as deer ticks) during their adult stage. These ticks are found in specific regions of the United States, such as the northeastern, mid-Atlantic, and north-central states (Battur et al. 2009).

### 2.2.2 Habitat and Behavior of Ticks

Ticks are ectoparasitic arthropods that play a significant role in the transmission of various diseases to humans, and livestock. Understanding the habitat preferences and the behavior of adult ticks is crucial for effective tick control and prevention strategies.

#### 2.2.2.1 Habitat

The habitat of ticks varies according to tick species, the environmental conditions, the available host species and/or vectors, and the evolutive phases of the parasitic cycle. Adult ticks can be found in a wide range of habitats, including forests, grasslands, and urban green spaces associate to warm-blooded mammals acting as hosts for these ectoparasites (Fig. 2.3). This provides ticks with essential resources and protection to carry out complete multiplication cycles (Hansford et al. 2023).

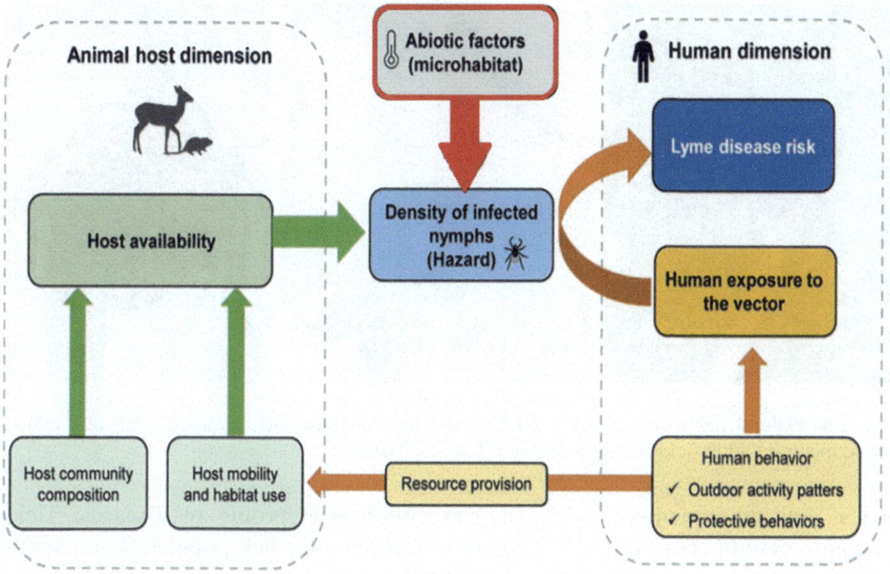


**Fig. 2.3** Tick population dynamics, microhabitat, and tick-borne diseases triggered by various abiotic factors (Diuk-Wasser et al. 2021)

Forests and woodlands are particularly favorable habitats for ticks as they support high populations of wildlife hosts, such as deer and rodents. These hosts not only serve as blood sources for the ticks but also act as reservoirs for tick-borne diseases (Gregory et al. 2022). The typical example of ticks colonizing these regions is the well-known *Ixodes* spp. associated to vegetation during an obligate part of its multiplication cycle (Fig. 2.3) (Diuk-Wasser et al. 2021).

Grasslands and meadows also offer suitable conditions for adult ticks, especially in areas where there is a high abundance of small mammals and birds. These hosts provide the necessary blood meals for the ticks to survive and reproduce (González et al. 2023). In open areas such as deserts, ticks seek out stones, the stems of desiccated plants and animal feeders to lay their eggs. Dromedary camels and wild small mammals are the main hosts of ticks in these areas. For example, *Hyalomma* spp. ticks infesting dromedary camels and *Rhipicephalus* spp. colonizing shepherd's hounds are commonly found in such zones.

Even in urban environments, ticks can thrive in green spaces, such as parks and gardens, if there are suitable hosts and adequate vegetation cover. The presence of these urban habitats can increase the risk of tick-borne disease transmission to human populations (Janzén et al. 2024).

The ability of ticks to inhabit such a wide range of environments highlights their adaptability and the challenges in effectively controlling their populations (Trout Fryxell et al. 2015). Today, with animal movements and intensive climate change, we are increasingly observing the phenomenon of the extension of the specific geographic range of these ticks, which will move into new areas, adapt to new animal

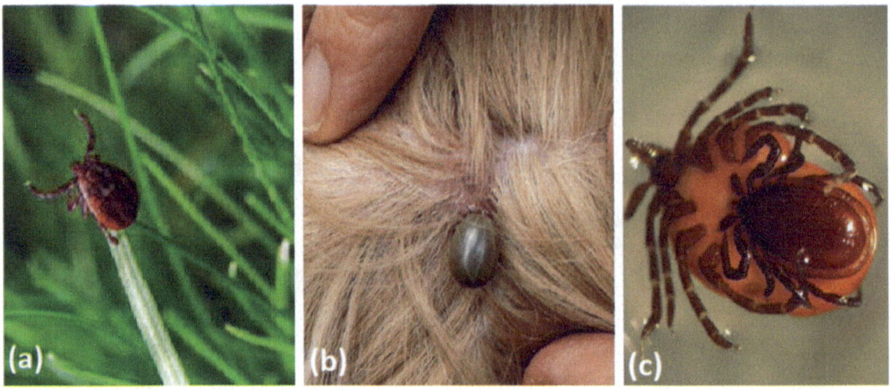


**Fig. 2.4** Natural behaviors of ticks: (**a**) host-seeking behavior; (**b**) engorged adult tick taking blood meal; (**c**) adult ticks mating (Vayssier-Taussat 2016)

hosts, and subsequently modify the epidemiological profile of diseases. Tick-mapping systems constitute an efficient tool to monitor tick population dynamics (Fig. 2.3) (Shah et al. 2023; Kopsco et al. 2023).

The continuous changes recorded on land use/cover, climate conditions, and forest fragmentation have globally impacted the microhabitat of ticks and subsequently the distribution of tick-borne diseases, including zoonotic pathogens (Diuk-Wasser et al. 2021).

### 2.2.2.2 Behavior

Ticks adopted various complex behaviors intricately tied to their parasitic lifestyle. Their questing and feeding processes as well as reproduction specificities are key areas of interest for veterinary public health researchers.

#### Host-Seeking Behavior or Questing Behavior

It is the active host-seeking behavior exhibited by adult ticks. To quest, ticks climb up onto vegetation, such as tall grasses or shrubs, and extend their front legs, known as the forelegs or "questing legs." They wait patiently for a suitable host to pass by using a variety of sensory cues, including thermal, olfactory, and vibrational stimuli, to detect the presence of potential hosts (Fig. 2.4a) (Vayssier-Taussat 2016). This natural behavior of ticks may be influenced by climatic changes, in particular increases in environmental temperature, low hygrometry, and forest fires (McClure and Diuk-Wasser 2019).

#### Blood Meal Behavior

Once a host is detected, the ticks latch onto the host's skin, often in areas with thin or delicate skin, such as the groin, armpits, or scalp. They then insert their specialized mouthparts, called the hypostome, into the host's skin to begin feeding on the blood (Fig. 2.4b). This blood meal is essential for the ticks' survival, oviposition, and successful cycle completion (Kopsco et al. 2023). Attached ticks extracted blood over extended periods, ranging from a few days to several weeks. This feeding process involves the secretion of saliva containing anticoagulants, immunomodulators, and anesthetics, which help them evade the host's immune response and ensure a steady flow of blood. Adult ticks are capable of enduring long periods of fasting between blood meals, lasting weeks or even months (Nuttall 2023). This ability to survive without a host allows ticks to persist in various environments and withstand seasonal fluctuations in host availability. During these fasting periods, ticks enter a state of reduced metabolism and activity, conserving energy until a suitable host is detected (Nuttall 2023).

**Ticks' Mating Behavior**

Blood meals completion initiates tick female to oviposition. Female ticks can lay thousands of eggs that vary according to tick species and climate conditions. The male attaches itself to the female at the gonopore and then detaches (Fig. 2.4c). The number of eggs and the success of the subsequent life cycle stages (larvae, nymph, and adult) depend significantly on the nutrients obtained from the blood meal (Kopsco et al. 2023). Each evolutive stage requires a blood meal to progress to the next step, making host availability a crucial factor in tick population dynamics (Vayssier-Taussat 2016).

### 2.2.3 Activity of Ticks

Tick activity can be defined as the evolution from one stage to another, the search for hosts, the blood meal, reproduction, the transmission of pathogens, that is, all activities related to the tick life cycle. On the contrary, ticks can have a silent phase during which their activities are stopped. This is an important aspect to consider when studying tick-borne diseases and their transmission dynamics. Tick activity is influenced by several biotic and abiotic factors, including tick species, developmental stage, hosts availability, and environmental temperature and hygrometry (season) (Zając et al. 2021, 2023). Regarding tick species, the blacklegged tick (*Ixodes scapularis*) activity is highly triggered by ambient temperature. It begins seeking for a host when the temperature rises by 4 degrees Celsius or above, and continues during winter, even when there is still snow on the ground. However, the immature stage of this tick specie acquires progressive activity in late spring and commonly extended throughout the summer season (Burtis et al. 2023). The American dog tick (*Dermacentor variabilis*) begins questing as the days get longer, so with the rise in temperature, in the spring and early summer activity decreases as days shorten in the late summer and fall (Kirby et al. 2023; Petrović et al. 2023).

Additionally, *Ixodes ricinus*, the most widespread tick species in Europe, has been found to be active in a temperature range of 7.5–28.8 °C and optimal humidity level of 70% (Probst et al. 2023). Its activity showed a peak in the Western Carpathians and foothill area of Poland recorded in June–July. In contrast, the peak activity of *I. ricinus* ticks in eastern Poland occurs in May–June (Probst et al. 2023).

These variations in activity patterns can be attributed to the differences in local climate and environmental conditions.

Tick activity is also influenced by the availability of suitable hosts. Ticks require hosts for feeding and reproduction, and their activity is often synchronized with the activity patterns of their preferred hosts. For example, the activity of *I. ricinus* nymphs in forest habitats has been found to be higher at night, which is also higher during the day than in open meadow habitats. Several tick species extended their host ranges to be adapted to other alternative animals as small mammals, reptiles, and birds (O'Neill et al., 2023). This suggests that ticks may exhibit different activity patterns depending on the availability and behavior of their preferred hosts.

Understanding tick activity is crucial for assessing the risk of tick exposure in different environments, including urban parks. Urban parks can serve as habitats for ticks and potential sources of tick-borne diseases. Assessing tick density and activity in urban parks, along with studying visitor behaviors, can help in evaluating the risk of tick exposure to park visitors (Hassett et al. 2022; Zając et al. 2021, 2023).

### 2.2.4 Host Preference

Ticks exhibit various behaviors, including host preference, which refers to their tendency to prefer certain hosts over others. Host specialization of tick species is influenced particularly by ecological and climatic contexts, which allows understanding tick population dynamics, the evolution of tick biodiversity, and the circulation and evolution of associated pathogens (McCoy et al. 2013). Spengler and Estrada-Peña (2018) focused on the host preferences of the *Hyalomma* genus ticks, which are known to be the main vectors of the notified disease Crimean-Congo hemorrhagic fever. The immature stage of *Hyalomma* ticks preferentially infest species from the orders Rodentia, Lagomorpha, and Aves, while adult ticks concentrate mainly on the family Bovidae (Spengler and Estrada-Peña 2018). These host preferences contribute to the maintenance and transmission of pathogens. Furthermore, specific preferences for attachment sites were evidenced within ticks parasitizing humans in New York. For example, *Amblyomma americanum* preferentially bites the inguinal area, while *Ixodes scapularis* and *Dermacentor albipictus* primarily bite the chest and axillary region (Fig. 2.5) (Hart et al. 2022). These preferences may contribute to developing strategies for tick bite prevention, especially for professionally exposed persons.

## 2.3 Anatomy and Physiology of Ticks

### 2.3.1 External Anatomy

Ticks are ubiquitous and some of the most important blood-sucking arthropods globally. They are characterized by various morphological traits and physiological mechanisms that contribute to host selection, blood ingestion, mating, survival, and

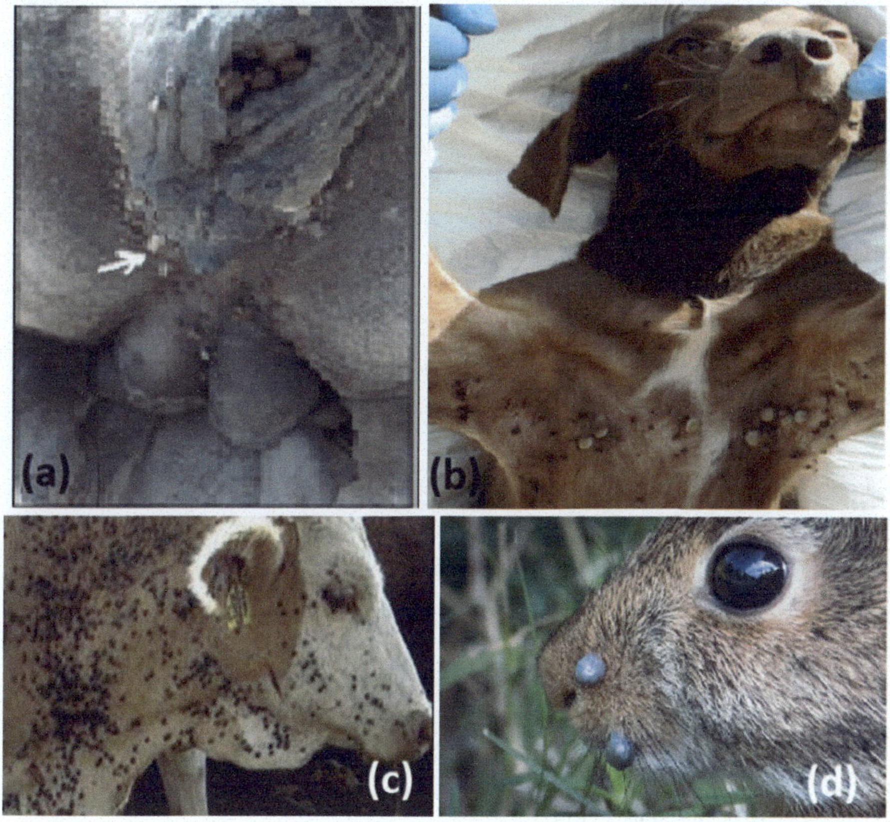


**Fig. 2.5** Ticks infesting animals' bodies: (**a**) dromedary camel; (**b**) dog; (**c**); cattle; (**d**) hare

reproduction (Anderson and Magnarelli 2008). Recognizing these external morphological particularities of ticks allowed implementing effective control strategies through the developing of active anti-ticks' substances. Some of the key aspects of the external anatomy of ticks are as follows.

#### 2.3.1.1 Carapace

The carapace is the hard, protective outer covering of a tick's body. It serves as a critical component of the tick's exoskeleton, providing structural support and safeguarding the tick from environmental threats and potential predators (Intirach et al. 2023). The carapace is composed of a tough, chitinous material that forms a rigid exoskeleton around the tick's body. This exoskeleton not only protects the tick but also helps maintain its body shape and prevent desiccation (Horak et al. 2002; Pacheco et al. 2020). The size, shape, and ornamentation of the carapace can vary significantly between different tick species. Some ticks, such as the hard ticks (family Ixodidae), have a conspicuous, sclerotized carapace that covers most of their dorsal surface (Figs. 2.6 and 2.7).

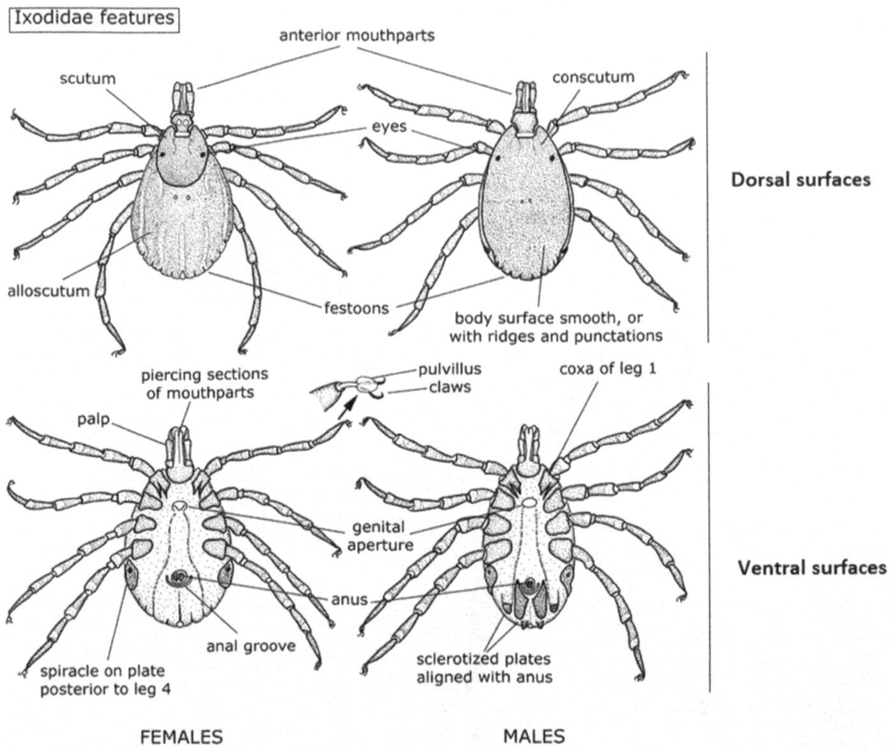


**Fig. 2.6** Schematic illustrations of dorsal and ventral features of hard ticks (Ixodidae) in males and females (Barker and Walker 2014)

In contrast, soft ticks (family Argasidae) have a more leathery, wrinkled carapace that is less extensive, leaving parts of the tick's body exposed (Horak et al. 2002). The variation in carapace morphology can be used as a key identifying feature for different tick species. For example, the carapace of *Ixodes* ticks is typically more rounded, while the carapace of *Dermacentor* ticks is often more elongated (Intirach et al. 2023; Pacheco et al. 2020).

#### 2.3.1.2 Legs

Adult ticks possess four pairs of legs, which are essential for their mobility and ability to locate and attach to hosts (Figs. 2.6 and 2.7). Each of the tick's eight legs is equipped with specialized structures that enhance their functionality (Intirach et al. 2023). These anatomic parts are covered in a dense array of sensory hairs and setae, which act as important tactile and chemosensory organs. These sensory structures allow ticks to detect physical and chemical cues in their environment, such as the presence of potential hosts, changes in temperature and humidity, and vibrations in the surrounding area (Radhakrishnan et al. 2016).

At the end of each leg, ticks have adhesive pads called pulvilli. The pulvilli are composed of sticky, suction-cup-like structures that enable the tick to cling to

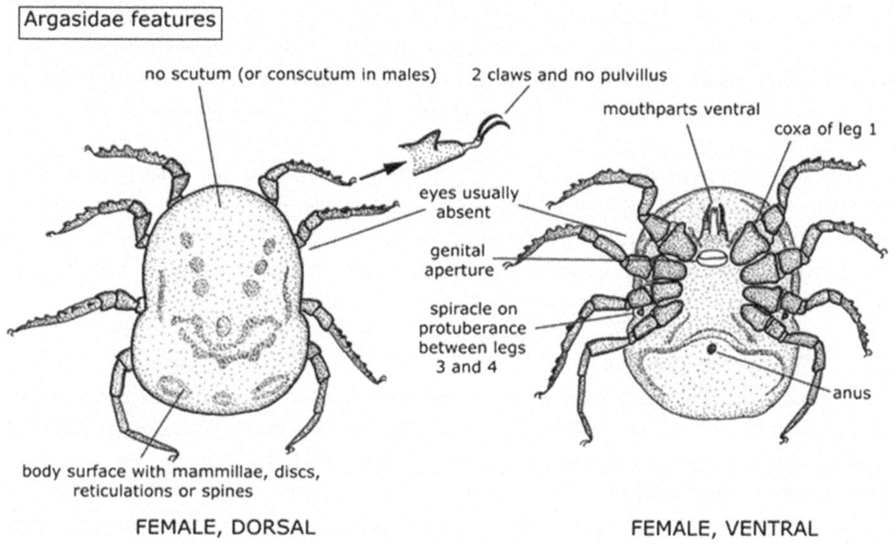


**Fig. 2.7** Schematic illustrations of dorsal and ventral features of soft ticks (Argasidae) in males and females (Barker and Walker 2014)

smooth surfaces, including the skin of its host. This allows the tick to firmly attach to the host and resist being dislodged during the feeding process (Radhakrishnan et al. 2016).

Additionally, the legs of ticks play a key role in the tick's locomotion. These arthropods use their legs to climb, crawl, and even jump short distances to reach and access their hosts. The length and arrangement of the legs, as well as the presence of claws, facilitate the tick's movement across a variety of substrates, including vegetation, soil, and the host's body (Radhakrishnan et al. 2016; Intirach et al. 2023).

#### 2.3.1.3 Mouthparts

Tick's mouthparts constitute a key route for both saliva pathogen transmission and acquisition through blood-sucking process. A lot of knowledge has been developed and learned about the basic anatomy of the tick's mouthparts and in the broad outlines of how they function. These anatomical parts allow the tick to locate, attach to, and feed on their specific hosts (Vancová et al. 2020).

The central structure of the tick's mouthparts is the hypostome, a barbed, harpoon-like structure that the tick uses to penetrate the host's skin and anchor itself in place. The hypostome is covered in sharp, backward-facing projections that help the tick firmly embed itself into the host's flesh and resist being dislodged (Vancová et al. 2020).

Surrounding the hypostome are the chelicerae, which act as a pair of scissors. The chelicerae cut into the host's skin, creating an opening through which the tick can insert its hypostome and feed on the host's blood (Vancová et al. 2020).

The final key components of the tick's mouthparts are the palps (Figs. 2.6 and 2.7). These appendages help the tick locate and grasp the host, acting as sensory organs to detect chemical and physical cues. The palps also assist in manipulating the host's skin and guiding the hypostome into the proper feeding position (Vancová et al. 2020).

Together, the hypostome, chelicerae, and palps form a highly effective feeding apparatus that allows ticks to latch onto their hosts and extract blood meals. Understanding the structure and function of the tick's mouthparts is essential for developing strategies to prevent tick-borne diseases as the mouthparts are the primary means by which ticks transmit pathogens to their hosts.

#### 2.3.1.4 Sensory Organs

Ticks possess a remarkable array of sensory organs that allow them to detect and locate potential hosts, as well as perceive their environment. These sophisticated sensory capabilities are critical adaptations that enable ticks to thrive as successful parasites (Carr et al. 2017).

The Haller's organ, located on the first pair of legs, is perhaps the most renowned of the tick's sensory structures. This specialized organ is extremely sensitive to heat, carbon dioxide, and movement—all important cues that ticks use to identify the presence and proximity of a potential host (Carr and Salgado 2019). In addition to the Haller's organ, ticks also possess a rudimentary visual system, with simple eyes that can detect light and movement. While their visual acuity is limited, these eyes play a role in the tick's orientation and host-seeking behaviors (Limas and Arimar 2021).

Ticks are also equipped with a diverse array of chemoreceptors, which allow them to sense a wide range of chemical stimuli from their environment and hosts. These chemosensory organs enable ticks to detect host-derived compounds, such as pheromones and kairomones, as well as environmental cues like humidity and the presence of other organisms (Josek et al. 2018).

### 2.3.2 Internal Anatomy of Ticks

Ticks have a complex and specific internal anatomy consisting of various body regions and organ systems. Unfortunately, there are a limited number of dissections guides available providing a detailed view of tick internal anatomy. Topography and anatomical differences between the internal organs of male, unfed, and gravid adult females are required to be studied to adopt specific strategies of measure control (Tidwell et al. 2021). This section will provide an overview of the internal anatomy of ticks, including the head, thorax, abdomen, digestive system, respiratory system, and nervous system (Fig. 2.8).

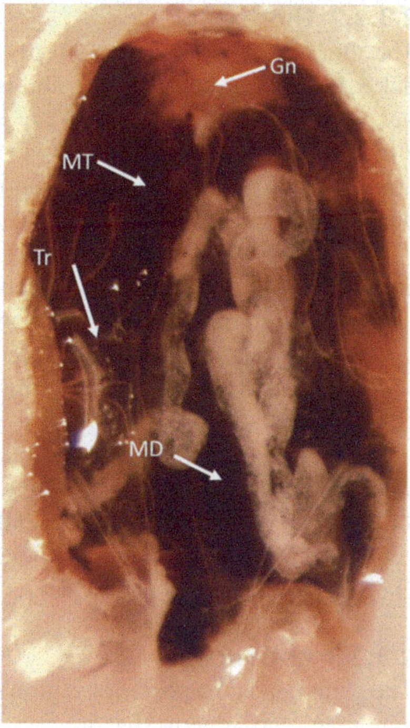


**Fig. 2.8** Dorsal view of the internal anatomical organs of hard ticks, example of *Rhipicephalus microplus*. MT: Malpighian tubes; Gn: gene gland; MD: midgut; Tr: trachea. 4× magnification. (Courtesy of Dr. Raquel Cossío-Bayúgar and Dr. César Arreguin Perez)

#### 2.3.2.1 Head

The head of a tick is a highly specialized structure that is central to the tick's parasitic lifestyle. It contains the essential sensory organs and mouthparts that allow the tick to detect and feed on its host.

The most notable feature of the tick's head is the presence of the Haller's organ, a highly sensitive structure located on the first pair of legs. As mentioned earlier, the Haller's organ is specialized for detecting heat, carbon dioxide, and movement—all critical cues that ticks use to identify and locate potential hosts (Edwards et al. 2015; Tidwell et al. 2021).

In addition to the Haller's organ, the tick's head also houses other important sensory structures, such as chemoreceptors that allow the tick to perceive various chemical stimuli from the environment and the host. These chemosensory organs play a crucial role in host-seeking behavior, enabling ticks to detect host-derived compounds like pheromones and kairomones (Fig. 2.8) (Edwards et al. 2015; Tidwell et al. 2021).

Integrated within the tick's head are the mouthparts, which are essential for the feeding process. The hypostome, chelicerae, and palps that make up the mouthparts are all concentrated in the head region, allowing the tick to effectively penetrate the host's skin and extract a blood meal (Edwards et al. 2015; Tidwell et al. 2021).

#### 2.3.2.2 Thorax

The thorax is the middle region of the tick's body and plays a critical role in the tick's locomotion and feeding abilities. The thorax is the primary location of the tick's four pairs of legs, which are essential for the tick's mobility and ability to cling to hosts. The leg muscles, tendons, and other associated structures are all housed within the thorax, allowing the tick to crawl, climb, and even jump short distances to access potential hosts (Edwards et al. 2015; Tidwell et al. 2021).

In addition to the legs, the thorax also contains the tick's salivary glands, which are vital for the feeding process. These specialized glands produce a complex mixture of saliva that the tick injects into the host during feeding. The saliva contains various enzymes, anticoagulants, and other compounds that facilitate blood meal acquisition and prevent host immune responses (Edwards et al. 2015; Tidwell et al. 2021).

The internal anatomy of the thorax also includes other important organs and systems, such as the tick's digestive and respiratory systems. These physiological structures enable the tick to efficiently take in and process a blood meal, as well as exchange gases and maintain homeostasis during the feeding process (Edwards et al. 2015; Tidwell et al. 2021).

#### 2.3.2.3 Abdomen

The abdomen is the posterior region of the tick's body and houses a variety of internal organs and systems that are critical for the tick's survival and reproduction. The abdomen is the primary location of the tick's reproductive organs. In female ticks, the abdomen contains the ovaries, where eggs are produced and stored. During the feeding and mating process, these eggs will be fertilized and eventually deposited by the female tick (Fig. 2.8) (Edwards et al. 2015; Tidwell et al. 2021).

In addition to the reproductive organs, the tick's abdomen also contains other important internal structures, such as the digestive system, excretory system, and respiratory system. These physiological systems are responsible for processing the blood meal, regulating waste and water balance, and facilitating gas exchange during the tick's parasitic life cycle (Edwards et al. 2015; Tidwell et al. 2021).

The expansive nature of the tick's abdomen allows it to dramatically increase in size during the blood-feeding process. As the tick engorges on its host's blood, the abdomen can swell to many times its original size, enabling the tick to obtain a substantial blood meal that provides the necessary resources for egg production and future survival (Edwards et al. 2015; Tidwell et al. 2021). The anatomy of the tick's abdomen, with its versatile internal structures and capacity for expansion, is a testament to the tick's evolutionary adaptations as a successful parasite.

#### 2.3.2.4 Digestive System

The digestive system of ticks is a complex and highly specialized structure that enables these parasites to efficiently extract nutrients from the blood meals they obtain from their hosts. The digestive system begins with the mouthparts, which the tick uses to penetrate the host's skin and access the blood supply. The blood is then drawn up through the esophagus and into the midgut, which is the primary site of digestion and nutrient absorption (Fig. 2.8) (Edwards et al. 2015; Tidwell et al. 2021).

The midgut, also known as the digestive diverticula or gastric caeca, is a large, sac-like structure that can dramatically expand in size as the tick engorges on its blood meal. This expansion allows the midgut to store large volumes of blood, which are then gradually digested, and the nutrients absorbed (Edwards et al. 2015; Tidwell et al. 2021).

The digestive process in the midgut is facilitated by a complex array of enzymes and other biomolecules produced by specialized cells lining the gut. These enzymes break down the blood components, such as proteins and lipids, into smaller molecules that can be more easily absorbed and utilized by the tick (Fig. 2.8) (Edwards et al. 2015; Tidwell et al. 2021).

Once the nutrients have been extracted, the waste products are passed through the hindgut and eventually excreted by the tick. This efficient digestive system allows ticks to obtain maximum nutritional benefit from their blood meals, which is essential for sustaining their parasitic lifestyle and successful reproduction (Edwards et al. 2015; Tidwell et al. 2021).

Understanding the structure and function of the tick's digestive system is crucial for developing effective control strategies as disrupting this system could impair the tick's ability to feed and reproduce, ultimately reducing tick populations.

#### 2.3.2.5 Respiratory System

Unlike many other arthropods, ticks do not possess lungs or a circulatory system to transport oxygen. Instead, they have a unique respiratory system based on a network of small, branching tubes called tracheae. The tracheal system in ticks originates from a series of openings on the body surface called spiracles. These spiracles allow air to enter and exit the tracheal network, which then distributes oxygen directly to the tick's tissues and organs (Fig. 2.8) (Edwards et al. 2015; Tidwell et al. 2021). The tracheal tubes branch extensively throughout the tick's body, with the smallest branches, called tracheoles, delivering oxygen right to the individual cells. This direct delivery of oxygen eliminates the need for a complex circulatory system and allows the tick's respiration to be highly efficient (Edwards et al. 2015; Tidwell et al. 2021). The spiracles are strategically located on the tick's body, typically along the sides and underside, to facilitate gas exchange. The spiracles can be opened and closed by specialized muscles, allowing the tick to regulate its oxygen intake and carbon dioxide release as needed (Edwards et al. 2015; Tidwell et al. 2021). This tracheal respiratory system is well suited to the tick's parasitic lifestyle as it allows the tick to obtain sufficient oxygen even while embedded in the host's skin or fur.

#### 2.3.2.6 Nervous System

The nervous system of ticks is a complex and highly coordinated network that enables these parasites to perceive and respond to their environment, as well as regulate their various physiological processes. The tick's nervous system is composed of a central nervous system and a peripheral nervous system. The central nervous system includes a primitive brain-like structure called the synganglion, which is in the anterior region of the tick's body. This synganglion serves as the integration and processing center for sensory information and motor control (Edwards et al. 2015; Tidwell et al. 2021).

Extending from the synganglion is a network of nerves and ganglia that make up the peripheral nervous system. These nerves innervate the tick's various organs, muscles, and sensory structures, allowing for the coordination of feeding, reproduction, and other vital functions (Edwards et al. 2015; Tidwell et al. 2021).

The tick's nervous system is responsible for processing a variety of sensory inputs, such as temperature, humidity, vibration, and chemical cues. This allows the tick to detect and respond to the presence of potential hosts, as well as regulate its own physiological state and behaviors, such as host-seeking, attachment, and feeding (Edwards et al. 2015; Tidwell et al. 2021). Additionally, the nervous system plays a crucial role in the tick's reproductive activities. It coordinates the release of hormones and other chemical signals that regulate mating, egg production, and other reproductive processes (Edwards et al. 2015; Tidwell et al. 2021).

## 2.4 Economic Importance of Ticks

### 2.4.1 Disease Transmission

Ticks play a significant role in the transmission of various diseases, including Lyme disease, Rocky Mountain spotted fever, and ehrlichiosis. These diseases have important economic implications due to their impact on human health and healthcare costs (Rajput et al. 2006).

#### 2.4.1.1 Lyme Disease

Lyme disease is the most reported vector-borne disease in the United States, caused by the bacterium *Borrelia burgdorferi* transmitted by ticks. According to recent research by the Centers for Disease Control and Prevention (CDC), the economic burden of Lyme disease in the United States ranges from $345 million to $968 million annually. The average patient cost for Lyme disease is approximately $1200 per infection, with higher costs for patients in later stages of the disease (Zhang et al. 2006).

The wide range in the estimated economic burden reflects the challenges in accurately quantifying the full impact of Lyme disease, which can include direct medical costs, lost productivity, and long-term complications. Nonetheless, these figures underscore the significant financial strain that Lyme disease places on the healthcare system and society (Hook et al., 2022).

#### 2.4.1.2 Rocky Mountain Spotted Fever (RMSF)

RMSF is a serious tick-borne illness caused by the bacterium *Rickettsia rickettsii*. It is transmitted by several tick species, including *Dermacentor variabilis*, *D. andersoni*, and *Rhipicephalus sanguineus* sensu lato. RMSF can have severe health consequences if not treated promptly, potentially leading to complications such as organ failure, neurological problems, and even death (Drexler et al. 2015).

While there is limited recent research specifically focusing on the economic impact of RMSF, it is known to be a significant public health concern in certain regions of the United States. These high-risk areas include Oklahoma, Missouri, Arkansas, North Carolina, Virginia, and Tennessee (Drexler et al. 2015).

#### 2.4.1.3 Ehrlichiosis

Ehrlichiosis is a tick-borne disease caused by various species of *Ehrlichia* bacteria. It can lead to flu-like symptoms such as fever, headache, and fatigue, and if left untreated, can cause severe complications, including organ failure, neurological problems, and even death (Singh et al. 2022).

The economic importance of ehrlichiosis has not been extensively studied compared to the detailed research available on the economic burden of Lyme disease and Rocky Mountain spotted fever. However, ehrlichiosis is recognized as a significant tick-borne disease in the United States, particularly in regions where the causative *Ehrlichia* species are endemic (Singh et al. 2022).

**Warning** While the specific economic impact of ehrlichiosis has not been quantified in recent studies, the potential costs associated with this disease can include direct medical costs related to the diagnosis, treatment, and management of ehrlichiosis, including hospitalization and outpatient care. There are also indirect costs, such as lost productivity and wages due to illness, hospitalization, and recovery time for patients, as well as caregiver time and lost productivity (Singh et al. 2022).

Finally, long-term consequences, such as severe complications like organ damage or neurological sequelae, can lead to ongoing medical expenses and reduced quality of life. In rare cases, ehrlichiosis can result in fatality, with significant emotional and financial implications for affected families (Singh et al. 2022).

### 2.4.2 Damage to Livestock and Pets

Ticks pose a significant threat to livestock and pets, causing various detrimental effects on their health and well-being. The economic impact of ticks on livestock and pets includes anemia, weight loss, and even death.

#### 2.4.2.1 Anemia

Ticks are blood-feeding parasites that can cause anemia in infested animals. As they feed on the host's blood, they can lead to a decrease in red blood cell count and hemoglobin levels. This anemia can result in symptoms such as weakness, fatigue, and reduced productivity in livestock (Salih et al. 2023).

For example, in cattle, severe tick infestations can lead to a substantial reduction in milk production and weight gain, negatively impacting the economic value of the animals. The constant blood loss and stress on the animal's body due to the tick infestation can cause a decrease in appetite and impaired nutrient absorption, resulting in poor weight gain or even weight loss (Brites-Neto et al. 2015; Salih et al. 2023). This directly affects the animals' market value and profitability for livestock producers.

The anemia caused by ticks can have a significant economic impact on livestock operations. Reduced milk production and weight gain translate to lower yields and reduced revenue for farmers and ranchers.

#### 2.4.2.2 Weight Loss

In addition to anemia, heavy tick infestations can also cause significant weight loss in livestock and pets. The constant blood loss and stress on the animal's body can lead to a decrease in appetite and impaired nutrient absorption, resulting in poor weight gain or even weight loss (Brites-Neto et al. 2015).

This can be particularly problematic for livestock producers as it directly affects the animals' market value and profitability. Reduced weight gain or weight loss in livestock, such as cattle, sheep, or pigs, can significantly lower the animals' sale price and overall economic value.

For example, a dairy cow that experiences substantial weight loss due to a severe tick infestation may produce less milk, which reduces the farm's milk yield and revenue. Similarly, beef cattle that fail to gain weight as expected can be worth less when sold, cutting into the producer's profits (Brites-Neto et al. 2015; Salih et al. 2023).

The impact of weight loss extends beyond just livestock. Companion animals, such as dogs and cats, can also suffer from reduced body condition and weight loss due to heavy tick infestations. This can negatively impact the overall health and well-being of these pets, requiring additional veterinary care and treatment, which can be costly for pet owners.

#### 2.4.2.3 Death

In severe cases, tick-borne diseases and the cumulative effects of heavy tick infestations can lead to the death of livestock and pets. Certain tick-borne pathogens, such as *Babesia* and *Theileria* species, can cause life-threatening illnesses in animals, leading to organ failure and mortality (Brites-Neto et al. 2015; Salih et al. 2023).

The loss of valuable livestock or companion animals can have a significant financial impact on farmers, ranchers, and pet owners. For livestock producers, the death of animals represents a direct economic loss as these animals represent a significant investment in terms of feed, veterinary care, and the time and resources used to raise them.

In the case of dairy or beef cattle, the death of an animal can mean the loss of a productive asset that was generating revenue for the farm. For smaller livestock like sheep or goats, the loss of even a single animal can be devastating as these animals may have a higher individual value.

Similarly, the death of a beloved companion animal can be emotionally and financially devastating for pet owners. Beyond the sentimental value, the costs associated with the loss of a pet, such as veterinary bills, cremation or burial expenses, and the potential need to acquire a replacement animal, can be substantial (Brites-Neto et al. 2015; Salih et al. 2023).

## 2.5 Conclusion

The fundamental biology of ticks, as outlined in this chapter, reveals their remarkable adaptations and the intricate role they play in various ecosystems. From their four-stage life cycle to their specialized sensory abilities, ticks have evolved to thrive as prolific parasites, seeking out a diverse range of host species. Their capacity to transmit an array of pathogens, including those responsible for Lyme disease and Rocky Mountain spotted fever, underscores the critical need for further research and understanding of tick biology.

As we continue to explore the multifaceted dimensions of tick ecology, it becomes increasingly evident that mitigating the threat posed by these arachnids requires a multipronged approach. Advancements in tick control strategies, enhanced public awareness, and the continued study of tick–host–pathogen interactions will be essential in safeguarding both human and animal health (Janzén et al. 2024). By deepening our comprehension of the basic biology of ticks, we can develop more effective measures to manage their impact and maintain the delicate balance of the ecosystems they inhabit.

## References

Anderson JF, Magnarelli LA (2008) Biology of ticks. Infect Dis Clin N Am 22(2):195–215, v. https://doi.org/10.1016/j.idc.2007.12.006

Barker SC, Walker AR (2014) Ticks of Australia. The species that infest domestic animals and humans. Zootaxa 18(3816):1–144. https://doi.org/10.11646/zootaxa.3816.1.1

Battur B, Boldbaatar D, Umemiya-Shirafuji R, Liao M, Battsetseg B, Taylor D et al (2009) LKR/SDH plays important roles throughout the tick life cycle including a long starvation period. PLoS One 4(9):e7136. https://doi.org/10.1371/journal.pone.0007136

Benelli G (2020) Pathogens manipulating tick behavior-through a glass, darkly. Pathogens 9(8):664. https://doi.org/10.3390/pathogens9080664. PMID: 32824571; PMCID: PMC7459789

Boulanger N, Wikel S (2021) Induced transient immune tolerance in ticks and vertebrate host: a keystone of tick-borne diseases? Front Immunol 12:625993. https://doi.org/10.3389/fimmu.2021.625993. PMID: 33643313; PMCID: PMC7907174

Brites-Neto J, Duarte KM, Martins TF (2015) Tick-borne infections in human and animal population worldwide. Vet World 8(3):301–315. https://doi.org/10.14202/vetworld.2015.301-315. Epub 2015 Mar 12. PMID: 27047089; PMCID: PMC4774835

Brunner J, Cheney L, Keesing F, Killilea M, Logiudice K, Previtali A, Ostfeld R (2011) Molting success of *ixodes scapularis* varies among individual blood meal hosts and species 48:860–866. https://doi.org/10.1603/ME10256

Burtis JC, Bjork J, Johnson TL, Schiffman E, Neitzel D, Eisen RJ (2023) Seasonal activity patterns of host-seeking *Ixodes scapularis* (Acari: Ixodidae) in Minnesota, 2015–2017. J Med Entomol 60(4):769–777

Cadenas F, Rais O, Humair P, Douet V, Moret J, Gern L (2007) Identification of host Bloodmeal source and *Borrelia burgdorferi* Sensu Lato in field-collected *Ixodes ricinus* ticks in Chaumont

(Switzerland). 44:1109–1117. https://doi.org/10.1603/0022-2585(2007)44[1109:IOHBSA]2.0.CO;2

Carr AL, Salgado VL (2019) Ticks home in on body heat: a new understanding of Haller's organ and repellent action. PLoS One 14(8):e0221659. https://doi.org/10.1371/journal.pone.0221659

Carr AL, Mitchell RD III, Dhammi A, Bissinger BW, Sonenshine DE, Roe RM (2017) Tick Haller's organ, a new paradigm for arthropod olfaction: how ticks differ from insects. Int J Mol Sci 18(7):1563. https://doi.org/10.3390/ijms18071563. PMID: 28718821; PMCID: PMC5536051

Chen Z, Yu Z, Yang X, Zheng H, Liu J (2009) The life cycle of *Hyalomma asiaticum kozlovi Olenev*, 1931 (Acari: Ixodidae) under laboratory conditions. Vet Parasitol 160(1–2):134–137. https://doi.org/10.1016/j.vetpar.2008.10.028

Costa GC, Soares AC, Pereira MH, Gontijo NF, Sant'Anna MR, Araujo RN (2015) Life cycle of *Ornithodoros rostratus* (Acari: Argasidae) ticks feeding on mice under laboratory conditions. Exp Appl Acarol 66(1):53–61. https://doi.org/10.1007/s10493-015-9888-1. Epub 2015 Feb 26

Dautel H, Knülle W (2010) Embryonic diapause and cold hardiness of *Ixodes ricinus* eggs (Acari: Ixodidae). In: Sabelis M, Bruin J (eds) Trends in acarology. Springer, Dordrecht. https://doi.org/10.1007/978-90-481-9837-5_52

Deshpande G, Beetch JE, Heller JG, Naqvi OH, Kuhn KG (2023) Assessing the influence of climate change and environmental factors on the top tick-borne diseases in the United States: a systematic review. Microorganisms 12(1):50. https://doi.org/10.3390/microorganisms12010050. PMID: 38257877; PMCID: PMC10821204

Dipeolu OO (1991) Laboratory studies on the oviposition, egg sizes and shapes and embryonic development of *Dermacentor variabilis*. *Rhipicephalus sanguineus* and *Amblyomma maculatum*, Acarologia 32(3):p233–p244

Diuk-Wasser MA, VanAcker MC, Fernandez MP (2021) Impact of land use changes and habitat fragmentation on the eco-epidemiology of tick-borne diseases. J Med Entomol 58(4):1546–1564. https://doi.org/10.1093/jme/tjaa209

Drexler NA, Traeger MS, McQuiston JH, Williams V, Hamilton C, Regan JJ (2015) Medical and indirect costs associated with a Rocky mountain spotted fever epidemic in Arizona, 2002-2011. Am J Trop Med Hyg 93(3):549–551. https://doi.org/10.4269/ajtmh.15-0104. Epub 2015 Jun 1. PMID: 26033020; PMCID: PMC4559696

Economic Burden of Reported Lyme Disease in High-Incidence Areas United States (2022) 2014–2016 Emerging Infectious Diseases 28(6) https://doi.org/10.3201/eid2806.211335

Edwards KT, Goddard J, and Varela-Stokes AS (2015) Examination of the internal morphology of the Ixodid tick, *Amblyomma maculatum* Koch, (Acari: Ixodidae); a "How-to" Pictorial Dissection Guide. Midsouth Entomologist; ISSN 1936–6019

Elhachimi L, Valcárcel F, Olmeda AS, Elasatey S, Khattat SE, Daminet S, Sahibi H, Duchateau L (2021) Rearing of *Hyalomma marginatum* (Acarina: Ixodidae) under laboratory conditions in Morocco. Exp Appl Acarol 84(4):785–794. https://doi.org/10.1007/s10493-021-00641-3. Epub 2021 Jul 6. PMID: 34231094; PMCID: PMC8367888

Espinaze M, Hellard É, Horak I, Cumming G (2015) Analysis of large new south African dataset using two host-specificity indices shows generalism in both adult and larval ticks of mammals. Parasitology 143:366–373. https://doi.org/10.1017/S0031182015001730

Estrada-Peña A, Ayllón N, de la Fuente J (2013) Impact of climate trends on tick-borne pathogen transmission. Front Physiol 3:64. https://doi.org/10.3389/fphys.2012.00064. PMID: 22470348; PMCID: PMC3313475

Fourie L, Horak I (2004) The life cycle of *Ixodes rubicundus* (Acari: Ixodidae) and its adaptation to a hot, dry environment. Exp Appl Acarol 18:23–35. https://doi.org/10.1007/BF00051400

GarciaGuizzo M, Meneses C, Amado Cecilio P et al (2023) Optimizing tick artificial membrane feeding for *Ixodes scapularis*. Sci Rep 13:16170. https://doi.org/10.1038/s41598-023-43200-z

Gherman CM, Mihalca AD, Dumitrache MO, Györke A, Oroian I, Sandor M, Cozma V (2012) CO2 flagging—an improved method for the collection of questing ticks. Parasit Vectors 5:125. https://doi.org/10.1186/1756-3305-5-125. PMID: 22720872; PMCID: PMC3461486

González J, Fonseca DM, Toledo A (2023) Seasonal dynamics of tick species in the ecotone of parks and recreational areas in Middlesex County (New Jersey, USA). Insects 14(3):258. https://doi.org/10.3390/insects14030258. PMID: 36975943; PMCID: PMC10057079

Gregory N, Fernandez MP, Diuk-Wasser M (2022) Risk of tick-borne pathogen spillover into urban yards in New York City. Parasit Vectors 15:288. https://doi.org/10.1186/s13071-022-05416-2

Hadi UK, Adventini M (2015) Fecundity, oviposition and egg incubation period of female *Rhipicephalus sanguineus* Latreille (Acari: Ixodidae) ticks in Indonesia. J Vet Med Res 2(5):1036

Hart C, Schad LA, Bhaskar JR et al (2022) Human attachment site preferences of ticks parasitizing in New York. Sci Rep 12:20897. https://doi.org/10.1038/s41598-022-25486-7

Hansford KM, Gillingham EL, Vaux AGC, Cull B, McGinley L, Catton M, Wheeler BW, Tschirren B, Medlock JM (2023) Impact of green space connectivity on urban tick presence, density and *Borrelia* infected ticks in different habitats and seasons in three cities in southern England, Ticks Tick-borne Dis,14(2):102103, https://doi.org/10.1016/j.ttbdis.2022.102103

Hassett E, Diuk-Wasser M, Harrington L et al (2022) Integrating tick density and park visitor behaviors to assess the risk of tick exposure in urban parks on Staten Island, New York. BMC Public Health 22:1602. https://doi.org/10.1186/s12889-022-13989-x

Hofmeester TR, Krawczyk AI, van Leeuwen AD et al (2018) Role of mustelids in the life-cycle of ixodid ticks and transmission cycles of four tick-borne pathogens. Parasit Vectors 11:600. https://doi.org/10.1186/s13071-018-3126-8

Hoogstraal H (1956) Africain Ixodidae. Ticks of the sudan (with spécial reference to Equatoria province and with preliminary reviews of the genera *Boophilus Margoropus* and *Hyalomma*) Washington. 1101

Hook SA, Jeon S, Niesobecki SA, Hansen AP, Meek JI, Bjork JKH, Dorr FM, Rutz HJ, Feldman KA, White JL, Backenson PB, Shankar MB, Meltzer MI, Hinckley AF (2022) Economic Burden of Reported Lyme Disease in High-Incidence Areas, United States, 2014-2016. Emerg Infect Dis. 28(6):1170–1179. https://doi.org/10.3201/eid2806.211335

Horak IG, Camicas JL, Keirans JE (2002) The Argasidae, Ixodidae and Nuttalliellidae (Acari: Ixodida): a world list of valid tick names. Exp Appl Acarol 28(1–4):27–54. https://doi.org/10.1023/a:1025381712339

Intirach J, Lv X, Han Q, Lv ZY, Chen T (2023) Morphological and molecular identification of hard ticks in Hainan Island, China. Genes (Basel) 14(8):1592. https://doi.org/10.3390/genes14081592. PMID: 37628643; PMCID: PMC10454830

Janzén T, Choudhury F, Hammer M et al (2024) Ticks, public health risks in urban green spaces. BMC Public Health 24:1031. https://doi.org/10.1186/s12889-024-18540-8

Josek T, Allan BF, Alleyne M (2018) Morphometric analysis of chemoreception organ in male and female ticks (Acari: Ixodidae). J Med Entomol 55(3):547–552. https://doi.org/10.1093/jme/tjx232

Keesing F, Mowry S, Bremer W, Duerr S, Evans AS Jr, Fischhoff IR, Hinckley AF, Hook SA, Keating F, Pendleton J, Pfister A, Teator M, Ostfeld RS (2022) Effects of tick-control interventions on tick abundance, human encounters with ticks, and incidence of tickborne diseases in residential neighborhoods, New York, USA. Emerg Infect Dis 28(5):957–966. https://doi.org/10.3201/eid2805.211146. PMID: 35447066; PMCID: PMC9045441

Kirby AM, Evans EP, Bishop SJ, Lloyd VK (2023) Establishment and range expansion of Dermacentor variabilis in the northern Maritimes of Canada: community participatory science documents establishment of an invasive tick species. PLoS One 18(10):e0292703. https://doi.org/10.1371/journal.pone.0292703. PMID: 37831710; PMCID: PMC10575507

Kiszewski A, Matuschka F, Spielman A (2001) Mating strategies and spermiogenesis in ixodid ticks. Annu Rev Entomol 46:167–182. https://doi.org/10.1146/ANNUREV.ENTO.46.1.167

Kopsco HL, Gronemeyer P, Mateus-Pinilla N, Smith RL (2023) Current and future habitat suitability models for four ticks of medical concern in Illinois, USA. Insects 14(3):213. https://doi.org/10.3390/insects14030213. PMID: 36975898; PMCID: PMC10059838

Leschnik M, Feiler A, Duscher G, Joachim A (2013) Effect of owner-controlled acaricidal treatment on tick infestation and immune response to tick-borne pathogens in naturally infested dogs from eastern Austria. Parasit Vectors 6:62–62. https://doi.org/10.1186/1756-3305-6-62

Limas L, Arimar J (2021) Phototransduction components in the visual system of hard-bodied ticks. Honors Undergraduate Theses. 1004. https://stars.library.ucf.edu/honorstheses/1004

McClure M, Diuk-Wasser MA (2019) Climate impacts on blacklegged tick host-seeking behavior. Int J Parasitol 49(1):37–47. https://doi.org/10.1016/j.ijpara.2018.08.005. Epub 2018 Nov 15. PMID: 30447202; PMCID: PMC6339851

McCoy KD, Léger E, Dietrich M (2013) Host specialization in ticks and transmission of tick-borne diseases: a review. Front Cell Infect Microbiol 3:57. https://doi.org/10.3389/fcimb.2013.00057. PMID: 24109592; PMCID: PMC3790072

Nuttall PA (2023) Tick saliva and its role in pathogen transmission. Wien KlinWochenschr 135(7–8):165–176. https://doi.org/10.1007/s00508-019-1500-y. Epub 2019 May 6. PMID: 31062185; PMCID: PMC10118219

O'Neill X, White A, Gortázar C, Ruiz-Fons F (2023) The Impact of Host Abundance on the Epidemiology of Tick-Borne Infection Abstract Bulletin of Mathematical Biology 85(4) https://doi.org/10.1007/s11538-023-01133-8. PMID: 36892680; PMCID: PMC9998325.

Olegário M, Gerardi M, Tsuruta S, Szabó M (2011) Life cycle of the tick *Amblyomma parvum* Aragão, 1908 (Acari: Ixodidae) and suitability of domestic hosts under laboratory conditions. Vet Parasitol 179(1–3):203–208. https://doi.org/10.1016/j.vetpar.2011.01.056

Ouhelli H, Pandey VS (1984) Development of *Hyalomma lusitanicum* under laboratory conditions. Vet Parasitol 15(1):57–66, ISSN 0304-4017,. https://doi.org/10.1016/0304-4017(84)90110-9

Pacheco I, Acevedo P, Prado E, Mihalca AD, de la Fuente J (2020) Targeting the exoskeleton elementome to track tick geographic origins. Front Physiol 11:572758. https://doi.org/10.3389/fphys.2020.572758. PMID: 33071826; PMCID: PMC7538837

Park JM, Oliva Chávez AS, Shaw DK (2021) Ticks: more than just a pathogen delivery service. Front Cell Infect Microbiol 11:739419. https://doi.org/10.3389/fcimb.2021.739419

Petrović A, Stanić K, Popović A, Ivanović I, Supić D, Marinković D, Bursić V (2023) Seasonal dynamics and physiological age of Ixodid ticks collected from dogs. Animals 13:3026. https://doi.org/10.3390/ani13193026

Price K, Khalil N, Witmier B, Coder B, Boyer C, Foster E, Eisen R, Molaei G (2023) Evidence of protozoan and bacterial infection and co-infection and partial blood feeding in the invasive tick *Haemaphysalis longicornis* in Pennsylvania. J Parasitol 109:265–273. https://doi.org/10.1645/22-122

Probst J, Springer A, Anna-Katharina T, Bröker M, Williams H, Dautel H, Kahl O, Strube C (2023) Winter activity of questing ticks (*Ixodes ricinus* and *Dermacentor reticulatus*) in Germany – evidence from quasi-natural tick plots, field studies and a tick submission study. Ticks Tick Borne Dis 14(6):102225. https://doi.org/10.1016/j.ttbdis.2023.102225

Radhakrishnan S, Agarwal DC, Marigeri MV (2016) Missed retained tick: "Look for the legs". Med J Armed Forces India 72(1):94–95. https://doi.org/10.1016/j.mjafi.2015.08.005. Epub 2015 Oct 17. PMID: 26900234; PMCID: PMC4723703

Rajput ZI, Hu SH, Chen WJ, Arijo AG, Xiao CW (2006) Importance of ticks and their chemical and immunological control in livestock. J Zhejiang Univ Sci B 7(11):912–921. https://doi.org/10.1631/jzus.2006.B0912. PMID: 17048307; PMCID: PMC1635821

Salih O, Chitanga S, Govinder K, Mukaratirwa S (2023) Modelling the burden of disease for cattle-a case of ticks and tick-borne diseases in cattle in a rural set-up in South Africa. PLoS One 18(10):e0293005. https://doi.org/10.1371/journal.pone.0293005. PMID: 37862337; PMCID: PMC10588883

Sasakawa K (2007) Laboratory studies on larval feeding habits of *Amara macronota* (Coleoptera: Carabidae: Zabrini). Appl Entomol Zool 42:669–674. https://doi.org/10.1303/AEZ.2007.669

Shah T, Li Q, Wang B, Baloch Z, Xia X (2023) Geographical distribution and pathogenesis of ticks and tick-borne viral diseases. Front Microbiol 14:1185829. https://doi.org/10.3389/fmicb.2023.1185829

Singh K, Kumar S, Sharma AK, Jacob SS, RamVerma M, Singh NK, Shakya M, Sankar M, Ghosh S (2022) Economic impact of predominant ticks and tick-borne diseases on Indian dairy production systems. Exp Parasitol 243:108408. https://doi.org/10.1016/j.exppara.2022.108408. Epub 2022 Nov 4

Spengler JR, Estrada-Peña A (2018) Host preferences support the prominent role of *Hyalomma* ticks in the ecology of Crimean-Congo hemorrhagic fever. PLoSNegl Trop Dis 12(2):e0006248. https://doi.org/10.1371/journal.pntd.0006248. PMID: 29420542; PMCID: PMC5821391

Tidwell JP, Treviño DE, Thomas DB, Mitchell RD 3rd, Heerman MC, Pérez de León A, Lohmeyer KH (2021) Pictorial dissection guide and internal anatomy of the cattle tick, *Rhipicephalus* (*Boophilus*) *microplus* (Canestrini). Ticks Tick Borne Dis 12(3):101685. https://doi.org/10.1016/j.ttbdis.2021.101685. Epub 2021 Feb 2

Trout Fryxell RT, Moore JE, Collins MD, Kwon Y, Jean-Philippe SR, Schaeffer SM, Odoi A, Kennedy M, Houston AE (2015) Habitat and vegetation variables are not enough when predicting tick populations in the southeastern United States. PLoS One 10(12):e0144092. https://doi.org/10.1371/journal.pone.0144092. PMID: 26656122; PMCID: PMC4676690

Vancová M, Bílý T, Šimo L, Touš J, Horodyský P, Růžek D, Novobilský A, Salát J, Strnad M, Sonenshine DE, Grubhoffer L, Nebesářová J (2020) Three-dimensional reconstruction of the feeding apparatus of the tick *Ixodes ricinus* (Acari: Ixodidae): a new insight into the mechanism of blood-feeding. Sci Rep 10(1):165. https://doi.org/10.1038/s41598-019-56811-2. PMID: 31932602; PMCID: PMC6957509

Vayssier-Taussat M (2016) Ticks: infection, co-infections and prevention. Bull Acad Natl Méd 200:1337–1348

Vechtova P, Fussy Z, Cegan R et al (2020) Catalogue of stage-specific transcripts in *Ixodes ricinus* and their potential functions during the tick life-cycle. Parasit Vectors 13:311. https://doi.org/10.1186/s13071-020-04173-4

Zając Z, Kulisz J, Bartosik K et al (2021) Environmental determinants of the occurrence and activity of *Ixodes ricinus* ticks and the prevalence of tick-borne diseases in eastern Poland. Sci Rep 11:15472. https://doi.org/10.1038/s41598-021-95079-3

Zając Z, Kulisz J, Woźniak A, Bartosik K, Foucault-Simonin A, Moutailler S, Cabezas-Cruz A (2023) Tick activity, host range, and tick-borne pathogen prevalence in mountain habitats of the Western Carpathians, Poland. Pathogens 12(9):1186. https://doi.org/10.3390/pathogens12091186. PMID: 37764994; PMCID: PMC10534405

Zhang X, Meltzer MI, Peña CA, Hopkins AB, Wroth L, Fix AD (2006) Economic impact of Lyme disease. Emerg Infect Dis 12(4):653–660. https://doi.org/10.3201/eid1204.050602. PMID: 16704815; PMCID: PMC3294685

# Acaricide Chemistry and Modes of Action

# 3

Imtiaz Ahmad, Fayaz Asad, Adil Khan, Murad Khan, Haseeb Ullah Khan, and Bader S. Alotaibi

**Abstract**

This chapter covers the complex chemistry and diverse mechanisms of acaricides that are important in managing the ticks and mites. Ticks and mites are ectoparasites that adversely affect the animal and human health. The chapter also provides an overview of the advantages and disadvantages of different acaricides. It also provides a comprehensive classification of acaricides, categorizing them into mineral source acaricides, organochlorine acaricides, pyrethroid, carbamates, natural sulfur insecticides, amidine acaricides, organotin acaricide, organic phosphorus acaricide, heterocyclic acaricide, microbial acaricide, and botanical acaricides. This classification system aims to facilitate the understanding and selection of acaricides, enabling the development of effective integrated pest management strategies against ticks and mites. It then explores their modes of action, highlighting how they disrupt essential physiological processes in mites and ticks. Key mechanisms include the inhibition of acetylcholinesterase, modulation of sodium channels, and interference with mitochondrial function. Through a detailed understanding of acaricide chemistry and modes of action, this chapter provides valuable insights for the development of novel acaricides and the sustainable management of acaricide resistance, aiming to enhance both crop protection and animal health.

**Keywords**

Acetylcholinesterase · Botanical acaricides · Carbamates · Pyrethroid · Ticks

---

I. Ahmad (✉) · F. Asad · A. Khan · M. Khan · H. U. Khan
Department of Botany and Zoology, Bacha Khan University, Charsadda, Pakistan
e-mail: drimtiazahmad@bkuc.edu.pk

B. S. Alotaibi
Department of Clinical Laboratory Sciences, College of Applied Medical Sciences, Al-Quwayiyah, Shaqra University, Riyadh, Saudi Arabia


S. Kumar et al. (eds.), *Acaricides Resistance in Ticks*,
https://doi.org/10.1007/978-981-97-7411-1_3

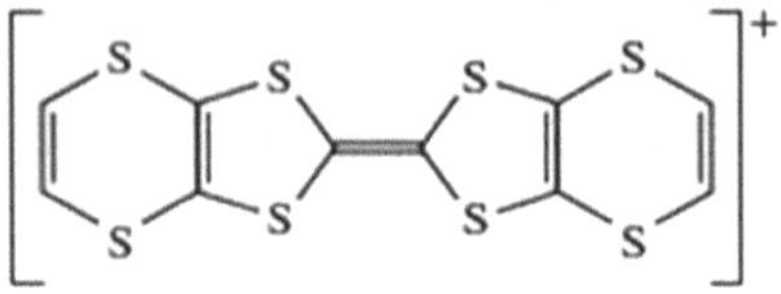


**Fig. 3.1** BEDT-TTF cation

## 3.1 Overview of Acaricides Classification

Based on their chemical makeup, acaricides fall into the following main categories.

### 3.1.1 Mineral Source Acaricides

This category includes inorganic substances such as compounds containing copper, arsenide, and sulfides. Certain inorganic substances with high boiling and melting points as well as low solubility in fats and water make up these acaricides (Agwunobi et al. 2021).

#### 3.1.1.1 Sulfide

Sulfide is an inorganic anion of sulfur or a compound having one or more ions of $S^{2-}$. Aliphatic disulfides are more potent insecticides. However, diaryl and aryl benzyl sulfides, which are aromatic sulfides, have moderate insecticidal and high acaricidal effects. Certain aromatic series of mixed sulfides and disulfides are employed as particular acaricides in agriculture. 4-Chlorobenzyl 4′-fluorophenyl sulfide and 4-chlorobenzyl 4′-chlorophenyl sulfides from the sulfide series are used in agriculture. The most active compounds are those that are 4,4′-substituted; fewer active compounds are created when substituents are added to other benzene ring locations. With respect to the initial sulfide, the sulfoxides and sulfones have nearly the same action. The related phenyl benzyl ethers have the highest activity in 4-chlorophenyl 4′-chlorobenzyl ether, and they are also acaricides. The thioacetals and the sulfide may also be somewhat connected. Methylenebis (4-chlorophenyl sulfides) is a chemical that is specifically employed as an acaricide (Ma et al. 2022) (Fig. 3.1).

#### 3.1.1.2 Arsenide

Arsenide (Fig. 3.2) is a compound of arsenic with one or more less electronegative elements. Arsenides are binary compounds composed of arsenic that are formed by many different metals. The first extensively used acaricide to prevent ticks and diseases caused by ticks was arsenic. Before the earliest reports of their use as acaricides to manage ticks on cattle in southern Africa and Australia in the years 1893 and 1895, arsenical solutions were applied to control sheep parasites. It is thought to be more affordable, stable, soluble in water, and effective overall (Obaid et al. 2022b).

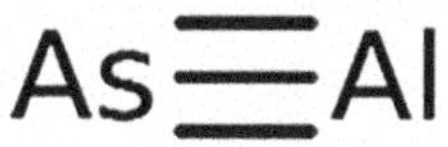


**Fig. 3.2** Aluminum arsenide

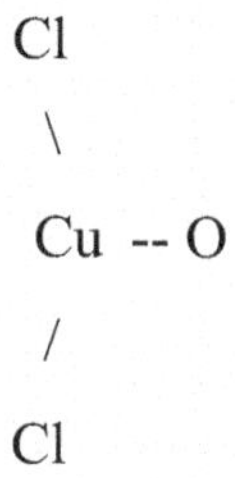


**Fig. 3.3** Copper oxychloride

#### 3.1.1.3 Copper-Containing Acaricide

Copper oxychloride (Fig. 3.3) is a commonly used copper compound. An acaricide used to manage mites and ticks is copper oxychloride, a chemical based on copper. Formulations containing copper oxychloride are frequently used in agriculture to manage mite infestations on crops, ornamentals, fruits, and vegetables (Roeber and Webster 2021).

#### 3.1.1.4 Sulfur-Containing Acaricides

Because sulfur can suppress a variety of mites and ticks, it has been utilized as an acaricide for millennia in agriculture, and sulfur-based acaricides are frequently used to manage mite infestations on crops such as citrus fruits, grapes, and strawberries. Sulfur is also utilized in several formulations for treating mites and ticks in cattle and pests (Zhu et al. 2022). It was the sole substance used to treat grape powdery mildew for a very long time. More than 70 years have passed since the adverse effects on phytophagous mites were first documented. Until approximately 1920, sulfur was the sole acaricide used to manage mites, although it has long been a useful fungicide, pesticide, and acaricide. When used as an acaricide, sulfur has several benefits, including minimal toxicity to users and applicators, low cost, availability in most places, etc. One drawback is that sulfur may be poisonous to a wide variety of plant species (Poché et al. 2023).

### 3.1.2 Organochlorine Acaricides

These include dichloro diphenyl trichloroethane (DDT), its analogs, cyclodienes and hexachlorocyclohexane, and its derivatives, urea and sulfamines. Organochlorine acaricides exhibit low water solubility, a high melting point, and low volatility and vapor pressure. They do not easily degrade the body's enzymes, have a stable chlorobenzene structure, and are soluble in many organic solvents but are almost insoluble in water. They have a lengthy residual duration before they gradually vanish from the body (Orgiazzi et al. 2022). Unfortunately, because of issues with resistance, residue, and pollution, this kind of acaricide is no longer manufactured.

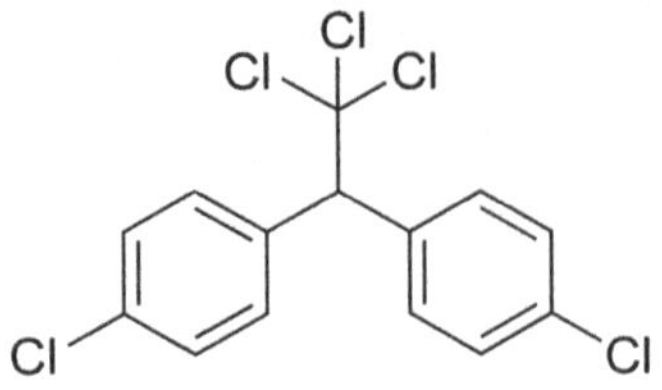

**Fig. 3.4** Dichlorodiphenyltrichloroethane

Among this group, DDT and benzene hexachloride were of particular concern. This class of chemicals also includes dieldrin, aldrin, cyclodiene compounds, and the polychloroterpene derivative toxaphene, which are widely employed to control ticks in cattle. In 1962, the use of any organochlorines against ticks was prohibited because of their low biodegradability and affinity for lipids, which left residues in meat, milk, and the environment (Alimi et al. 2021).

#### 3.1.2.1 Dichlorodiphenyltrichloroethane

1,1,1-Trichloro-2,2-bis(4-chlorophenyl) ethane (**DDT**) (Fig. 3.4) is a colorless, tasteless, and almost odorless crystalline chemical compound with the empirical formula $C_{14}H_9Cl_5$. DDT is a common synthetic insecticide used to control ticks, mites, and mosquitoes. The acaricidal qualities of DDT effectively destroy ticks, mites, and other acari, including *Rhipicephalus sanguineus*, as well as mites (*Demodex* species, *Sarcoptes scabiei*, etc.) (Menon et al. 2023). The greatest advancement in the history of pest management was most likely the discovery of the insecticidal qualities of DDT by the Swiss chemist Paul Mueller in 1939. DDT pesticides are among the most effective pesticides ever created. However, the excessive DDT use in the 1950s and 1960s led to the development of broad target site and metabolic resistance in many insect species, which poses a serious risk to the continued widespread use of pesticides in many pest control programs. Since the 1970s, most governments have restricted or outright prohibited the use of DDT and most other chlorinated hydrocarbon chemicals in agriculture, in part because of its unacceptable long-term persistence in the environment. DDT is still used, albeit sparingly, to control insect vectors for public health purposes (Shankar et al. 2021).

#### 3.1.2.2 Cyclopentadiene

Cyclopenta-1,3-diene (cyclopentadiene) (Fig. 3.5) is a colorless liquid possessing a terpene-like irritating odor. Cyclodienes are extremely toxic to ticks, mites, and other insects. Cyclodienes function long after application because of their extended residual activity. They are effective against ticks, mites, and spiders, among other acari species. Some cyclodienes are systemic, meaning that they are absorbed by the plant and dispersed throughout its tissues to protect it from the acari that feeds on it. Some cyclodienes are volatile, which allows them to seep through the soil to acari that are in the soil or on plant roots (Hamamoto et al. 2023).

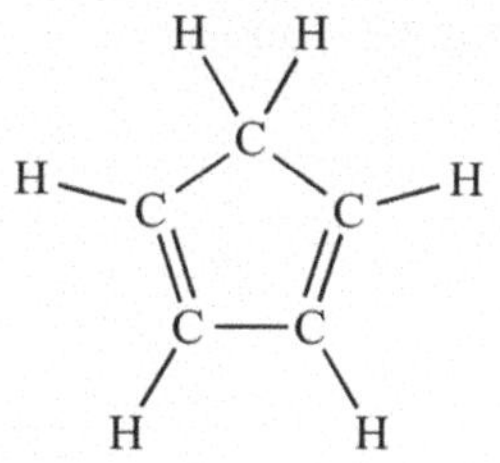


**Fig. 3.5** Cyclopenta-1,3-diene

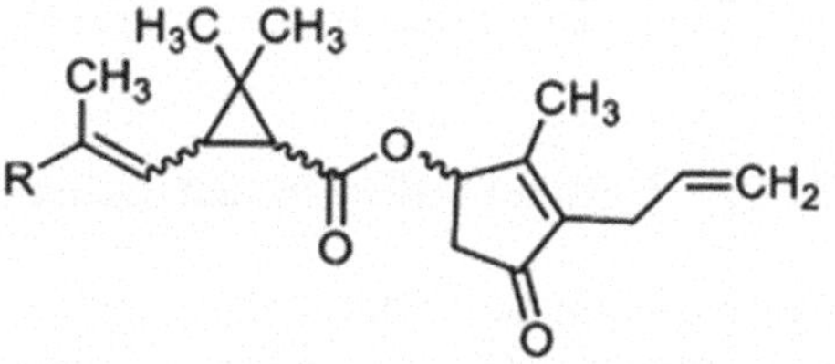


**Fig. 3.6** Pyrethroid

### 3.1.3 Pyrethroid

Pyrethroids (Fig. 3.6) are synthetic derivatives of pyrethrin insecticides isolated from flower extracts of *Chrysanthemum cinerariaefolium* flowers. The chemical structure of natural pyrethrin is used to create pyrethroid acaricides. These compounds are synthetically comparable to the naturally occurring insecticidal esters of pyrethric acid (pyrethrin II) and chrysanthemic acid (pyrethrin I), which were initially found in the flowers of several plants. The three naturally occurring pyrethrin series variants that are produced from the alcohol moiety of pyrethrins are Pyrethrin I and II, Jasmolin I and II, and Cinerin I and II. This type of acaricide has a high melting and boiling temperature, low vapor pressure, high density, weak water solubility, and high melting and boiling points; however, it is soluble in most organic solvents (Li et al. 2023). These acaricides are highly effective at killing acarians, have a potent knockdown effect, are not toxic to larger animals, and degrade readily in the environment. A wide range of synthetic pyrethroids are currently widely used for crop protection, animal health, and the control of insects that pose a health concern to humans, with annual sales reaching \$1.5 billion (Roeber and Webster 2021).

### 3.1.4 Carbamates

Organic substances called carbamates are produced from carbamic acid ($NH_2COOH$). Carbamate esters (Fig. 3.7) are the functional group found in carbamate insecticides. Carbamate acaricides have low boiling and vapor pressures, a high melting point, and are soluble in water (Liao et al. 2023). Most of them are soluble in organic solvents and are based on contact. Most types do not damage larger animals and are readily broken down by other species and the environment. Fish are not chronically harmed by this kind of acaricide. With respect to hazardous consequences measured

**Fig. 3.7** Carbamate

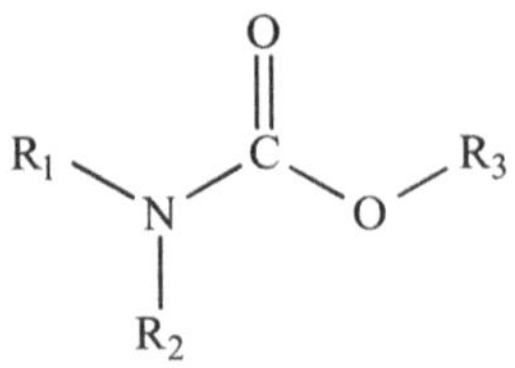


using multiple methods and criteria, only a few carbamates (CMs) have been carefully examined for their immunotoxic potential (Sabová et al. 2022).

### 3.1.5 Natural Sulfur Insecticides

Organic sulfur acaricides include sulfites, thiourea, ethers, thioethers, hydrazines, and sulfonates. Organic sulfur acaricides are characterized by high melting and boiling temperatures, low vapor pressures, and densities greater than one.

The active component of organic sulfur acaricides, a kind of pesticide, is sulfur. In addition to other insects, they are used to control acari or ticks and mites (Morfin et al. 2022). Sulfur, also known as sulfiram, sulfuraphos, Di thiocarbamates, thiuram, lime sulfur, and calcium polysulfide are a few examples of organic sulfur acaricides. Most of the species are soluble in organic solvents but insoluble in water. Most of them have little toxicity to larger animals and mostly use contact killing. Organic sulfur acaricides function by disrupting the nervous system, respiratory system, and cuticle (Gonzaga et al. 2022).

### 3.1.6 Amidine Acaricides

The major acaricides of this group include the compounds cymiazole (Fig. 3.8a) and amitraz (Fig. 3.8b). Amitraz is a white crystalline substance that is insoluble in water. Chlordimeform (Fig. 3.8c) is a colorless crystalline substance with an amine-like odor. Cymiazole is a white crystalline substance that is sparingly soluble in water at room temperature. Amidine acaricides exhibit strong contact effects on mites and eggs, a fumigating effect, a prolonged duration, minimal toxicity, and low accumulation in mammals. Ticks, especially bovine ticks, and phytophagous and parasitic mites are important target groups in agricultural practice. This kind of acaricide is safe for use on people, animals, and plants and does not cause chronic poisoning. The natural enemies of pests are amidine acaricides (Malik et al. 2021). The fact that the numerous acarines that have grown exceedingly resistant to carbamate, organophosphate, and chlorinated hydrocarbon insecticides are typically just as sensitive, if not more sensitive, to formamidines is a very important general characteristic of the amidine group in most of these applications (Williams and Linske 2024).

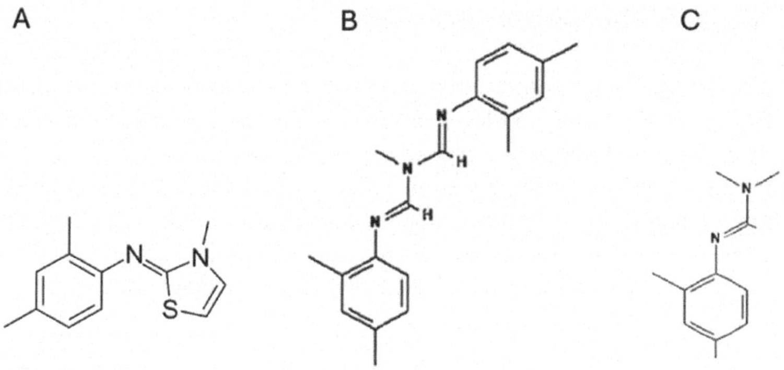


**Fig. 3.8** Amidine acaricides. (**a**) Cymiazole, (**b**) amitraz, (**c**) chlordimeform

### 3.1.7 Organotin Acaricide

Organotin-selective acaricides are employed in spider mite integrated pest management (IPM). Since OTs efficiently eliminate spider mites and are only mildly to moderately toxic to predatory phytoseiid mites that regulate many phytophagous mite species, they are beneficial for integrated pest management (IPM). There are four major forms of organotin: triazolyltin, phen butyl tin, triphosphorous tin, and tricyclotin. They are not the predominant type of acaricide. Organotin acaricides are organic substances that contain tin (Adesanya et al. 2021). Organotin displays low vapor pressure, poor water solubility, insolubility in water, high-fat solubility, and solubility in most organic solvents, in addition to their substantial contact and killing effects. This pesticide has strong acaricidal activity, causes gastric distress, and has unique effects on resistant acarids. It also has an antifeeding effect but no egg-killing effect (Carneiro et al. 2022).

Organotin acaricides are agents that change with temperature. Plictran, which is the forerunner of this class of miticides, is sometimes referred to as tri cyclohexyl hydroxy tin. One distannoxane is Vendex. The acid anhydride moiety of R-28627 is tri cyclohexyl tin, a di-n-propyl phosphorodithioate. Notable acaricidal activity is exhibited by these three organotins. Plicontran is a white, crystalline powder that is currently the sole organotin used for mite control (Selles et al. 2021). Trisubstituted organotins, including Plictran and Du-Ter, have been linked, at least partially, to the suppression of oxidative phosphorylation. In mice and house flies, ATPases are inhibited by both Du-Ter and Plictran. Furthermore, Plictran is a superb inhibitor of the fish brain and spider mite oligomycin-sensitive (mitochondrial) $Mg^{2+}$ ATPase.

Research utilizing Plictran-119Sn revealed that it broke down into inorganic tin compounds, namely, stannic acid, most likely through a series of decyclohexylation reactions (Schulze and Jordan 2021).

### 3.1.8 Organic Phosphorus Acaricide

Organic phosphorus, a neurotoxin that can also be used as an acaricide, can inhibit acetylcholinesterase (AChE) in blood and tissues. Organophosphorus acaricides are characterized by a high refractive index, high MW (200–400), low vapor pressure, significant air volatility, extremely high melting and boiling temperatures, and a density of less than 1. This type of acaricide has varying solubility levels in different solvents. Most of them are hazardous to the gastrointestinal tract and have intermediate toxicity; they also degrade at 200 °C and are not resistant to high heat (Cardoso et al. 2023).

### 3.1.9 Heterocyclic Acaricide

These kinds consist of derivatives of hydrazine, nitrophenol, and azobenzene. Heterocyclic acaricides often exhibit modest toxicity, clearly visible systemic effects, and contact toxicity. There are various types of acaricides that can be distinguished, such as those that demonstrate neurotoxicity, growth-regulating properties, and respiratory metabolism regulatory properties. Eggs are efficiently destroyed by growth-regulating acaricides, which are highly soluble in fat. These acaricides, which include pyrazole, triazole, oxazole, and thiazole, have distinct ring structures (Arshed et al. 2021).

### 3.1.10 Microbial Acaricide

Mite pathogenic bacteria and their metabolites are employed as acaricidal agents in microbial acaricides. They are selective and adept at using the cover that their natural adversaries afford. They are safe for people and animals, have high specificity, can protect bugs from their natural enemies, and can prevent pests from rapidly becoming resistant to medications. Because they do not contaminate the environment, they help protect water resources and improve the ecosystem. Since microbes have greater acaricidal potential than other acaricide classes, they are the main source of acaricides (Moudgil et al. 2023).

### 3.1.11 Botanical Acaricides

Plant-derived acaricides are low-molecular-weight secondary metabolites that, when applied in small amounts, can repel, prevent eating, regulate growth and development, and poison plants. When used on animals and humans, most acaricides derived from plants are harmless and have minimal toxicity to mammals. Typically, composed of many components, botanical acaricides are less prone to develop drug resistance (Schödl et al. 2022). A major source of natural compounds with acaricidal activity is essential oils, which are secondary metabolites obtained from different parts of aromatic plants, primarily from a few families (*Asteraceae*, *Apiaceae*, *Lamiaceae*, *Myrtaceae*, and *Rutaceae*). Terpenoids (monoterpenes and sesquiterpenes) and related aromatic chemicals make up the complex combinations of essential oils. The primary function of many essential oils and their components, especially monoterpenes, is that of fumigants (Arbabi and Khani 2021).

Certain components of essential oils have been proposed to have neurotoxic effects, that is, to inhibit acetylcholinesterase (AChE) and antagonize octopaminergic receptors. Essential oils may have multiple sites of action because they are complex combinations. The principal active ingredient found in extracts, oils, and other products derived from the seeds of *Azadirachta indica*, also known as Indian neem, is the triterpenoid azadirachtin. This compound has been utilized for the past 20 years as a botanical insecticide (Mitton et al. 2022).

## 3.2 Mechanisms of Action for Different Acaricides

Chemicals called acaricides are used to eradicate or manage acari, a group of mites and ticks. The modes of action of acaricides can differ based on the chemical compound they employ. Nonetheless, a few typical modes of operation are as follows.

### 3.2.1 Sulfide

Synthetic acaricide sulfides work by blocking essential enzymes that are involved in the manufacture of chitin, which prevents the creation of the tick's exoskeleton. The tick eventually dies because of this disruption to chitin manufacturing, which also inhibits development and molting. Furthermore, sulfides may interfere with neurotransmitter signaling pathways in the nervous system of ticks, impairing or paralyzing their movement. Sulfides have been shown to be effective in suppressing tick infestations in recent studies, highlighting their potential as useful tools in tick management efforts (Ayub et al. 2023).

### 3.2.2 Arsenide

The synthetic acaricide arsenide targets ticks through a variety of mechanisms. It causes metabolic malfunction and cellular death by interfering with important enzymatic pathways that are essential for cellular respiration and energy production. Moreover, arsenide disrupts the neurological system of ticks, resulting in paralysis or reduced motor capability (Alimi et al. 2022). Recent studies have demonstrated how effective arsenide is at reducing tick infestations. Similarly, research by White et al. has clarified the usefulness of arsenide for tick control. Taken together, these results highlight the potential of arsenide as a useful weapon for fighting tick infestations and preserving animal health (Kumar et al. 2022).

### 3.2.3 Copper-Containing Acaricide

Acaricides containing copper affect the vital physiological functions of ticks through a variety of methods. The tick dies because of cellular damage caused mostly by the disruption of enzyme activities involved in oxidative stress responses and cellular respiration by copper ions. Furthermore, ion channels and neurotransmitter receptors in the tick nervous system are disrupted by copper ions, leading to paralysis and reduced motor performance. Acaricides containing copper have been shown to be effective in tick control programs in recent research (da Silva et al. 2021). Similarly, studies have further bolstered the effectiveness of copper-based formulations for the management of tick infestations. These results emphasize the value of acaricides containing copper as effective instruments for tick management planning and safeguarding animal health (Bravo-Ramos et al. 2021).

### 3.2.4 Sulfur-Containing Acaricide

Acaricides containing sulfur work by obstructing ticks' essential metabolic functions. Sulfur chemicals specifically cause metabolic dysfunction and eventual death in ticks by interfering with enzymatic pathways that are essential for cellular respiration and energy production. Furthermore, acaricides based on sulfur injure ticks physically and impede normal growth and development by breaking down the tick cuticle and interfering with the molting process (Alborzi et al. 2023). Recent research has demonstrated how well acaricides containing sulfur work to manage tick infestations. In a similar vein, research has further highlighted the effectiveness of formulations based on sulfur in tick control programs (Eisen 2024).

### 3.2.5 Organochlorine Acaricides

The main way that organochlorine acaricides work is by attacking the neurological system of ticks. They interfere with regular neurotransmission processes by acting as agonists or antagonists at neuronal receptors. In particular, in tick neurons, organochlorines such as DDT and dieldrin target GABA-gated chloride channels and voltage-gated sodium channels, causing hyperexcitation or suppression of neuronal activity. The ticks eventually become paralyzed and die because of this disruption (Keve et al. 2024). Both improved metabolic detoxification processes and mutations in target receptor genes can result in resistance to organochlorine acaricides. These alterations may result in insensitivity to the actions of the acaricide, making therapy ineffective against populations of resistant ticks (Osikowicz et al. 2024).

### 3.2.6 Dichlorodiphenyltrichloroethane

The main way that dichlorodiphenyltrichloroethane (DDT) kills ticks is by attacking their nervous system. It interferes with normal neuronal function by binding to voltage-gated sodium channels on axons. Because of this binding, sodium channels cannot close after depolarization, resulting in a constant sodium input into the neuron and prolonged membrane depolarization. Ticks ultimately die from hyperexcitation, paralysis, or this disturbance in neural signaling (Shiri et al. 2024). Mutations in the amino acid sequence of the target sodium channel can increase the resistance of tick populations to DDT, reducing their susceptibility to chemical effects. Ticks exposed to the acaricide can survive because these alterations lessen the affinity of DDT for its target location (Gryczyńska et al. 2024).

### 3.2.7 Cyclodiene

Cyclodiene, which includes substances such as dieldrin, works against ticks by specifically targeting their gamma-aminobutyric acid (GABA) receptor. By attaching to GABA-gated chloride channels on tick nerve cells, these acaricides function as GABA agonists. Cyclodienes alter the channel's characteristics by attaching to these receptors and preventing chloride ions from entering nerve cells. This inhibition causes hyperexcitation, which in turn causes the ticks to become paralyzed and die (Harman et al. 2024). This disruption of normal nervous system activity results from this inhibition. Alterations in the expression of GABA-gated chloride channel genes in ticks can result in resistance to Cyclodienes, including dieldrin. These changes, which include single nucleotide polymorphisms (SNPs), change the way in which chloride channels function or are shaped, which decreases the affinity of cycloidians for binding and decreases their ability to regulate tick populations (Chikufenji et al. 2024).

### 3.2.8 Pyrethroid

A class of synthetic acaricides known as pyrethroids works by selectively binding to voltage-gated sodium channels in the nervous system of ticks. These acaricides attach to these channels and alter their function, keeping them open for an extended period following activation. Consequently, nerve cells experience a prolonged influx of sodium ions, which causes hyperexcitation and aperiodic neuronal firing. Eventually, the disruption of normal nerve function causes ticks to become paralyzed and die (Pérez-Otáñez et al. 2024). Mutations in tick voltage-gated sodium channel genes are related to resistance to pyrethroids. These changes, which can affect different regions of the channel protein, decrease the sensitivity of the channels to pyrethroids and the ability of acaricides to regulate tick populations (Chaisri et al. 2024).

### 3.2.9 Carbamates

The acaricidal effects of carbamates, a type of synthetic acaricide, are achieved by blocking the activity of acetylcholinesterase (AChE), an enzyme essential to tick nervous system function. Carbamates inhibit the degradation of acetylcholine, a neurotransmitter important in nerve signal transmission, by binding to the active site of AChE (Gupta et al. 2024). Acetylcholine builds up in the synaptic cleft because of this suppression of AChE, which causes constant nerve stimulation and excessive nervous system excitation. Tick resistance to carbamates can result from several different pathways, such as changes to the AChE target site, mutations to the genes encoding carboxylesterase (CE), and metabolic detoxifying procedures. The effectiveness of these acaricides in tick control programs is decreased by these resistance mechanisms, which allow ticks to tolerate the harmful effects of carbamates (Benito-Murcia et al. 2024).

### 3.2.10 Organic Sulfur Acaricides

Organic sulfur acaricides function by interfering with the essential metabolic functions of ticks. These substances usually target pathways or enzymes necessary for tick survival, which disrupts cellular processes and ultimately results in death. The suppression of enzymes involved in tick energy metabolism or respiration is one theory for this mode of action. Organic sulfur acaricides cause death by interfering with vital metabolic pathways; thus, organic sulfur compounds may affect the composition and operation of tick cell membranes, impairing cellular homeostasis and membrane integrity. Cell death may result from this disruption, which can also hinder communication within cells and cause content leakage (van Dalen and Jansen van Rensburg 2024).

### 3.2.11 Amidine Acaricides

The primary mechanism by which amidine acaricides cause acaricide effects in ticks is by interfering with their essential physiological functions. These substances cause paralysis and eventually death by targeting receptors or enzymes necessary for tick survival (Malak et al. 2024). One theory for how it works is that it interferes with ticks' neurological systems by attaching to receptors, such as octopamine receptors. Amidine acaricides prevent neural signaling by inhibiting these receptors, which causes the tick to become paralyzed and die. Amidine acaricides may disrupt other physiological functions in ticks, such as cellular respiration or metabolism, although more research is needed to determine the precise underlying mechanisms involved (Habeeba et al. 2024).

### 3.2.12 Organotin Acaricide

Organotin acaricides work by focusing on physiological functions in ticks, causing paralysis and death as a result. Although the precise targets and routes may differ, the mechanism of action of organotin chemicals involves interfering with vital cellular operations. Tick-induced impairment of mitochondrial function is one theory. It has been demonstrated that organotin chemicals prevent the synthesis of ATP and mitochondrial respiration, which causes cellular malfunction and ultimately kills the tick. Additionally, it is possible that organotin acaricides interfere with tick ion channels or receptors, impairing neural signaling and resulting in paralysis (Anholeto et al. 2024).

### 3.2.13 Organic Phosphorus Acaricide

To cause paralysis and death in ticks, organic phosphorus acaricides target physiological processes and metabolic pathways in ticks. Acetylcholinesterase (AChE), an enzyme necessary for the termination of nerve impulses in the tick nervous system, is inhibited as part of the mechanism of action. Acetylcholine (ACh) is a neurotransmitter that is not hydrolyzed by AChE due to the irreversible binding of organophosphate acaricides to its active site (Bai et al. 2024). Consequently, ACH builds up at neuron synapses, causing postsynaptic receptors to be continuously stimulated and nerve transmission to be prolonged. Ticks suffer from paralysis and eventually die because of this overstimulation of their neurological system (Adenubi et al. 2024).

### 3.2.14 Heterocyclic Acaricide

To cause paralysis and death in ticks, heterocyclic acaricides target physiological processes and biochemical pathways. The mechanism of action involves interfering with the regular operation of the tick nerve system. By interfering with neurotransmission, especially by targeting neurotransmitter receptors or enzymes involved in neurotransmitter metabolism, these acaricides usually function as neurotoxins. For example, certain heterocyclic acaricides may inhibit the enzyme acetylcholinesterase (AChE), which is necessary for the termination of nerve impulses. This could result in the buildup of acetylcholine (ACh) at nerve synapses and ongoing stimulation of the nerves. Ticks that experience this disturbance in neurotransmission eventually become paralyzed and die (Alimi et al. 2024).

### 3.2.15 Microbial Acaricides

Microbial acaricides are a class of insecticides that are generated by microorganisms such as bacteria, fungi, or viruses. They work by disrupting the physiology or life cycle of ticks, among other methods. Among these mechanisms, microbial acaricides can enter the tick body through ingestion, contact, or cuticle penetration. After inside the tick, the pathogenic agent multiplies and interferes with vital physiological functions, causing illness and death. Ticks are hazardous to several microbial acaricides due to their production of toxins or secondary metabolites (Shah et al. 2023). These toxins can harm tick cells, paralyze them, or even kill them by targeting metabolic processes or cellular components. Certain microbial acaricides weaken the immune system of ticks, increasing their vulnerability to illnesses and environmental stresses.

Microbial agents can aid in tick colonization and proliferation by weakening the tick immune response. Microbial acaricides have the potential to impede the reproduction of ticks, including egg production, hatching, and larval development. Microbial agents can suppress tick populations and stop new infestations by interfering with the ability of ticks to reproduce (de la Fuente et al. 2023).

### 3.2.16 Botanical Acaricides

Ticks, which are made from plants and plant extracts, are the target of botanical acaricides and work against them in a variety of ways. Numerous botanical acaricides contain substances that cause the malfunction of the nerve system of ticks, paralyzing or killing the insect. These substances might disrupt ion channels, neurotransmission, or other neurological functions necessary for tick survival. Certain plant-based insecticides deter ticks by releasing scents or substances that are unpleasant. Botanical acaricides can decrease tick infestations and stop the spread of diseases carried by ticks by discouraging ticks from approaching or feeding on treated surfaces. Some botanical acaricides include antifeedant qualities that prevent ticks from feeding on victims or obtaining nutrients necessary for their existence (Sparks and Bryant 2022).

Botanical acaricides can disturb the life cycle and population dynamics of ticks by decreasing their feeding activity. Botanical acaricides can pierce the cuticle of a tick, which is the outermost layer of protection, and interfere with vital physiological functions necessary for the tick to survive. Ticks exposed to botanical acaricides may experience dehydration, desiccation, or other negative consequences due to a compromised cuticle (Jeschke 2021). Certain botanical acaricides cause the release of reactive oxygen species or disrupt antioxidant defense systems, which causes oxidative stress in ticks. In ticks, oxidative stress can result in cellular damage, malfunction, and eventually death. The effectiveness, safety, and mechanism of action of botanical acaricides have been the subject of recent research, which highlights their potential as supplemental or alternative options for tick control in integrated pest management programs (Sparks et al. 2023).

## 3.3 Advantages and Disadvantages of Different Acaricides

Acaricides have benefits and drawbacks, much like any other type of pest control. This is an overview.

### 3.3.1 Advantages

Since the late nineteenth century, arsenicals have proven effective in suppressing ticks and diseases transmitted by ticks, making them the first acaricides to be used worldwide. Arsenicals were once thought to be affordable, stable, and water soluble, and they offered tick control methods that were also reasonably priced. It is widely used to control *Boophilus* ticks in several countries, including Brazil, South Africa, Australia, and others. The first synthetic family of organic insecticides to be commercialized for the control of ticks was organochlorines, which provide long-lasting residual activity, broad-spectrum action, and increased efficiency. They are more affordable and less poisonous than arsenicals, which makes them appealing alternatives for managing tick populations. Particularly efficient against ticks are substances such as DDT and benzene hexachloride, which offer important control in several areas (Chagas 2023). Synthetic compounds are often present in the active ingredients of products that are registered as tick toxicants or repellents by the EPA, such as skin repellents such as N,N-diethyl-meta-toluamide, and picaridin; clothing treatment products such as permethrin; and host-seeking tick products such as various carbamates and pyrethroids. Synthetic acaricides are easy to use, readily available, versatile in application, offer persistent activity, and have broad-spectrum efficacy. They are also effective in quickly eliminating tick populations, which lowers the risk of tick-borne diseases (Kasheverov et al. 2022). They have the potential to effectively mitigate tick infestations and reduce losses associated with tick-borne diseases in the livestock industry. Their ability to limit the number of ticks on migrating birds may slow the spread of diseases such as *T. gondii,* which is carried by ticks. Active sampling efforts are needed to control tick populations, thereby assisting in the detection of tick-borne pathogens. Synthetic acaricides can effectively reduce tick populations on domesticated animals, thereby mitigating the risk of tick-borne diseases and their transmission to humans. Acaricides reduce tick populations on hosts, thereby decreasing the risk of tick-borne disease transmission to humans and animals (Kem et al. 2022). Acaricides work well to reduce tick infestations and related problems in cattle, including diseases caused by ticks and monetary losses. In resource-constrained farming communities, the effective treatment of ticks and tick-borne illnesses is essential for preserving the health and production of livestock. Although synthetic acaricides effectively reduce tick populations and diseases caused by ticks, they may be hazardous to people, animals, and the environment. It offers efficient and economical tick population suppression, which is essential for reducing livestock industry financial losses and managing tick-borne illnesses. Successful management of parasites such as *Varroa destructor* in honeybee colonies, reducing financial losses for the beekeeping sector (Jeschke 2023). Management of tick species such as *Rhipicephalus (Boophilus) decoloratus* can assist in reducing financial losses in the cattle sector and reducing the spread of diseases such as *Babesia bigemina.* In the past, efficient tick control was applied, helping to manage diseases caused by ticks and decreasing financial losses in the cattle industry. To effectively reduce tick infestations and mitigate the spread of infections, two regularly used interventions for managing tick-borne diseases, such as East Coast fever, are cypermethrin and deltamethrin (Venkatesan et al. 2022). This reduces economic losses in the livestock industry. To prevent infections in humans and livestock, cypermethrin and chlorpyrifos are useful for managing tick infestations and decreasing the spread of pathogens carried by ticks. It has long been known to be successful in controlling ticks. Frequently applied techniques, such as spot-ons and dipping tanks, offer prompt relief from tick infestations. Although they provide efficient tick control, synthetic acaricides such as ivermectin, alpha-cypermethrin, and amitraz have drawbacks, including resistance development and environmental damage. They are efficient at limiting the spread of illnesses caused by ticks and managing tick populations. They are efficient at halting the spread of illnesses caused by ticks and lowering tick populations (Bickerton et al. 2023).

The following are the advantages of some synthetic acaricide classes.

#### 3.3.1.1 Organophosphates

Organophosphates were created as substitutes for organochlorines and provided efficient tick control, especially against *Boophilus* ticks that were resistant to organochlorines. With the introduction of organophosphates, carbamates offer more tick management alternatives due to their comparable modes of action. In different areas, organophosphates and carbamates were effective at managing tick populations, but they were not as durable as organochlorines. The class of substances known as organophosphates (OPs) comprises malathion, diazinon, and chlorpyrifos. These enzymes cause target pests to become paralyzed and die by blocking acetylcholinesterase, an enzyme required for nerve signal transmission. Organophosphates (OPs) are a versatile option for pest management because they exert rapid knockdown effects on target pests, resulting in quick control of acarine and insects. With their efficacy against a wide range of pest species, including mites and ticks, OPs are often less expensive than some alternative classes of acaricides, making them cost-effective pest control alternatives in agricultural and public health applications (Zhang et al. 2022).

#### 3.3.1.2 Carbamates

A few examples of carbamate acaricides are propoxur and carbaryl carbamate. Unlike organophosphates, they also inhibit acetylcholinesterase, but their mode of action is distinct. When applied to pests of interest, carbamates respond quickly to knockdown and provide control, and tend to be less persistent in the environment than certain other chemical types, which lowers the possibility of environmental buildup. When handled properly, carbamates have a limited impact on nontarget organisms and are specific, so they can be successfully incorporated into IPM programs (Lionello et al. 2023).

#### 3.3.1.3 Synthetic Pyrethroids

Synthetic pyrethroids, such as deltamethrin and permethrin, have been shown to have a knockdown effect on arachnids and effectively control ticks that are resistant to other chemical classes. Compared to certain other kinds of acaricides, pyrethroids are less hazardous to mammals and birds in the short term. These are artificial forms of pyrethrins, which are naturally occurring substances present in *Chrysanthemum* blossoms. Permethrin, cypermethrin, and deltamethrin are examples of synthetic pyrethroids that cause paralysis and death in pests by interfering with their neurological systems. Because they quickly eradicate pests, synthetic pyrethroids are useful for emergency pest management. Compared to certain other classes, these acaricides have a longer residual action that offers greater protection against reinfestation. The effectiveness of synthetic pyrethroids against a variety of arthropod pests, such as ticks and mites, increases their usefulness in pest management (Martínez et al. 2021).

#### 3.3.1.4 Formamidines

Formamidines, such as amitraz, have proven to be effective against tick strains that are resistant to other pesticides, providing an alternative to ineffective organophosphates and carbamates. Despite concerns about resistance development, amitraz was found to be especially effective in eradicating infestations of *R. microplus* and has continued to be used. In veterinary medicine, amitraz is a formamidine acaricide used to eradicate mites, ticks, and other pests. It functions by upsetting the nervous system of bugs. Amitraz is a formamidine that has proven to be highly effective in reducing tick infestations in a variety of contexts, including veterinary and agricultural settings. The rapid knockdown of formamidines in ticks causes the parasites to quickly become immobile and die. Certain acaricides based on formamidine have residual activity, which offers extended defense against tick reinfestation. Formamidines are useful in pest management programs because they may have broad-spectrum efficacy against different kinds of ticks and mites (Chandi and Kaur 2021).

#### 3.3.1.5 Benzoylphenylureas (BPUS)

One BPU acaricide that inhibits chitin production and disrupts insect molting and growth is fenoxycarb. This compound functions as a growth regulator for insects. BPUs, such as lufenuron and diflubenzuron, have proven to be highly effective against a variety of arthropod pests, such as insects, mites, and ticks. BPUs have an acaricidal effect on arthropods by preventing the production of chitin, which hinders growth, molting, and development. Because of their low toxicity to nontarget animals and negligible effects on beneficial arthropods and natural predators, BPUs are regarded as environmentally friendly. Certain BPUs have residual activity that lasts for a long time after treatment, which prolongs protection against arthropod pest reinfestation (Yan and Xia 2021).

#### 3.3.1.6 Spinosyns

A naturally occurring substance called spinosad is produced when the soil actinomycete *Saccharopolyspora spinosa* ferments. It affects the neurological systems of pests, leading to hyperexcitation and ultimately death. Spinosyns are adaptable choices for pest control since they exhibit broad-spectrum activity against a variety of arthropod pests, such as ticks, mites, and insects. Spinosyns exhibit great efficacy at low application rates, minimizing their environmental impact and lowering the amount of active component needed for successful pest control. Because spinosyns are less harmful to mammals, including humans, they are safer alternatives for controlling pests in homes and farms. Spinosyns have a rapid knockdown effect on their intended pests, resulting in rapid death and efficient infestation management (Krol et al. 2023).

#### 3.3.1.7 Tetronic and Tetramic Acid Derivatives

This class includes the bacteria *Streptomyces avermitilis*, from which abamectin is produced. It causes paralysis and death in pests by interfering with their neurotransmission. Derivatives of tetronic and tetrameric acids reduce ecological risks by exhibiting strong selectivity toward target pests and negligible influence on nontarget organisms. These compounds frequently have several mechanisms of action, such as interfering with neurotransmitters or insect growth regulators, which effectively control target pests and delay the emergence of resistance. Derivatives of tetronic and tetramic acid are often less harmful to animals, which makes them safer alternatives for controlling pests in homes and farms. When coupled with other active substances, these derivatives may show synergistic effects that increase their efficacy against target pests while lowering the likelihood of resistance development (Obaid et al. 2022b).

#### 3.3.1.8 Nereistoxin Analogs

Nereistoxin analog acaricides, such as cartap and bensultap, work on the neurological system of insects by obstructing the nicotinic acetylcholine receptor. Analogs of nereistoxin have demonstrated excellent efficacy in managing specific pests, such as mites and insects. They are adaptable for pest management since they have wide-ranging activity against a variety of pest species. By acting as acetylcholinesterase inhibitors, they can effectively manage pests by disrupting their neurological systems. Nereistoxin analogs frequently have a fast start of action, which causes target pests to quickly succumb to application. Certain analogs may exhibit comparatively low mammalian toxicity, hence mitigating application-related risk to both people and animals (Nasreen et al. 2020).

#### 3.3.1.9 Pyrroles

The pyrrole acaricide chlorfenapyr disrupts the cellular respiration of pests, ultimately resulting in their death. Pyrroles are effective against a variety of arthropod pests, including ticks and mites, and have broad-spectrum effects. Pyrroles are safer for use in veterinary and agricultural applications since they frequently show low toxicity to mammals (Jack and Ellis 2021).

#### 3.3.1.10 Isoxazolines

This relatively recent class of acaricides contains substances such as afoxolaner and fluralaner that cause paralysis and death by disrupting the neurological system of pests. Isoxazolines are flexible choices for pest control because of their broad-spectrum action against a variety of tick and flea species. Because isoxazolines are highly effective at low dosages and are rapidly metabolized in mammals, there is little chance that they will contaminate the environment. The convenience of isooxazolines for pet owners and veterinarians is increased by their availability of a variety of formulations for simple administration, such as oral tablets and topical spot-on treatments (Rochlin et al. 2022).

The following are the disadvantages of synthetic acaricides.

### 3.3.2 Disadvantages

The emergence of resistance in tick populations, such as *R. microplus*, resulted in decreased effectiveness and eventual prohibition of the use of organochlorines. Regulations were imposed because of their residual impact on meat, milk, and the environment, as well as worries about their poor biodegradability and poor lipid affinity. A few years after widespread use, field failures due to tick resistance started to occur, which resulted in decreased efficacy. Synthetic organic pesticides replaced them after World War II due to several factors, including the evolution of tick resistance, the need to prevent toxic residues in animal tissues, and the limited safety margins between dangerous concentrations for cattle and effective concentrations for tick control (Mirza et al. 2023). Overuse can result in resistance, be expensive, disturb natural ecosystems, leave residues, endanger the environment and human health, and be subject to regulations. These include the risk of environmental contamination, harm to nontarget organisms, and the development of resistance in tick populations over time. These factors may also reduce the long-term effectiveness of tick control methods. The ecological effects on organisms that are not the intended targets and the emergence of resistance in tick populations could jeopardize the efficacy of tick control methods in passive sampling initiatives. Environmental pollution and the emergence of acaricide resistance in tick populations can eventually decrease the effectiveness of these pesticides, increasing the need for alternate control measures. Acaricide resistance may cause environmental contamination and aid in tick populations, requiring the investigation of alternate and integrated pest management techniques (Ortíz-Giraldo et al. 2021). Acaricide misuse can result in low effectiveness, which feeds a cycle of overuse and the emergence of resistance in tick populations. The issues posed by the widespread evolution of acaricide resistance call for the creation of novel control measures to counter resistant phenotypes and reduce harm to ecosystems and public health. Due to the buildup of hazardous residues in the environment and the resistance of tick populations caused by the widespread use of synthetic acaricides, researchers are investigating natural alternatives such as lemongrass essential oil. Many tick species have developed resistance because of prolonged use of synthetic acaricides, making it more difficult to control tick populations and requiring the investigation of alternate tactics (Malak et al. 2022). Long-term exposure to synthetic acaricides such as tau-fluvalinate and coumaphos can cause residues to accumulate in beehive matrices, which may have an adverse effect on the general health of the hive and perhaps cause long-term health problems in honeybee populations. This causes tick populations to become resistant, which reduces the effectiveness of control measures and makes the search for alternate tick management strategies necessary. Tick populations have become resistant because of the extensive use of synthetic acaricides, making it more difficult to manage tick populations and requiring the investigation of alternate strategies such as extracts derived from plants (Shyma et al. 2022). Synthetic acaricide overuse can cause tick populations to become resistant, making it more difficult to control tick populations and perhaps increasing financial losses for the livestock industry. Synthetic acaricide overuse can cause resistance in tick populations, which makes it more difficult to control tick populations and may eventually decrease the effectiveness of these treatments. Synthetic acaricides have the drawback of possibly causing target insect populations to quickly acquire resistance (Abdel-Ghany et al. 2021). Synthetic acaricide overuse can cause tick populations to become resistant, which makes it difficult to control tick populations over the long term and forces the exploration of alternate approaches to controlling tick infestations. Their short-term efficacy in controlling tick populations is hampered by their single mode of action, environmental contamination, and the ease with which acaricidal resistance can be induced. Synthetic acaricide use without consideration has resulted in the growth of resistant tick populations, environmental pollution, and hazardous residues in animal byproducts, all of which pose threats to the environment and public health (Abdel-Shafy et al. 2020). It provides excellent tick control, but ticks also face issues related to resistance development and environmental harm. Although synthetic acaricides are effective at controlling tick populations, they are becoming less effective and pose risks to people, animals, and the environment. These include threats to nontarget organisms, potential for resistance to develop, and effects on the environment. Hazards to nontarget creatures, potential harm to the environment, and evolution of resistance. Risk to nontarget organisms, potential for environmental damage, and development of resistance. Danger to nontarget creatures, potential harm to the environment, and the evolution of resistance can occur (Srisanyong et al. 2021).

The following are the disadvantages of some synthetic acaricide classes.

#### 3.3.2.1 Organophosphates

Over time, the efficacy of antimicrobial agents has decreased in tick species that have developed resistance to organophosphates and carbamates, including *R. microplus*. Carbamates are not as widely used as organophosphates because they are more costly and somewhat more hazardous to mammals. Because of their nonspecific toxicity, organophosphates can harm a broad variety of species, including beneficial insects, birds, and mammals, which can cause ecological imbalances and a decline in biodiversity. Long-term ecological harm and negative effects on nontarget species can result from the long-term persistence of organophosphates in the environment, which can contaminate soil, water bodies, and plants (Patoliya et al. 2022). Long-term exposure to OPs can cause target pests to become resistant, which eventually decreases the efficiency of these chemicals and calls for increased treatment rates or different forms of management. Humans, particularly farmworkers, people living near treated regions, and people who consume contaminated food products, are at serious risk of developing acute and long-term health impacts that include neurotoxicity, respiratory problems, and cancer from exposure to organic pollutants (OPs). Owing to the possible risks they pose to human health and the environment, OPs may be subject to legislative limitations or outright prohibitions in some nations. This would restrict their availability and use and force alternative approaches to pest management to be developed (Kumar et al. 2022).

#### 3.3.2.2 Carbamates

Because carbamates cause nervous system disruption, they can be harmful to non-target creatures such as beneficial insects, birds, and mammals. Compared to other synthetic acaricides, carbamates sometimes have shorter residual activity, necessitating more frequent applications to preserve efficacy. Over time, the efficiency of carbamates may decrease because target pest populations develop resistance to carbamates because of prolonged or frequent treatment. After application, carbamates may linger in the environment and endanger ecosystems, as well as contaminating water sources through runoff. Humans who are exposed to carbamates by ingestion, inhalation, or skin contact may experience acute poisoning symptoms such as nausea, vertigo, and respiratory distress. Carbamates may be subject to regulatory restrictions or bans in some places due to possible health and environmental concerns, which limits their use in pest control measures (dos Rosário et al. 2023).

#### 3.3.2.3 Synthetic Pyrethroids

Due to concerns about environmental pollution and possible harm to aquatic creatures, the widespread use of pyrethroids has necessitated careful application practices. Reports of the development of resistance to permethrin and deltamethrin have increased globally, which has limited the long-term effectiveness of these pyrethroids. The long-term environmental persistence of synthetic pyrethroids following application may result in their accumulation in soil, water, and sediment, which could be harmful to nontarget organisms such as fish and aquatic invertebrates (Shanmuganath et al. 2021). Synthetic pyrethroids can nevertheless be dangerous to nontarget organisms, particularly aquatic species and beneficial insects such as bees and butterflies, even if they are usually thought to be harmless to mammals, birds, and humans at low levels. Synthetic pyrethroid resistance in target pest populations can result from prolonged or repeated use, which eventually reduces compound activity and calls for the deployment of alternate control strategies (Lima et al. 2020). Humans who are exposed to synthetic pyrethroids by ingestion, dermal contact, or inhalation may experience adverse health effects, such as headaches, dizziness, and irritation of the skin and eyes. Through direct contact with contaminated prey or ingestion, synthetic pyrethroids may unintentionally affect wildlife, resulting in population losses and ecological changes. Certain synthetic pyrethroids have been subject to legislative limits or bans in certain places due to potential health and environmental hazards, which has limited their usage in pest management and agriculture (Muhanguzi et al. 2022).

#### 3.3.2.4 Formamidines

The long-term effectiveness of formamidines, such as amitraz, has been limited by reports of resistance that have surfaced from different places. The extensive application of macrocyclic lactones in tick control programs has been limited by their high cost. Formamidines are a class of acaricides that may become less effective over time due to the development of resistance in tick populations because of prolonged and extensive use. If used incorrectly or in excess, formamidine-based acaricides may be harmful to nontarget creatures and environmental ecosystems. It is crucial to handle and store formamidine-based acaricides properly since improper application or inadvertent consumption can be unsafe for humans, pets, and cattle. Since formamidines usually target physiological pathways in ticks, their effectiveness against specific tick species or stages may be limited, requiring the use of alternate control methods (Khan et al. 2023).

#### 3.3.2.5 Benzoylphenylureas (BPUS)

Since formamidines usually target physiological pathways in ticks, in comparison to other acaricides, BPUs usually have a delayed onset of action, meaning that it takes longer for target pests to experience these effects. Although BPUs work well against immature tick stages, their effectiveness against adult ticks may be restricted, requiring the use of additional control techniques. Long-term BPU use may cause arthropod populations to become resistant, which eventually decreases the efficacy of these acaricides. Because BPUs mainly target the synthesis of chitin in arthropods, their effectiveness against specific pest species or stages may be limited, requiring the use of integrated pest management techniques. Their effectiveness against specific tick species or stages may be limited, requiring the use of alternate control methods (Hakami et al. 2023).

#### 3.3.2.6 Spinosyns

Ecological imbalances may result from the impact of spinosyns on nontarget animals, such as beneficial insects and natural predators, preventing their efficacy against target pests. The extended use of spinosyn may cause target pest populations to become resistant, eventually decreasing the efficacy of these acaricides. Following their application, spinosyns may linger in the environment and have an impact on ecosystems and nontarget creatures. Compared to other synthetic acaricides, spinosyn-based formulations may be less readily available, which could limit their usage in some areas or applications (Aziz et al. 2023).

#### 3.3.2.7 Tetronic and Tetramic Acid Derivatives

Compared to those of other synthetic acaricides, the availability of commercial formulations, including derivatives of tetronic and tetramic acids, may be restricted, which could limit their use in specific areas or applications. After application, tetronic and tetramic acid derivatives may linger in the environment and have an impact on ecosystems and nontarget animals. Over time, target pest populations may become resistant to tetronic and tetramic acid derivatives due to prolonged use, which decreases the efficiency of these acaricides.

#### 3.3.2.8 Nereistoxin Analogs

Through inadvertent exposure or toxicity, they may present threats to nontarget creatures, such as beneficial insects and wildlife. The long-term use of nereistoxin analogs may cause target insect populations to become resistant, eventually decreasing their effectiveness. There could be long-term ecological effects from some nereistoxin analogs. Pyrroles can linger in the environment, which could raise ecological issues such as exposure to nontarget organisms and buildup in soil and water systems. Pyrroles, like many other synthetic acaricides, are susceptible to resistance in target insect populations, which can eventually decrease their efficacy (Eltaly et al. 2023).

#### 3.3.2.9 Isoxazolines

The target pest populations are at risk of developing isoxazoline resistance over time; therefore, cautious management techniques are needed. Because isoxazoline products can be more costly than conventional acaricides, some pet owners may not be able to afford them. Although isoxazolines are usually well tolerated, certain animals may experience negative side effects, such as neurological symptoms or gastrointestinal disturbances (Jain et al. 2021).

## References


Abdel-Ghany HSM, Abdel-Shafy S, Abuowarda MM, El-Khateeb RM, Hoballah EM, Fahmy MM (2021) Acaricidal activity of some medicinal plant extracts against different developmental stages of the camel tick *Hyalomma dromedarii*. Adv Anim Vet Sci 9(5):722–733

Abdel-Shafy S, Alanazi AD, Gabr HS, Allam AM, Abou-Zeina HA, Masoud RA, Alshahrani MY (2020) Efficacy and safety of ethanolic *Curcuma longa* extract as a treatment for sand tampan ticks in a rabbit model. Vet World 13(4):812

Adenubi OT, Salihu T, Akande FA, Adekoya OA, Mshelbwala FM, Afolabi TA, Olukunle JO (2024) Acaricidal activities of the essential oils of six ethnoveterinary plants used by Fulani Herdsmen in Nigeria. Egypt J Vet Sci 55(4):1007–1019

Adesanya AW, Lavine MD, Moural TW, Lavine LC, Zhu F, Walsh DB (2021) Mechanisms and management of acaricide resistance for *Tetranychus urticae* in agroecosystems. J Pest Sci 94:639–663

Agwunobi DO, Yu Z, Liu J (2021) A retrospective review on ixodid tick resistance against synthetic acaricides: implications and perspectives for future resistance prevention and mitigation. Pestic Biochem Physiol 173:104776

Alborzi A, Larki S, Sefidi JG, Khodadad H (2023) Anti-tick effect of aqueous, aqueous-alcoholic and alcoholic extracts of *Moringa olifera* on hatching eggs process and the growth of *Hyalomma anatolicum anatolicum* larvae by Immersion test method. Vet Res Biol Prod 36(2):22–31

Alimi D, Hajri A, Jallouli S, Sebai H (2021) *In vitro* acaricidal activity of essential oil and crude extracts of *Laurus nobilis*, (Lauraceae) grown in Tunisia, against arthropod ectoparasites of livestock and poultry: *Hyalomma scupense* and *Dermanyssus gallinae*. Vet Parasitol 298:109507

Alimi D, Hajri A, Jallouli S, Sebai H (2022) Phytochemistry, anti-tick, repellency and anti-cholinesterase activities of *Cupressus sempervirens* L. and *Mentha pulegium* L. combinations against *Hyalomma scupense* (Acari: Ixodidae). Vet Parasitol 303:109665

Alimi D, Trabelsi N, Hajri A, Amor MB, Mejri A, Jallouli S, Sebai H (2024) Laboratory assessment of the acaricidal, repellent and anti-cholinesterase effects of *Melaleuca alternifolia* and *Chamaemelum nobile* essential oils against *Hyalomma scupense* ticks. Vet Res Commun 48:1379–1391

Anholeto LA, Brancaglion GA, Dos Santos DM, Kapritchkoff RTI, de Carvalho Castro KN, Canuto KM, Pastre JC (2024) Acaricidal activity of synthetic spilanthol derivative against ticks of medical and veterinary importance. Vet Parasitol 327:110137

Arbabi M, Khani M (2021) Comparative effects of botanical and synthetic pesticides in the control of tomato russet mite, *Aculops lycopersici* (Acari: Eriophyidae). BioControl Plant Protect 8(2):83–92

Arshed M, Nasir S, Hussain T, Babar MI, Imran M (2021) Comparison efficacy of synthetic chemicals and plant extracts for tick control. Slov Vet Res 58(1):13–23

Ayub S, Malak N, Cossío-Bayúgar R, Nasreen N, Khan A, Niaz S, Ben Said M (2023) *In vitro* and *in silico* protocols for the assessment of anti-tick compounds from *Pinus roxburghii* against *Rhipicephalus* (*Boophilus*) *microplus* ticks. Animals 13(8):1388

Aziz AAA, Abdelfattah AM, Khalil WF, Mahmoud AE, Abouelhassan EM (2023) *In vitro* and *in vivo* evaluation of the efficacy of phoxim and deltamethrin against life stages of *Rhipicephalus sanguineus* (brown dog tick). J Adv Vet Res 13(5):827–832

Bai L, Gao Z, Xu X, Lv W, Wang Y, Dong K, Yang X (2024) The acaricidal activity and enzymatic targets of the essential oils of *Cinnamomum cassia* and *Cinnamomum camphora* and their major components against *Physalis longicornis* (Acari: Ixodidae). Ind Crop Prod 209:117967

Benito-Murcia M, Botías C, Martín-Hernández R, Higes M, Soler F, Pérez-López M, Martínez-Morcillo S (2024) Biomarker responses and lethal dietary doses of tau-fluvalinate and coumaphos in honeybees: implications for chronic acaricide toxicity. Environ Toxicol Pharmacol 105:104330

Bickerton M, González J, Egizi A, Toledo A (2023) Baseline susceptibility of *Physalis longicornis* to organophosphate, carbamate, and pyrethroid acaricides. Pest Manag Sci 79(11):4328–4334

Bravo-Ramos JL, Flores-Primo A, Paniagua-Vega D, Sánchez-Otero MG, Cruz-Romero A, Romero-Salas D (2021) Acaricidal activity of the hexanic and hydroethanolic extracts of three medicinal plants against southern cattle tick *Rhipicephalus* (*Boophilus*) *microplus* (Acari: Ixodidae). Exp Appl Acarol 85(1):113–129

Cardoso ERN, Carvalho SF, Dias SA, Santos RA, Tavares MA, Neves LC, Krawczak FDS (2023) Susceptibility of *Amblyomma sculptum*, vector of *Rickettsia rickettsii*, ticks from a National Park and an experimental farm to different synthetic acaricides. Pathogens 12(11):1304

Carneiro ADS, Mesquita E, Meirelles LN, Bittencourt VREP, Golo PS (2022) Compatibility of different *Metarhizium* spp. propagules with synthetic acaricides for controlling *Rhipicephalus microplus*. Rev Bras Parasitol Vet 31:e018221

Chagas RC (2023) Métodos de criação de Chrysoperla externa (Hagen) (Neuroptera: Chrysopidae) em laboratório e seu uso no controle de artrópodes-praga em cultivos de coqueiro e algodoeiro

Chaisri W, Aneknan T, Khonkarn R, Tiwananthagorn S, Suriyasathaporn W, Pangprasit N, Pikulkaew S (2024) Self-emulsifying drug delivery systems (SEDDS) containing *Cymbopogon citratus* essential oil: enhancing the stability and acaricide efficacy against *Rhipicephalus* (*Boophilus*) *microplus*. Vet Parasitol 328:110171

Chandi AK, Kaur A (2021) Hormone analogs and chitin synthesis inhibitors. In: Molecular approaches for sustainable insect pest management. Springer, Cham, pp 253–282

Chikufenji B, Chatanga E, Galon EM, Mohanta UK, Mdzukulu G, Ma Y, Xuan X (2024) First report of dog ticks and tick-borne pathogens they are carrying in Malawi. J Vet Med Sci 86(2):150–159

da Silva GD, de Lima HG, de Freitas HF, da Rocha Pita SS, dos Santos Luz Y, de Figueiredo MP, Botura MB (2021) *In vitro* and i*n silico* studies of the larvicidal and anticholinesterase activities of berberine and piperine alkaloids on *Rhipicephalus microplus*. Ticks Tick-Borne Dis 12(2):101643

de la Fuente J, Estrada-Peña A, Rafael M, Almazán C, Bermúdez S, Abdelbaset AE, Dahal A (2023) Perception of ticks and tick-borne diseases worldwide. Pathogens 12(10):1258

dos Rosário CJR, Lima AS, de JS Mendonça C, Soares IS, Júnior EB, Gomes MN, da Rocha CQ (2023) Essential oil A*geratum conyzoides* chemotypes and anti-tick activities. Vet Parasitol 319:109942

Eisen L (2024) Efficacy of unregulated minimum risk products to kill and repel ticks. Emerg Infect Dis 30(1):1

Eltaly RI, Baz MM, Radwan IT, Yousif M, Abosalem HS, Selim A, Khater HF (2023) Novel acaricidal activity of *Vitex castus* and *Zingiber officinale* extracts against the camel tick, *Hyalomma dromedarii*. J Vet Sci 12(2):255–259

Gonzaga BCF, de Moraes NR, Gomes GW, Coutinho AL, Vale FL, Sousa LJMP, Monteiro C (2022) Combination of synthetic acaricides with (E)-cinnamaldehyde to control *Rhipicephalus microplus*. Exp Appl Acarol 88(2):191–207

Gryczyńska A, Polaczyk J, Welc-Falęciak R (2024) Toxoplasma gondii infection in ticks infesting migratory birds: the blackbird (*Turdus merula*) and the song thrush (*Turdus philomelos*). Exp Appl Acarol 92:233–240

Gupta S, Sangwan N, Sangwan AK, Gupta S, Kumar A, Maan S, Kumar S (2024) Acaricide resistance status of deltamethrin and coumaphos in *Hyalomma anatolicum* ticks collected from different districts of Haryana. Exp Appl Acarol 92:809–833

Habeeba S, Bensalah OK, Ibrahim A, Al Muhairi S, Al Hammadi Z, Commey A, Shah A (2024) Acaricide resistance in ticks from livestock farms in Abu Dhabi, United Arab Emirates. Acarologia 64(1):138–145

Hakami MA, Malak N, Khan A, Ullah H, Cossío-Bayúgar R, Nasreen N, Chen CC (2023) *In silico* exploration and experimental validation of *Camellia sinensis* extract against *Rhipicephalus microplus* and *Sarcoptes scabiei:* an integrated approach. Life 13(10):2040

Hamamoto I, Kawaguchi M, Nakamura T, Yano M, Koizumi K, Takahashi J (2023) Discovery of a novel acaricide, acynonapyr. J Pestic Sci 48(4):202–210

Harman PR, Mendell NL, Harman MM, Draney PA, Boyle AT, Gompper ME, Hanley KA (2024) Science abhors a surveillance vacuum: detection of ticks and tick-borne pathogens in southern New Mexico through passive surveillance. PLoS One 19(1):e0292573

Jack CJ, Ellis JD (2021) Integrated pest management control of *Varroa destructor* (Acari: Varroidae), the most damaging pest of (*Apis mellifera* L. (Hymenoptera: Apidae)) colonies. J Insect Sci 21(5):6

Jain P, Satapathy T, Pandey RK (2021) Acaricidal activity and biochemical analysis of *Citrus limetta* seed oil for controlling Ixodid Tick *Rhipicephalus microplus* infesting cattle. Syst Appl Acarol 26(7):1350–1360

Jeschke P (2021) Status and outlook for acaricide and insecticide discovery. Pest Manag Sci 77(1):64–76

Jeschke P (2023) Recent developments in fluorine-containing pesticides. Pest Manag Sci 80:3065–3087

Kasheverov I, Kudryavtsev D, Shelukhina I, Nikolaev G, Utkin Y, Tsetlin V (2022) Marine origin ligands of nicotinic receptors: low molecular compounds, peptides and proteins for fundamental research and practical applications. Biomolecules 12(2):189

Kem WR, Andrud K, Bruno G, Xing H, Soti F, Talley TT, Taylor P (2022) Interactions of nereistoxin and its analogs with vertebrate nicotinic acetylcholine receptors and molluskan ACh binding proteins. Mar Drugs 20(1):49

Keve G, Csörgő T, Kováts D, Hornok S (2024) Long term evaluation of factors influencing the association of ixodid ticks with birds in Central Europe, Hungary. Sci Rep 14(1):4958

Khan A, Taj S, Malak N, Swelum AA, Khan A, Nasreen N, Wu WF (2023) Integrating *in vitro* and *in silico* approaches to assess *Monotheca buxifolia* plant extract against *Rhipicephalus (Boophilus) microplus* and *Sarcoptes scabiei*. Molecules 28(19):6930

Krol L, Dunker FH, LaDouceur E, Biswell E, Dilly GF, Delbeek JC, Hill J (2023) Milbemycin oxime (interceptor) treatment of pycnogonid sea spider infestation in three species of corals. J Zoo Wildl Med 54(2):292–300

Kumar B, Shukla PK, Sharma AK, Rawat AKS, Rawat YS, Ghosh S, Srivastava S (2022) Anti-tick potential and intraspecific chemical variations in *Ageratum conyzoides* L. collected from Indus plain and Central India. Pharmacogn Mag 18(77):226–232

Li T, Lv M, Wen H, Xu H (2023) Discovery of 3-formyl-N-(un) substituted benzylindole pyrimidines as an acaricidal agent and their mechanism of action. J Agric Food Chem 71(45):17036–17045

Liao F, Han C, Deng Q, Zhou Z, Bao T, Zhong M, Hu Y (2023) Natural products as mite control agents in animals: a review. Molecules 28(19):6818

Lima HGD, Santos FO, Santos ACV, Silva GDD, Santos RJD, Carneiro KDO, Botura MB (2020) Anti-tick effect and cholinesterase inhibition caused by *Prosopis juliflora* alkaloids: *in vitro* and *in silico* studies. Rev Bras Parasitol Vet 29:e019819

Lionello FCP, Rotundo S, Bruno G, Marino G, Morrone HL, Fusco P, Torti C (2023) Touching base with some Mediterranean diseases of interest from paradigmatic cases at the "Magna Graecia" university unit of infectious diseases: a didascalic review. Diagnostics 13(17):2832

Ma Y, Huang Y, Song Y, Yao M (2022) A novel copper oxychloride@HKUST-1 composite: enhanced catalytic activity in thermal decomposition of ammonium perchlorate. J Hazard Mater 427:128111

Malak N, Niaz S, Wadood A, Nasreen N, Ali I, Iqbal J, Khan A (2022) *In silico* approaches to develop herbal acaricides against *R.* (*Boophilus*) *microplus* and i*n vitro* anti-tick activities of selected medicinal plants. Saudi J Biol Sci 29(6):103302

Malak N, Niaz S, Miranda-Miranda E, Cossío-Bayúgar R, Duque JE, Amaro-Estrada I, Zając Z (2024) Current perspectives and difficulties in the design of acaricides and repellents from plant-derived compounds for tick control. Exp Appl Acarol 93:1–16

Malik A, Afshan K, Razzaq A, Fatima Z, Hussain M, Firasat S (2021) Comparative efficacy of synthetic acaricides against tick infestations in goats. Kafkas Üniv Vet Fakül Dergisi 27(2):159–164

Martínez LC, Plata-Rueda A, Serrão JE (2021) Effect of benzoylphenyl ureas on survival and reproduction of the lace bug, Leptopharsa gibbicarina. Insects 12(1):34

Menon AG, Bhaskar H, Subramanian SM, Gopal KS (2023) Acaricidal effects of two native isolates of entomo-pathogenic bacteria *Photorhabdus luminescens* (Thomas & Poinar) against spider mite, *Tetranychus truncatus* Ehara (Acari: Tetranychidae). Int J Acarol 49(7-8):395–399

Mirza JH, Kamran M, Alatawi FJ (2023) Taxonomy of the family teneriffiidae (Acari: Prostigmata: Anystoidea): generic synonymies with the key to world species of the family. Animals 13(23):3736

Mitton GA, Meroi Arcerito F, Cooley H, Fernandez de Landa G, Eguaras MJ, Ruffinengo SR, Maggi MD (2022) More than sixty years living with *Varroa destructor*: a review of acaricide resistance. Int J Pest Manag. https://doi.org/10.1080/09670874.2022.2094489

Morfin N, Rawn D, Petukhova T, Kozak P, Eccles L, Chaput J, Guzman-Novoa E (2022) Surveillance of synthetic acaricide efficacy against Varroa destructor in Ontario, Canada. Can Entomol 154(1):e17

Moudgil AD, Daundkar PS, Nehra AK, Vohra S, Gupta S, Sharma D (2023) Molecular characterization of *Hyalomma dromedarii* and evaluation of acaricidal potential of herbal methanolic extracts against *H. dromedarii* larvae in comparison to synthetic acaricides. Exp Appl Acarol 89(1):141–156

Muhanguzi D, Ndekezi C, Nkamwesiga J, Kalayou S, Ochwo S, Vuyani M, Kimuda MP (2022) Anti-tick vaccines: current advances and future prospects. In: Vaccine design: methods and protocols, volume 2. Vaccines for veterinary diseases. Springer, Cham, pp 253–267

Nasreen N, Niaz S, Khan A, Zaman MA, Ayaz S, Naeem H, Elgorban AM (2020) The potential of *Allium sativum* and *Cannabis sativa* extracts for anti-tick activities against *Rhipicephalus* (*Boophilus*) *microplus*. Exp Appl Acarol 82:281–294

Obaid MK et al (2022b) Acaricides resistance in ticks: selection, diagnosis, mechanisms, and mitigation. Front Cell Infect Microbiol 12:941831

Orgiazzi A, Panagos P, Fernández-Ugalde O, Wojda P, Labouyrie M, Ballabio C, Jones A (2022) LUCAS soil biodiversity and LUCAS soil pesticides, new tools for research and policy development. Eur J Soil Sci 73(5):e13299

Ortíz-Giraldo M, Tobón-Escobar WD, Velásquez-Guarín D, Usma-Marín MF, Ossa-López PA, Ramírez-Chaves HE, Rivera-Páez FA (2021) Ticks (Acari: Ixodoidea) associated with mammals in Colombia: a historical review, molecular species confirmation, and establishment of new relationships. Parasitol Res 120:383–394

Osikowicz LM, Rizzo MR, Hojgaard A, Maes SE, Eisen RJ (2024) Detection of sensu lato species in host-seeking Ixodes species ticks in the United States. Ticks Tick-Borne Dis 15(1):102270

Patoliya P, Raval K, Upadhyaya V, Dewry RK, Maiti S, Mondal G, Bhakat M (2022) Tick infestation and its herbal treatment approach in India: a review. Pharma Innov J 11:1323–1339
Pérez-Otáñez X, Vanwambeke SO, Orozco-Alvarez G, Arciniegas-Ortega S, Ron-Garrido L, Rodríguez-Hidalgo R (2024) Widespread acaricide resistance and multiresistance in *Rhipicephalus microplus* in Ecuador and associated environmental and management risk factors. Ticks Tick-Borne Dis 15(1):102274
Poché DM, Smith Z, Poché RM (2023) Efficacy of a federally approved flea bait, orally administered to white-footed mice (*Peromyscus leucopus*), against blood feeding Ixodes scapularis larvae under simulated field conditions. Int J Parasitol 21:33–42
Rochlin I, Egizi A, Lindström A (2022) The original scientific description of the lone star tick (*Amblyomma americanum*, Acari: Ixodidae) and implications for the species' past and future geographic distributions. J Med Entomol 59(2):412–420
Roeber F, Webster M (2021) Protecting dogs and cats against the Australian paralysis tick, *Ixodes holocyclus* (Acari: Ixodidae): a review of the Australian acaricide registration process. Curr Res Parasitol Vector-Borne Dis 1:100054
Sabová L, Maruščáková IC, Koleničová S, Mudroňová D, Holečková B, Sabo R, Ratvaj M (2022) The adverse effects of synthetic acaricide tau-fluvalinate (tech.) on winter adult honeybees. Environ Toxicol Pharmacol 92:103861
Schödl I, Odemer R, Becher MA, Berg S, Otten C, Grimm V, Groeneveld J (2022) Simulation of *Varroa* mite control in honeybee colonies without synthetic acaricides: demonstration of good beekeeping practice for Germany in the BEEHAVE model. Ecol Evol 12(11):e9456
Schulze TL, Jordan RA (2021) Synthetic pyrethroid, natural product, and entomopathogenic fungal acaricide product formulations for sustained early season suppression of host-seeking *Ixodes scapularis* (Acari: Ixodidae) and *Amblyomma americanum* nymphs. J Med Entomol 58(2):814–820
Selles SMA, Kouidri M, González MG, González J, Sánchez M, González-Coloma A, Valcárcel F (2021) Acaricidal and repellent effects of essential oils against ticks: a review. Pathogens 10(11):1379
Shah T, Li Q, Wang B, Baloch Z (2023) Geographical distribution and pathogenesis of ticks and tick-borne viral diseases. Front Microbiol 14:1185829
Shankar S, Jaiswal L, Rhim JW (2021) New insight into sulfur nanoparticles: synthesis and applications. Crit Rev Environ Sci Technol 51(20):2329–2356
Shanmuganath C, Kumar S, Singh R, Sharma AK, Saminathan M, Saini M, Ghosh S (2021) Development of an efficient antitick natural formulation for the control of acaricide-resistant ticks on livestock. Ticks Tick-Borne Dis 12(3):101655
Shiri A, Kheirandish F, Sazmand A, Kayedi MH, Hosseini-Chegeni A (2024) Molecular identification of hemoparasites in ixodid ticks in Iran. Vet Parasitol 47:100967
Shyma KP, Singh V, Parsani HR, Solanki V, Pawar MM, Srivastava AK, Gupta JP (2022) Acaricidal properties of herbal extracts against deltamethrin resistant multihost cattle tick *Hyalomma anatolicum*. Indian J Anim Res 56(5):613–618
Sparks TC, Bryant RJ (2022) Innovation in insecticide discovery: approaches to the discovery of new classes of insecticides. Pest Manag Sci 78(8):3226–3247
Sparks TC, Sparks JM, Duke SO (2023) Natural product-based crop protection compounds—origins and future prospects. J Agric Food Chem 71(5):2259–2269
Srisanyong W, Bunyaluk D, Srinontong P, Chitsanoor S (2021) Acaricidal activity of phenolic crude extract from *Artocapus lakoocha* leaves against cattle tick *Rhipicephalus* (*Boophilus*) *microplus*. J Vet Sci 10(4):307–311
van Dalen EM, Jansen van Rensburg C (2024) Competitive displacement and acaricide resistance of two *Rhipicephalus* (*Boophilus*) species collected on commercial farms in South Africa. Exp Appl Acarol 92(1):135–149
Venkatesan T, Chethan BR, Mani M (2022) Insecticide resistance and its management in the insect pests of horticultural crops. In: Trends in horticultural entomology. Elsevier, Amsterdam, pp 455–490

Williams SC, Linske MA (2024) Late fall synthetic acaricide application is effective at reducing host-seeking adult and nymphal *Ixodes scapularis* (Ixodida: Ixodidae) abundances the following spring. J Med Entomol 61(4):965–974
Yan YS, Xia HY (2021) Recent advances in the research of milbemycin biosynthesis and regulation as well as strategies for strain improvement. Arch Microbiol 203(10):5849–5857
Zhang W, Ren H, Sun F, Shen T, Yuan S, Gao X, Tan Y (2022) Evaluation of the toxicity of chemical and biogenic insecticides to three outbreaking insects in desert steppes of northern China. Toxins 14(8):546
Zhu L et al (2022) Acaricidal activity and field efficacy analysis of the potential biocontrol agent *Bacillus vallismortis* NBIF-001 against spider mites. Microorganisms 10(9):1750

# Mechanisms of Acaricide Resistance

# 4

Jéssica Waldman, Luís Fernando Parizi, Abid Ali,
Carlos Termignoni, and Itabajara da Silva Vaz Junior

**Abstract**

Ticks transmit disease agents to humans and animals, causing health problems and economic losses. Tick control is currently based on synthetic acaricides; however, effective control and prevention of tick infestation remain distant goals. In recent decades, a progressive decrease in the efficiency of acaricides due to drug resistance has been observed. Tick resistance can be caused by two main mechanisms: (1) toxicodynamic resistance, where mutations in tick genes make them less susceptible to acaricides, involving changes in the target sites where acaricides bind or alterations in how these chemicals work within the tick; and (2) toxicokinetic resistance, where ticks develop ways to detoxify or eliminate acaricides more efficiently, involving increased activity of enzymes that break

J. Waldman · L. F. Parizi
Centro de Biotecnologia, Universidade Federal do Rio Grande do Sul, Campus do Vale, Porto Alegre, RS, Brazil

A. Ali
Department of Zoology, Abdul Wali Khan University, Mardan, Pakistan

C. Termignoni
Centro de Biotecnologia, Universidade Federal do Rio Grande do Sul, Campus do Vale, Porto Alegre, RS, Brazil

Departamento de Bioquímica, Universidade Federal do Rio Grande do Sul, Porto Alegre, RS, Brazil

I. da Silva Vaz Junior (✉)
Centro de Biotecnologia, Universidade Federal do Rio Grande do Sul, Campus do Vale, Porto Alegre, RS, Brazil

Faculdade de Veterinária, Universidade Federal do Rio Grande do Sul, Campus do Vale, Porto Alegre, RS, Brazil
e-mail: itabajara.vaz@ufrgs.br



S. Kumar et al. (eds.), *Acaricides Resistance in Ticks*,
https://doi.org/10.1007/978-981-97-7411-1_4

down acaricides or changes in how acaricides are transported within the tick's body. The widespread use of acaricides selects for resistant tick populations, which emphasizes the need for judicious use of these chemicals and the development of alternative tick control methods. Understanding the tick resistance mechanisms is crucial to overcoming this challenge and protecting human and animal health.

**Keywords**
Tick · Acaricide · Resistance · Mechanism

## 4.1 Introduction

Ticks are the source of important health problems for humans and animals and cause considerable economic burden on livestock. Pesticide resistance is defined as "*a heritable change in the sensitivity of a pest population that is reflected in the repeated failure of a product to achieve the expected level of control when used according to the label recommendation for that pest species*" (Sparks and Nauen 2015). Global tick resistance to acaricides is an increasing hindrance to tick control. The identification of new targets to reduce selection for resistance is a long and expansive endeavor. Additionally, legal restrictions for acaricide use add new difficulties for this strategy (Pesticide Residues in Food 2019—Joint FAO/WHO Meeting on Pesticide Residues. Evaluation Part I 2020).

Acaricide-resistant tick populations are usually observed after just a few years of tick interaction with the acaricide (Rodriguez-Vivas et al. 2011). These ectoparasites have remarkable adaptability, which confers their ability to survive in different niches and under harsh environmental conditions, including interactions with acaricides. The time taken to achieve resistance selection for a specific acaricide depends on the parasite anatomy, physiology, behavior, and management of the acaricide. Moreover, if a drug is intensively misused, the resistant population can quickly emerge, which occurs in a few years. Additionally, the intensive use of pesticides leads to the emergence of resistance in off-target species, potentially affecting several other arthropods (Van Lenteren et al. 2018).

It is alarming how tick-resistant populations to acaricides are spreading worldwide. The use and misuse of synthetic acaricides over time have led to an increase in reports on tick populations that are resistant to these drugs (Abbas et al. 2014). Indeed, resistant and multiresistant tick populations to all commercially available acaricides have already been reported (Reck et al. 2014). Therefore, comprehensive knowledge of tick metabolism, physiology, and the specific pathways influencing resistance selection can be helpful in the identification of potential novel acaricides. Additionally, this knowledge is pivotal for the development of innovative tick control strategies to effectively address growing resistance to acaricides.

Tick resistance can be split into two main mechanisms: toxicodynamic and toxicokinetic changes. Toxicodynamic changes occur as a consequence of point mutations at the pesticide binding site, decreasing the acaricide affinity to the biological mechanisms of the target tick. Another toxicodynamic mechanism involves gene amplification or gene silencing, which modifies the availability of tick proteins related to acaricide resistance. Toxicokinetic resistance primarily stems from variations in the expression of detoxification-related proteins caused by alterations in regulatory elements or through events such as gene duplication. These two mechanisms can be present in ticks in different combinations, showing protection levels that can result in additive, synergistic, or even antagonistic effects (Fotoukkiaii 2020). Other factors that affect acaricide resistance include physicochemical alterations in ticks, such as cuticle thickening, which can reduce acaricide penetration through the exoskeleton (Schnitzerling et al. 1983). However, in ticks, physiochemical alteration mechanisms are poorly understood.

## 4.2 Toxicodynamic Resistance

Target-site insensitivity occurs when one or multiple point mutations modify the amino acid sequence of the binding site of acaricidal molecules. This mechanism can confer resistance to different pesticide classes among tick populations (Guerrero et al. 2012). Herein, different types of resistance pathways associated with the occurrence of target-site insensitivity are discussed (Fig. 4.1).

### 4.2.1 Acetylcholinesterase (AChE)

Acetylcholinesterase (AChE) enzymes catalyze the hydrolysis of the neurotransmitter acetylcholine into choline and acetic acid, inactivating it (Colovic et al. 2013). The accumulation of these neurotransmitters due to AChE inhibition leads to overstimulation of the central nervous system (CNS) and death of the parasite (Casida and Durkin 2013; Guerrero et al. 2012). Since pesticides, such as organophosphates and carbamates, act by inhibiting this enzymatic activity, point mutations that produce a structurally modified AChE can prevent these chemicals from binding to the enzyme (Fig. 4.1).

Almost 60 years ago, tick populations susceptible and resistant to organophosphate and carbamate acaricides were shown to exhibit differences in their cholinesterase activities (Lee and Batham 1966). *Rhipicephalus sanguineus* sensu lato and *Rhipicephalus microplus* have three AchEs (BmAchE1, BmAchE2 and BmAchE3) (Baxter and Barker 1998; Hernandez et al. 1999; Lees et al. 2009; Temeyer et al. 2004). To date, single-nucleotide polymorphisms (SNPs) that confer organophosphate target insensitivity have been reported for BmAchE1 and BmAchE3 (Bendele et al. 2015; Temeyer 2018; Temeyer et al. 2010). Multiple amino acid substitutions were identified in BmAchE3, indicating its potential involvement in acaricide resistance (Jyoti Singh et al. 2016). However, increased AchE activity has been shown to be related to pesticide resistance to different classes (organophosphates and pyrethroids), suggesting that other mechanisms could be associated with this acaricide resistance (Gupta et al. 2023).

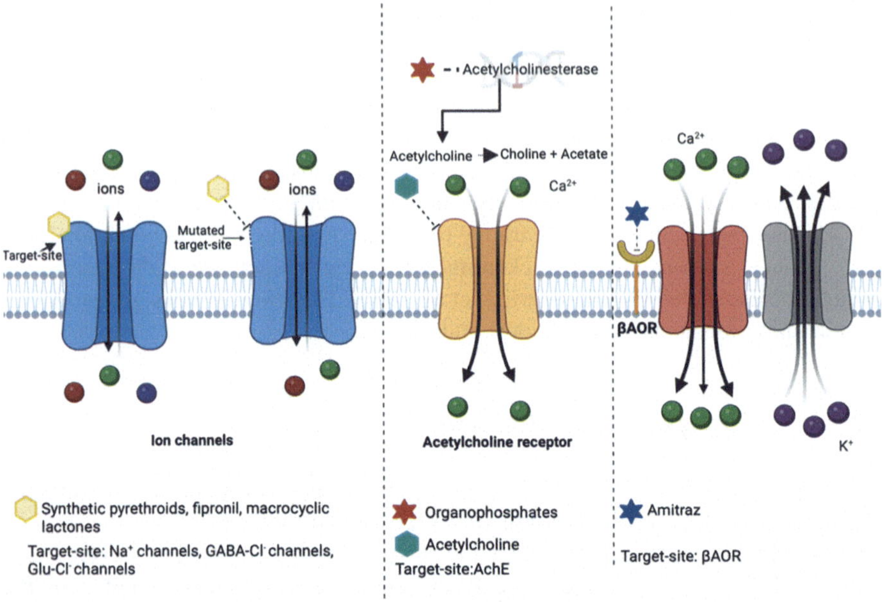


**Fig. 4.1** Toxicodynamic resistance. The main mechanisms of acaricide resistance interfere with the binding of acaricides to different channels or receptors in the cells of the tick's central nervous system. (Image created with BioRender)

## 4.2.2 Voltage-Gated Sodium Channels

Many widely used pesticides have neurotoxic effects on arthropod CNS ion channels (Narahashi 2002; Roma et al. 2014). Synthetic pyrethroids are a class of broad-spectrum acaricides that change the activation and inactivation characteristics of voltage-gated sodium channels ($Na^+$) (Soderlund 2012). The interaction of the acaricide on $Na^+$ channels prolongs the channel opening and closing time, leading to increased entry of $Na^+$ into the cell and consequently alternating the action potential (Narahashi 2001).

Arthropod $Na^+$ channels present four homologous domains (DI–DIV) and six transmembrane helices (S1–S6). Voltage-sensing domains are composed of helices S1 to S4 and a loop connecting S5 and S6. Changes in the interaction among these domains switch the channel from closed to open (Fig. 4.1). Therefore, a channel forms a pore connecting the intracellular and extracellular milieu (Auteri et al. 2018; Catterall 1995; Oliveira et al. 2013). Mutations in ion channels, called knockdown resistance (KDR), were reported for the first time in houseflies (Busvine 1951). In DII, nonsynonymous mutations have been described in different tick species (Janadaree Bandara and Parakrama Karunaratne 2017). Polymorphisms that replace a specific leucine, which is distinctive of susceptible isolates, with isoleucine were identified in pyrethroid-resistant *R. microplus* (Cruz-Valdés et al. 2023) and *Rhipicephalus appendiculatus* (Vudriko et al. 2018). In *R. sanguineus* s.l., a phenotypical association between pyrethroid resistance and an SNP with a phenylalanine replaced by a leucine in the DIIIS6 transmembrane segment was identified (Klafke et al. 2017). Additionally, a substitution of cytosine for thymine in the $Na^+$ channel, DIIISVI, has been reported in this tick species (Tucker et al. 2017). These mutations lead to a modification in the conformation of domain binding sites, inhibiting interactions with acaricides (Vudriko et al. 2018).

Another type of target-site resistance in $Na^+$ channels includes super KDR mutation (Stone et al. 2014). The emergence of *Rhipicephalus decoloratus* resistant to deltamethrin and cypermethrin has been reported (Vudriko et al. 2016). In addition, in *R. microplus*, multiresistant populations of all classes of commercially available acaricides were found (Reck et al. 2014). Therefore, super KDR mutations may occur in conjunction with other mechanisms that lead to resistance to more than one class of pesticides, and reversing the resistance process is difficult and time-consuming (Vudriko et al. 2017).

### 4.2.3 GABA-Gated Chloride Channels

The gamma-aminobutyric acid (GABA) receptor is a chloride channel ($Cl^-$). The binding of a neurotransmitter in this receptor allows this ion to enter the cell. $Cl^-$ channel antagonist drugs such as organochlorines (cyclodiene and lindane), phenylpyrazoles (fipronil), and isoxazolines inhibit the binding of GABA to their receptors, preventing the influx of $Cl^-$ and leading to CNS hyperexcitation and eventually parasite death (Bloomquist 1993, 1994, 2003; Matsumura and Ghiasuddin 1983; Zhou et al. 2022).

The *resistance to dieldrin* (*RDL*) gene was identified as a gamma-aminobutyric acid gated chloride channel (GABA-$Cl^-$) in arthropods and is associated with cyclodiene resistance in *Drosophila melanogaster* (Ffrench-Constant et al. 1991) and with fipronil and picrotoxinin resistance in *Dermacentor variabilis* (Zheng et al. 2003). In *R. microplus*, point mutations in *RDL* were reported in fipronil-resistant populations (Fig. 4.1) (Castro Janer et al. 2019). Mutations in particular alanine residues have already been described in other arthropods resistant to cyclodiene and phenylpyrazoles (Castro Janer et al. 2019). Moreover, a codon change causing the replacement of a threonine by a leucine was identified in *Rhipicephalus australis* (formerly *R. microplus*) resistant to dieldrin (Hope et al. 2010). However, similar mutations were not found in dieldrin-resistant Uruguayan and Brazilian *R. microplus* populations (Castro Janer et al. 2019).

### 4.2.4 Octopamine Receptor

Three octopamine receptors have been described: (1) α-adrenergic-like octopamine receptors (αAORs), (2) octopamine/tyramine receptors (OCT/TYRs), and (3) β-adrenergic-like octopamine receptors (βAORs). Formamidine pesticides bind to octopamine receptors, and this interaction culminates in $K^+$ efflux and decreased

$Ca^{2+}$ influx (Evans and Gee 1980). Tick resistance to formamides still emerged (Fig. 4.1), although it was not widespread due to the low selection pressure because of the lower usage of formamidines than of other pyrethroids (Gupta et al. 2022). In βAOR, an SNP in transmembrane region 1 (TM1) has been suggested to be the cause of the resistance to amitraz observed in *R. microplus* (Takata et al. 2020). Similarly, OCT/Tyr mutations from threonine to proline (T8P) and leucine to serine (L22S) in *R. microplus* are associated with amitraz (formamidine class) resistance and are present in tick populations at different locations, such as in India, Brazil, Zimbabwe, and South Africa (de La Canal et al. 2021; Jyoti Singh et al. 2021; Robbertse et al. 2016; Sungirai et al. 2018). Therefore, mutations in two octopamine receptors have been associated with acaricide resistance in ticks, suggesting that resistance to formamidines may be related to nonsynonymous mutations in more than one receptor (Waldman et al. 2023).

## 4.3 Toxicokinetic Resistance

Metabolic resistance to acaricide results from adaptation in metabolizing enzymatic systems, playing a role in the detoxification, sequestration, or excretion of foreign materials (Fig. 4.2) (De Rouck et al. 2023). Indeed, the ancestral ability to degrade dietary or environmental toxins is adapted to increase the degradation and excretion of parasiticidal molecules, leading to metabolic resistance (Dermauw et al. 2013).

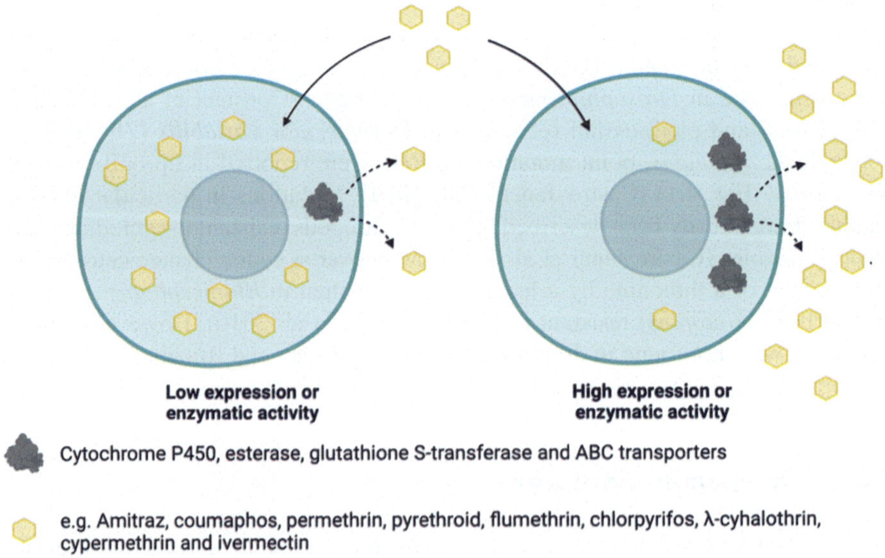


**Fig. 4.2** Toxicokinetic resistance. The main mechanisms of acaricide resistance that occur due to overexpression or increased activity of detoxification enzymes. This figure represents cytosolic enzymes, which can be located in other cellular compartments. (Image created with BioRender)

In arthropods, the detoxification process is understood as having three phases. Phase I and II comprise the toxicity reduction process mediated by cytochrome P450 (CYP450- phase I), esterases (phase I), and glutathione S-transferases (GSTs) (phase II), which leads to an increase in the hydrophilicity of toxic molecules (Agwunobi et al. 2020). In phase III, other proteins, such as ATP-binding cassette (ABC) transporters, contribute to detoxification processes by transporting biotransformed toxicants (phase I and II metabolites) out of cells (Pohl et al. 2012).

### 4.3.1 Cytochrome P450

Cytochrome P450 belongs to a superfamily of heme-containing enzymes that control the metabolism and detoxification of endogenous and exogenous cell-damaging compounds in arthropods (Fig. 4.2) (Kasai 2004). These enzymes are involved in metabolic resistance to toxins mainly through protein overexpression, which increases acaricide detoxification (Cossío-Bayúgar et al. 2018). Similar to insects, where the role of P450s in insecticide resistance is well described (Balabanidou et al. 2016; Daborn et al. 2007; Wang et al. 2020), the activities of these enzymes in tick detoxification have been documented (Cossío-Bayúgar et al. 2018; Eiden et al. 2017). In this way, when piperonyl butoxide (PBO), a P450 inhibitor, was applied to amitraz-resistant *R. microplus* or the pyrethroid *R. sanguineus* s.l., the toxicity of these acaricides increased, affecting tick survival (de La Canal et al. 2021; Eiden et al. 2017). These reports show a distinct metabolic activity of P450 in different tick populations, indicating that this enzyme plays a role in tick acaricide resistance mechanisms. Interestingly, fipronil-resistant *R. sanguineus* s.l. is not affected by PBO, indicating the existence of an alternative fipronil detoxification mechanism (Eiden et al. 2017).

Despite the metabolic resistance correlation of *P450* overexpression in drug-resistant tick populations, increased expression of these enzymes does not always occur, as in the case of some *R. microplus* populations in which *P450* expression decreases in tick populations exposed to deltamethrin (Nagar et al. 2021). This can be related to the acaricide activation and metabolization promoted by P450s, as shown in a population of *R. microplus* susceptible to acaricides, in which P450 enzymes are inhibited, resulting in a reduction in coumaphos toxicity (Li et al. 2003). Thus, a relationship between P450 expression levels in susceptible or resistant populations of ticks does not always occur, as observed for the organophosphate acaricide in *R. microplus* (Cossío-Bayúgar et al. 2008).

### 4.3.2 Esterases

Increased esterase activity is one of the most common types of metabolic resistance mechanisms found among ticks, mites, and insects (Fig. 4.2). Several studies have reported that an increase in esterase activity through gene amplification or upregulated transcription due to point mutations within esterase genes accounts for esterase-mediated pesticide resistance (Hemingway 2000; Shi et al. 2016). The mechanism of massive production of hydrolyzing enzymes by esterase and mediated acaricide resistance has been identified in several arthropods, including mosquitoes, aphids, and ticks (Rosario-Cruz 2009).

High levels of esterase activity were observed in *R. microplus* cell lines resistant to organophosphates after coumaphos exposure (Cossío-Bayúgar et al. 2002). In addition, increased carboxylesterase activity was detected in the integument of *R. microplus*, which is resistant to organophosphates (Villarino et al. 2003). In *R. sanguineus* s.l., metabolic resistance mediated by esterases was the most important resistance pathway related to permethrin-resistant tick strains. In contrast, the activity of enzymes is not modified in fipronil-resistant tick populations (Eiden et al. 2017). However, point mutations that replace glutamine with alanine in carboxylesterase were detected in the pyrethroid-resistant tick population. Other resistant strains did not present this substitution, showing that other mechanisms, such as metabolic detoxification, may also be involved in resistance to acaricides.

### 4.3.3 Glutathione S-Transferases

Glutathione S-transferases constitute an enzyme family of proteins ubiquitously found in eukaryotes that catalyze the nucleophilic conjugation of reduced glutathione (GSH) with a large variety of endogenous and exogenous electrophilic toxic complexes, including pesticides, decreasing the cell damage triggered by oxidative processes (Eaton 1999; Hayes and Pulford 1995). Groups of GSTs, which are classified as cytosolic, mitochondrial, or microsomal enzymes, have distinct structures and biochemical properties in ticks (Niranjan Reddy et al. 2011). Unlike in insects, where GSTs are well known as the main mechanism for eliminating insecticides, in ticks, the role of these enzymes in detoxification is less established. However, some studies have shown an association between tick GST overexpression and drug resistance (Fig. 4.2) (Becker et al. 2019; Gaudêncio et al. 2017). Furthermore, when GST transcription is blocked in *R. sanguineus* s.l. treated with permethrin, the susceptibility to this acaricide increases (Duscher et al. 2014). Similarly, increased susceptibility to flumethrin and chlorpyrifos was observed in *Haemaphysalis longicornis* larvae and adult males (Hernandez et al. 2018). In other works, high amounts of GST protein or transcripts were detected from different tick tissues when *H. longicornis* or *Hyalomma rufipes* were treated with chlorpyrifos (Xue et al. 2023) or cyhalothrin (Zhao et al. 2024), respectively, suggesting that GSTs play a role in the detoxification of these acaricides. Interestingly, different acaricide treatments can suppress (Vaz Junior et al. 2004a, b) or increase (Vaz Junior et al. 2004a, b; Enayati et al. 2010; Hernandez et al. 2018) the activity of tick GSTs. For example, GST activity in *R. microplus* increased in the presence of coumaphos (Vaz Junior et al. 2004a, b), which was correlated with *R. microplus* resistance to this acaricide (Gupta et al. 2023). Moreover, field populations of *Rhipicephalus bursa* susceptible to λ-cyhalothrin and cypermethrin showed enhanced GST activity (Enayati et al. 2010).

### 4.3.4 ABC Transporters

ATP-binding cassette transporters are membrane-integrated proteins present in several organisms (Lage 2003). These transporters regulate the excretion of endogenous and exogenous substances via an ATP-dependent pathway (Buss and Callaghan 2008; Higgins 2001). Several reports have correlated ABC transporters with transport and resistance to pesticides (Fig. 4.2) (Dermauw and Van Leeuwen 2014). The tick digestive process occurs intracellularly, in which the transport of heme from digestive cells to hemosomes is carried out by ABC transporters and is a crucial factor in heme detoxification. Amitraz detoxification is related to heme transport, suggesting that pesticide resistance can be associated with the detoxification mechanisms of endogenous compounds (Le Gall et al. 2018).

The contribution of ABC transporters to metabolic resistance to acaricides is reinforced in *R. microplus* because the transcription of these protein-encoding genes is increased in cells exposed to ivermectin. Additionally, tolerance to this acaricide is reduced in cells cotreated with an inhibitor of these transporters (Pohl et al. 2014). In contrast, transcriptional modulation of ABC transporter-encoded genes was not detected in *the Ixodes ricinus* cell line treated with ivermectin (Mangia et al. 2018), confirming that acaricide resistance involves several distinct mechanisms.

Detoxification mediated by ABC transporters and the use of compounds that act synergistically with pesticides were verified via in vivo tick assays. In *R. sanguineus* s.l., a lower concentration of ivermectin in combination with cyclosporine A (an inhibitor of ABC transporters) was required to reach the LC50 in ticks exposed (Cafarchia et al. 2015). Cyclosporine A had a similar dose-dependent effect on ivermectin-resistant *R. microplus* larvae (Pohl et al. 2011). Therefore, compounds that modulate the activity of these transporters can influence tick tolerance to acaricides.

## 4.4 Discussion

Despite advances in recent years in understanding the molecular mechanisms involved in tick resistance to synthetic acaricides, this field of research remains largely unknown. The limited knowledge of the molecular mechanisms enabling ticks to develop resistance to acaricides poses a significant challenge in devising strategies to overcome acaricide resistance (Kumar 2019; Waldman et al. 2023). Given that resistance to almost all acaricides already occurs in ticks globally, it is likely that similar resistance mechanisms evolve when new acaricides are introduced in the field (Obaid et al. 2022). Considering this, the judicious use of these compounds, coupled with other control strategies, can delay the proliferation of acaricide resistance in tick populations, allowing more time for the development of effective acaricidal solutions. Additionally, ticks residing in proximity to areas where acaricides are commonly used are quickly being selected for resistance to these chemicals (Higa et al. 2020). This crucial aspect needs to be considered in prevention campaigns to curb the spread of ticks and their associated pathogens into new areas, as recently predicted due to anthropogenic activities in the environment, including global warming, deforestation, and desertification (Bouchard et al. 2019; Gilbert 2021).

Most of the tick acaricide resistance knowledge pertains to economically or medically significant species such as *R. microplus* and *R. sanguineus* s.l. The large genomes of ticks introduce a layer of complexity regarding the understanding of potential molecular mechanisms through which they have evolved to endure exposure to acaricides (Heylen et al. 2024). This complexity is evident in certain homologous genes, such as *P450* or *GSTs*, which exhibit a variety of functions in arthropod physiology (Koirala et al. 2022; Nauen et al. 2022). Multiple physiological pathways can affect ectoparasiticide resistance. For instance, in *R. microplus*, it was confirmed that esterases and ABC transporters, as well as GSTs and CYP450, are associated with ivermectin resistance (Le Gall et al. 2018). The mechanisms of acaricide resistance discussed here, such as target-site insensitivity and metabolic detoxification (Table 4.1), represent only a subset of yet-documented factors. Other mechanisms, as observed in insects, may also play a role, including behavioral and morphological resistance mechanisms.

**Table 4.1** Toxicodynamic or toxicokinetic changes leading to acaricide resistance in different ticks

| Proteins | Name | Tick specie/acaricide | Modifications related to acaricide resistance | Reference |
|---|---|---|---|---|
| **Toxicodynamic resistance** | | | | |
| Acetylcholinesterase | BmAchE1 | *Rhipicephalus microplus*/coumaphos | Asp → Gly, Glu → Gly, Val → Ala, Phe → Ser, Asn → Asp, Pro → Ala | Bendele et al. (2015), Temeyer (2018), Temeyer et al. (2010) |
| Voltage-gated sodium channel | N.I. | *R. microplus*/pyrethroid | Leu → Ile in DII | Cruz-Valdés et al. (2023) |
| | N.I. | *Rhipicephalus appendiculatus*/ pyrethroid<br>*Rhipicephalus sanguineus* sensu lato/ pyrethroid<br>*R. sanguineus s.l.*/permethrin | Leu → Ile in DII, Phe → Leu in DIIIS6<br>Phe → Leu in DIIISVI | Vudriko et al. (2018), Klafke et al. (2017), Tucker et al. (2017) |
| GABA-gated chloride channels | N.I. | *R. microplus*/fipronil<br>*Rhipicephalus australis*/dieldrin | Ala→Ser/Leu in RDL<br>Thr → Leu | Castro Janer et al. (2019), Hope et al. (2010) |
| Octopamine receptor | OCT/Tyr | *R. microplus*/amitraz | Thr → Pro, Leu → Ser | de La Canal et al. (2021), Jyoti Singh et al. (2021), Robbertse et al. (2016), Sungirai et al. (2018) |
| **Toxicokinetic resistance** | | | | |
| Cytochrome P450 | N.I. | *R. microplus*/amitraz; *R. sanguineus s.l.*/pyrethroid | High P450 expression levels | de La Canal et al. (2021); Eiden et al. (2017) |
| | N.I. | *R. microplus*/deltamethrin | Low P450 expression levels | Nagar et al. (2021) |
| | N.I. | *R. microplus*/coumaphos | Low P450 expression levels | Li et al. (2003) |
| Esterases | N.I. | *R. microplus*/organophosphates | *R. microplus*/organophosphates | Cossio-Bayugar et al. (2002) |

(continued)

**Table 4.1** (continued)

| Proteins | Name | Tick specie/acaricide | Modifications related to acaricide resistance | Reference |
|---|---|---|---|---|
| | N.I. | *R. microplus*/organophosphates | Increased activity of carboxylesterase | Villarino et al. (2003) |
| | | *R. sanguineus* s.l./pyrethroid | Replacement of glutamine by alanine (carboxylesterase) | Eiden et al. (2017) |
| Glutathione S-transferases | N.I. | *R. sanguineus* s.l./permethrin | High GST expression levels | Duscher et al. (2014) |
| | N.I. | *Haemaphysalis longicornis*/flumethrin and chlorpyrifos | High GST expression levels | Hernandez et al. (2018), Xue et al. (2023) |
| | N.I. | *Hyalomma rufipes*/cyhalothrin | High GST expression levels | Zhao et al. (2024) |
| | N.I. | *R. microplus*/coumaphos | High GST activity | Vaz Junior et al. (2004a, b), Gupta et al. (2023) |
| | N.I. | *Rhipicephalus bursa*/cyhalothrin and cypermethrin | High GST activity | Enayati et al. (2010) |
| ABC transporters | N.I. | *R. microplus*/ivermectin | Increase in transcription of ABC transporters | Pohl et al. (2014) |

*N.I.* not identified

## References

Abbas RZ, Zaman MA, Colwell DD, Gilleard J, Iqbal Z (2014) Acaricide resistance in cattle ticks and approaches to its management: the state of play. Vet Parasitol 203(1–2):6–20

Agwunobi DO, Pei T, Yang J, Wang X, Lv L, Shen R, Yu Z, Liu J (2020) Expression profiles of glutathione S-transferases genes in semi-engorged *Haemaphysalis longicornis* (Acari: Ixodidae) exposed to cymbopogon citratus essential oil. Syst Appl Acarol 25(5):918–930

Auteri M, La Russa F, Blanda V, Torina A (2018) Insecticide resistance associated with *kdr* mutations in *Aedes albopictus*: an update on worldwide evidences. Biomed Res Int 2018:1–10

Balabanidou V, Kampouraki A, MacLean M, Blomquist GJ, Tittiger C, Juárez MP, Mijailovsky SJ, Chalepakis G, Anthousi A, Lynd A, Antoine S, Hemingway J, Ranson H, Lycett GJ, Vontas J (2016) Cytochrome P450 associated with insecticide resistance catalyzes cuticular hydrocarbon production in *Anopheles gambiae*. Proc Natl Acad Sci 113(33):9268–9273

Baxter GD, Barker SC (1998) Acetylcholinesterase cDNA of the cattle tick, *Boophilus microplus*: characterisation and role in organophosphate resistance. Insect Biochem Mol Biol 28(8):581–589

Becker S, Webster A, Doyle RL, Martins JR, Reck J, Klafke GM (2019) Resistance to deltamethrin, fipronil and ivermectin in the brown dog tick, *Rhipicephalus sanguineus* sensu stricto, Latreille (Acari: Ixodidae). Ticks Tick-Borne Diseases 10(5):1046–1050

Bendele KG, Guerrero FD, Miller RJ, Li AY, Barrero RA, Moolhuijzen PM, Black M, McCooke JK, Meyer J, Hill CA, Bellgard MI (2015) Acetylcholinesterase 1 in populations of organophosphate-resistant North American strains of the cattle tick, *Rhipicephalus microplus* (Acari: Ixodidae). Parasitol Res 114(8):3027–3040

Bloomquist JR (1993) Toxicology, mode of action and target site-mediated resistance to insecticides acting on chloride channels. Comp Biochem Physiol C: Pharmacol Toxicol Endocrinol 106(2):301–314

Bloomquist JR (1994) Cyclodiene resistance at the insect GABA receptor/chloride channel complex confers broad cross resistance to convulsants and experimental phenylpyrazole insecticides. Arch Insect Biochem Physiol 26(1):69–79

Bloomquist JR (2003) Chloride channels as tools for developing selective insecticides. Arch Insect Biochem Physiol 54(4):145–156

Bouchard C, Dibernardo A, Koffi J, Wood H, Leighton P, Lindsay L (2019) Increased risk of tick-borne diseases with climate and environmental changes. Can Commun Dis Rep 45(4):83–89

Buss DS, Callaghan A (2008) Interaction of pesticides with p-glycoprotein and other ABC proteins: a survey of the possible importance to insecticide, herbicide and fungicide resistance. Pestic Biochem Physiol 90(3):141–153

Busvine JR (1951) Mechanism of resistance to insecticide in houseflies. Nature 168(4266):193–195

Cafarchia C, Porretta D, Mastrantonio V, Epis S, Sassera D, Iatta R, Immediato D, Ramos RAN, Lia RP, Dantas-Torres F, Kramer L, Urbanelli S, Otranto D (2015) Potential role of ATP-binding cassette transporters against acaricides in the brown dog tick *Rhipicephalus sanguineus* sensu lato: ABC transporters in *R. sanguineus*. Med Vet Entomol 29(1):88–93

Casida JE, Durkin KA (2013) Neuroactive insecticides: targets, selectivity, resistance, and secondary effects. Annu Rev Entomol 58(1):99–117

Castro Janer E, Klafke GM, Fontes F, Capurro ML, Schumaker TSS (2019) Mutations in *Rhipicephalus microplus* GABA gated chloride channel gene associated with fipronil resistance. Ticks Tick-Borne Diseases 10(4):761–765

Catterall WA (1995) Structure and function of voltage-gated ion channels. Annu Rev Biochem 64(1):493–531

Colovic MB, Krstic DZ, Lazarevic-Pasti TD, Bondzic AM, Vasic VM (2013) Acetylcholinesterase inhibitors: pharmacology and toxicology. Curr Neuropharmacol 11(3):315–335

Cossío-Bayúgar R, Wagner GG, Holman PJ (2002) In vitro generation of organophosphate resistant *Boophilus microplus* (Acari: Ixodidae) cell lines. J Med Entomol 39(2):278–284

Cossío-Bayúgar R, Miranda-Miranda E, Ortiz-Najera AO-N, Neri-Orantes S, Olvera-Valencia F (2008) Cytochrome P-450 monooxygenase gene expression supports a multifactorial origin for acaricide resistance in *Ripicephalus microplus*. Res J Parasitol 3(2):59–66

Cossío-Bayúgar R, Martínez-Ibañez F, Aguilar-Díaz H, Miranda-Miranda E (2018) Pyrethroid acaricide resistance is proportional to P-450 cytochrome oxidase expression in the cattle tick *Rhipicephalus microplus*. Biomed Res Int 2018:1–6

Cruz-Valdés T, Grostieta E, Chagoya-Fuentes JL, Bravo-Ramos JL, Ojeda-Chi M, Lammoglia-Villagómez MA, Rojas-Ronquillo R, Cabrera-Núñez A, Aguilar-Tipacamú G, Colunga-Salas P, Becker I, Montes SS (2023) Identification of the G184C, C190A and T2134—A mutations in the Para-sodium channel gene of the southern cattle tick *Rhipicephalus* (*Boophilus*) *microplus* associated with resistance to cypermethrin in northern Veracruz, Mexico. Vet Parasitol 39:100838

Daborn PJ, Lumb C, Boey A, Wong W, ffrench-Constant, R. H., & Batterham, P. (2007) Evaluating the insecticide resistance potential of eight *Drosophila melanogaster* cytochrome P450 genes by transgenic over-expression. Insect Biochem Mol Biol 37(5):512–519

de La Canal LH, Dall'Agnol B, Webster A, Reck J, Martins JR, Klafke GM (2021) Mechanisms of amitraz resistance in a *Rhipicephalus microplus* strain from southern Brazil. Ticks Tick-Borne Diseases 12(5):101764

De Rouck S, İnak E, Dermauw W, Van Leeuwen T (2023) A review of the molecular mechanisms of acaricide resistance in mites and ticks. Insect Biochem Mol Biol 159:103981

Dermauw W, Van Leeuwen T (2014) The ABC gene family in arthropods: comparative genomics and role in insecticide transport and resistance. Insect Biochem Mol Biol 45:89–110

Dermauw W, Wybouw N, Rombauts S, Menten B, Vontas J, Grbić M, Clark RM, Feyereisen R, Van Leeuwen T (2013) A link between host plant adaptation and pesticide resistance in the polyphagous spider mite *Tetranychus urticae*. Proc Natl Acad Sci 110(2):E113

Duscher GG, Galindo RC, Tichy A, Hummel K, Kocan KM, de la Fuente J (2014) Glutathione S-transferase affects permethrin detoxification in the brown dog tick, *Rhipicephalus sanguineus*. Ticks Tick-Borne Diseases 5(3):225–233

Eaton D (1999) Concise review of the glutathione S-transferases and their significance to toxicology. Toxicol Sci 49(2):156–164

Eiden AL, Kaufman PE, Oi FM, Dark MJ, Bloomquist JR, Miller RJ (2017) Determination of metabolic resistance mechanisms in pyrethroid-resistant and fipronil-tolerant brown dog ticks. Med Vet Entomol 31(3):243–251

Enayati AA, Asgarian F, Amouei A, Sharif M, Mortazavi H, Boujhmehrani H, Hemingway J (2010) Pyrethroid insecticide resistance in *Rhipicephalus bursa* (Acari, Ixodidae). Pestic Biochem Physiol 97(3):243–248

Evans PD, Gee JD (1980) Action of formamidine pesticides on octopamine receptors. Nature 287(5777):60–62

FAO and WHO Pesticide residues in food 2019—Joint FAO/WHO Meeting on Pesticide Residues. Evaluation Part I: Residues (2020)

Ffrench-Constant RH, Mortlock DP, Shaffer CD, MacIntyre RJ, Roush RT (1991) Molecular cloning and transformation of cyclodiene resistance in *drosophila*: an invertebrate gamma-aminobutyric acid subtype A receptor locus. Proc Natl Acad Sci 88(16):7209–7213

Fotoukkiaii SM (2020) Genetic basis of acaricide resistance: identification and characterization of the risk and mechanisms of resistance to bifenazate, acequinocyl, and the novel acaricide pyflubumide. Tetranychus urticae. Universiteit van Amsterdam, New York

Gaudêncio FN, Klafke GM, Tunholi-Alves VM, Ferreira TP, Coelho CN, da Fonseca AH, da Costa Angelo I, Pinheiro J (2017) Activity of carboxylesterases, glutathione-S-transferase and monooxygenase on *Rhipicephalus microplus* exposed to fluazuron. Parasitol Int 66(5):584–587

Gilbert L (2021) The impacts of climate change on ticks and tick-borne disease risk. Annu Rev Entomol 66(1):373–388

Guerrero FD, Lovis L, Martins JR (2012) Acaricide resistance mechanisms in *Rhipicephalus* (*Boophilus*) *microplus*. Rev Bras Parasitol Vet 21(1):1–6

Gupta S, Gupta S, Kumar S (2022) Deltamethrin and coumaphos resistance and role of biochemical mechanisms in camel tick, *Hyalomma dromedarii* collected from Haryana state of India. Int J Trop Insect Sci 42(1):269–274

Gupta S, Sangwan N, Sangwan AK, Mann S, Gupta S, Kumar A, Kumar S (2023) Understanding the resistance mechanisms of *Rhipicephalus microplus* ticks to synthetic pyrethroids and organophosphates in south-west regions of Haryana, North India. Pesticide Biochem Physiol 196:105634

Hayes JD, Pulford DJ (1995) The glutathione s-transferase supergene family: regulation of GST and the contribution of the isoenzymes to cancer chemoprotection and drug resistance part I. Crit Rev Biochem Mol Biol 30(6):445–520

Hemingway J (2000) The molecular basis of two contrasting metabolic mechanisms of insecticide resistance. Insect Biochem Mol Biol 30(11):1009–1015

Hernandez R, He H, Chen AC, Ivie GW, George JE, Wagner GG (1999) Cloning and sequencing of a putative acetylcholinesterase cDNA from *Boophilus microplus* (Acari: Ixodidae). J Med Entomol 36(6):764–770

Hernandez EP, Kusakisako K, Talactac MR, Galay RL, Hatta T, Fujisaki K, Tsuji N, Tanaka T (2018) Glutathione S-transferases play a role in the detoxification of flumethrin and chlorpyrifos in *Haemaphysalis longicornis*. Parasit Vectors 11(1):460

Heylen DJA, Labuschagne M, Meiring C, Van Der Mescht L, Klafke G, Costa Junior LM, Strydom T, Wentzel J, Shacklock C, Halos L, Maree F, Fourie J, Madder M, Evans A (2024) Phenotypic and genotypic characterization of acaricide resistance in *Rhipicephalus microplus* field isolates from South Africa and Brazil. Int J Parasitol Drugs Drug Resist 24:100519

Higa LDOS, Barradas Piña FT, Rodrigues VDS, Garcia MV, Salas DR, Miller RJ, De Leon AP, Barros JC, Andreotti R (2020) Evidence of acaricide resistance in different life stages of *Amblyomma mixtum* and *Rhipicephalus microplus* (Acari: Ixodidae) collected from the same farm in the state of Veracruz, Mexico. Prevent Vet Med 174:104837

Higgins CF (2001) ABC transporters: physiology, structure and mechanism—an overview. Res Microbiol 152(3–4):205–210

Hope M, Menzies M, Kemp D (2010) Identification of a dieldrin resistance-associated mutation in *Rhipicephalus (Boophilus) microplus* (Acari: Ixodidae). J Econ Entomol 103(4):1355–1359

Janadaree Bandara KMU, Parakrama Karunaratne SHP (2017) Mechanisms of acaricide resistance in the cattle tick *Rhipicephalus (Boophilus) microplus* in Sri Lanka. Pestic Biochem Physiol 139:68–72

Jyoti Singh NK, Singh H, Singh NK, Rath SS (2016) Multiple mutations in the acetylcholinesterase 3 gene associated with organophosphate resistance in *Rhipicephalus (Boophilus) microplus* ticks from Punjab, India. Vet Parasitol 216:108–117

Jyoti Singh NK, Singh H, Singh NK, Rath SS (2021) Genotyping amitraz resistance profiles in *Rhipicephalus microplus* Canestrini (Acari: Ixodidae) ticks from Punjab, India. Ticks and Tick-Borne Diseases 12(1):101578

Kasai S (2004) Role of cytochrome P450 in mechanism of pyrethroid resistance. J Pestic Sci 29(3):220–221

Klafke GM, Miller RJ, Tidwell J, Barreto R, Guerrero FD, Kaufman PE, Pérez de León AA (2017) Mutation in the sodium channel gene corresponds with phenotypic resistance of *Rhipicephalus sanguineus* sensu lato (Acari: Ixodidae) to pyrethroids. J Med Entomol 54(6):1639–1642

Koirala BKS, Moural T, Zhu F (2022) Functional and structural diversity of insect glutathione s-transferases in xenobiotic adaptation. Int J Biol Sci 18(15):5713–5723

Kumar R (2019) Molecular markers and their application in the monitoring of acaricide resistance in *Rhipicephalus microplus*. Exp Appl Acarol 78(2):149–172

Lage H (2003) ABC-transporters: implications on drug resistance from microorganisms to human cancers. Int J Antimicrob Agents 22(3):188–199

Le Gall VL, Klafke GM, Torres TT (2018) Detoxification mechanisms involved in ivermectin resistance in the cattle tick, *Rhipicephalus (Boophilus) microplus*. Sci Rep 8(1):12401

Lee RM, Batham P (1966) The activity and organophosphate inhibition of cholinesterases from susceptible and resistant ticks (Acari). Entomol Exp Appl 9(1):13–24

Lees K, Woods DJ, Bowman AS (2009) Transcriptome analysis of the synganglion from the brown dog tick, *Rhipicephalus sanguineus*: tick synganglion transcriptome. Insect Mol Biol 19(3):273–282

Li AY, Davey RB, Miller RJ, George JE (2003) Resistance to coumaphos and diazinon in *Boophilus microplus* (Acari: Ixodidae) and evidence for the involvement of an oxidative detoxification mechanism. J Med Entomol 40(4):482–490

Mangia C, Vismarra A, Genchi M, Epis S, Bandi C, Grandi G, Bell-Sakyi L, Otranto D, Passeri B, Kramer L (2018) Exposure to amitraz, fipronil and permethrin affects cell viability and ABC transporter gene expression in an *Ixodes ricinus* cell line. Parasit Vectors 11(1):437

Matsumura F, Ghiasuddin SM (1983) Evidence for similarities between cyclodiene type insecticides and picrotoxinin in their action mechanisms. J Environ Sci Health 18(1):1–14

Nagar G, Upadhaya D, Sharma AK, Kumar R, Fular A, Ghosh S (2021) Association between overexpression of cytochrome P450 genes and deltamethrin resistance in *Rhipicephalus microplus*. Ticks Tick-Borne Diseases 12(2):101610

Narahashi T (2001) Handbook of pesticide toxicology. In: Neurotoxocology of pesticides, vol 1. Academic Press, Cambridge, pp 789–860

Narahashi T (2002) Nerve membrane ion channels as the target site of insecticides. Mini-Rev Med Chem 2(4):419–432

Nauen R, Bass C, Feyereisen R, Vontas J (2022) The role of cytochrome P450s in insect toxicology and resistance. Annu Rev Entomol 67(1):105–124

Niranjan Reddy BP, Prasad GBKS, Raghavendra K (2011) In silico analysis of glutathione S-transferase supergene family revealed hitherto unreported insect specific δ-and ϵ-GSTs and mammalian specific μ-GSTs in *Ixodes scapularis* (Acari: Ixodidae). Comput Biol Chem 35(2):114–120

Obaid MK, Islam N, Alouffi A, Khan AZ, da Silva Vaz I, Tanaka T, Ali A (2022) Acaricides resistance in ticks: selection, diagnosis, mechanisms, and mitigation. Front Cell Infect Microbiol 12:941831

Oliveira EE, Du Y, Nomura Y, Dong K (2013) A residue in the transmembrane segment 6 of domain I in insect and mammalian sodium channels regulate differential sensitivities to pyrethroid insecticides. Neurotoxicology 38:42–50

Pohl PC, Klafke GM, Carvalho DD, Martins JR, Daffre S, da Silva Vaz I, Masuda A (2011) ABC transporter efflux pumps: A defense mechanism against ivermectin in *Rhipicephalus* (*Boophilus*) *microplus*. Int J Parasitol 41(13–14):1323–1333

Pohl PC, Klafke GM, Júnior JR, Martins JR, da Silva Vaz I, Masuda A (2012) ABC transporters as a multidrug detoxification mechanism in *Rhipicephalus* (*Boophilus*) *microplus*. Parasitol Res 111(6):2345–2351

Pohl PC, Carvalho DD, Daffre S, da Silva Vaz I Jr, Masuda A (2014) In vitro establishment of ivermectin-resistant *Rhipicephalus microplus* cell line and the contribution of ABC transporters on the resistance mechanism. Vet Parasitol 204(3–4):316–322

Reck J, Klafke GM, Webster A, Dall'Agnol B, Scheffer R, Souza UA, Corassini VB, Vargas R, dos Santos JS, de Souza Martins JR (2014) First report of fluazuron resistance in *Rhipicephalus microplus*: a field tick population resistant to six classes of acaricides. Vet Parasitol 201(1–2):128–136

Robbertse L, Baron S, van der Merwe NA, Madder M, Stoltsz WH, Maritz-Olivier C (2016) Genetic diversity, acaricide resistance status and evolutionary potential of a *Rhipicephalus microplus* population from a disease-controlled cattle farming area in South Africa. Ticks Tick-Borne Diseases 7(4):595–603

Rodriguez-Vivas RI, Trees AJ, Rosado-Aguilar JA, Villegas-Perez SL, Hodgkinson JE (2011) Evolution of acaricide resistance: phenotypic and genotypic changes in field populations of *Rhipicephalus* (*Boophilus*) *microplus* in response to pyrethroid selection pressure. Int J Parasitol 41(8):895–903

Roma GC, Camargo Mathias MI, Nunes PH, Bechara GH (2014) Ultrastructure of the synganglion in the larvae and nymphs of tick *Rhipicephalus sanguineus* (Latreille, 1806) (Acari: Ixodidae). Int J Acarol 40(3):207–213

Rosario-Cruz R (2009) Genetic basis and impact of tick acaricide resistance. Front Biosci 14(7):2657–2665

Schnitzerling HJ, Nolan J, Hughes S (1983) Toxicology and metabolism of some synthetic pyrethroids in larvae of susceptible and resistant strains of the cattle tick *Boophilus microplus* (can.). Pestic Sci 14(1):64–72

Shi L, Wei P, Wang X, Shen G, Zhang J, Xiao W, Xu Z, Xu Q, He L (2016) Functional analysis of esterase TCE2 gene from *Tetranychus cinnabarinus* (Boisduval) involved in acaricide resistance. Sci Rep 6(1):18646

Soderlund DM (2012) Molecular mechanisms of pyrethroid insecticide neurotoxicity: recent advances. Arch Toxicol 86(2):165–181

Sparks TC, Nauen R (2015) IRAC: mode of action classification and insecticide resistance management. Pestic Biochem Physiol 121:122–128

Stone NE, Olafson PU, Davey RB, Buckmeier G, Bodine D, Sidak-Loftis LC, Giles JR, Duhaime R, Miller RJ, Mosqueda J, Scoles GA, Wagner DM, Busch JD (2014) Multiple mutations in the Para-sodium channel gene are associated with pyrethroid resistance in *Rhipicephalus microplus* from the United States and Mexico. Parasit Vectors 7(1):456

Sungirai M, Baron S, Moyo DZ, De Clercq P, Maritz-Olivier C, Madder M (2018) Genotyping acaricide resistance profiles of *Rhipicephalus microplus* tick populations from communal land areas of Zimbabwe. Ticks Tick-Borne Diseases 9(1):2–9

Takata M, Misato S, Ozoe F, Ozoe Y (2020) A point mutation in the β-adrenergic-like octopamine receptor: possible association with amitraz resistance. Pest Manag Sci 76(11):3720–3728

Temeyer KB (2018) Molecular biology of tick acetylcholinesterases. Front Biosci 23(4):1320–1337

Temeyer KB, Davey RB, Chen AC (2004) Identification of a third *Boophilus microplus* (Acari: Ixodidae) cDNA presumptively encoding an acetylcholinesterase. J Med Entomol 41(3):259–268

Temeyer KB, Pruett JH, Olafson PU (2010) Baculovirus expression, biochemical characterization and organophosphate sensitivity of rBmAChE1, rBmAChE2, and rBmAChE3 of *Rhipicephalus* (*Boophilus*) *microplus*. Vet Parasitol 172(1–2):114–121

Tucker NSG, Kaufman PE, Weeks ENI, Rowland J, Tidwell J, Miller RJ (2017) Characterization of a sodium channel mutation in permethrin-resistant *Rhipicephalus sanguineus* (Acari: Ixodidae). J Med Entomol 54(6):1633–1638

Van Lenteren JC, Bolckmans K, Köhl J, Ravensberg WJ, Urbaneja A (2018) Biological control using invertebrates and microorganisms: plenty of new opportunities. BioControl 63(1):39–59

Vaz Junior IS, Torino Lermen T, Michelon A, Sanchez Ferreira CA, Joaquim de Freitas DR, Termignoni C, Masuda A (2004a) Effect of acaricides on the activity of a *Boophilus microplus* glutathione S-transferase. Vet Parasitol 119(2–3):237–245

Vaz Junior IS, Imamura S, Ohashi K, Onuma M (2004b) Cloning, expression and partial characterization of a *Haemaphysalis longicornis* and a *Rhipicephalus appendiculatus* glutathione S-transferase. Insect Mol Biol 13(3):329–335

Villarino MA, Waghela SD, Wagner GG (2003) Biochemical detection of esterases in the adult female integument of organophosphate-resistant *Boophilus microplus* (Acari: Ixodidae). J Med Entomol 40(1):52–57

Vudriko P, Okwee-Acai J, Tayebwa DS, Byaruhanga J, Kakooza S, Wampande E, Omara R, Muhindo JB, Tweyongyere R, Owiny DO, Hatta T, Tsuji N, Umemiya-Shirafuji R, Xuan X, Kanameda M, Fujisaki K, Suzuki H (2016) Emergence of multi-acaricide resistant *Rhipicephalus* ticks and its implication on chemical tick control in Uganda. Parasit Vectors 9(1):4

Vudriko P, Umemiya-Shirafuji R, Okwee-Acai J, Tayebwa DS, Byaruhanga J, Jirapattharasate C, Liu M, Adjou Moumouni PF, Fujisaki K, Xuan X, Suzuki H (2017) Genetic mutations in sodium channel domain II and carboxylesterase genes associated with phenotypic resistance against synthetic pyrethroids by *Rhipicephalus* (*Boophilus*) *decoloratus* ticks in Uganda. Pestic Biochem Physiol 143:181–190

Vudriko P, Umemiya-Shirafuji R, Okwee-Acai J, Tayebwa DS, Byaruhanga J, Bbira JS, Fujisaki K, Xuan X, Suzuki H (2018) C190A knockdown mutation in sodium channel domain II of pyrethroid-resistant *Rhipicephalus appendiculatus*. Ticks Tick-Borne Diseases 9(6):1590–1593

Waldman J, Klafke GM, Tirloni L, Logullo C, Da Silva Vaz I (2023) Putative target sites in synganglion for novel ixodid tick control strategies. Ticks Tick-Borne Diseases 14(3):102123

Wang K, Liu M, Wang Y, Song W, Tang P (2020) Identification and functional analysis of cytochrome P450 CYP346 family genes associated with phosphine resistance in *Tribolium castaneum*. Pestic Biochem Physiol 168:104622

Xue X, Wang N, Ma J, Ji A, Wang H, Li M, Di X, Liu J, Wang H (2023) Effect of chlorpyrifos on the expression and regulation of salivary gland protein of *Haemaphysalis longicornis*. Int J Acarol 49(2):154–164

Zhao M, Gao Z, Ji X, Wang K, Zhang S, Shi Y, Song X, Yu Z, Yang X (2024) The diverse functions of mu-class glutathione S-transferase HrGSTm1 during the development of *Hyalomma rufipes* with a focus on the detoxification metabolism of cyhalothrin. Parasit Vectors 17(1):1

Zheng Y, Priest B, Cully DF, Ludmerer SW (2003) RdlDv, a novel GABA-gated chloride channel gene from the American dog tick *Dermacentor variabilis*. Insect Biochem Mol Biol 33(6):595–599

Zhou X, Hohman AE, Hsu WH (2022) Current review of isoxazoline ectoparasiticides used in veterinary medicine. J Vet Pharmacol Ther 45(1):1–15

# Monitoring Acaricide Resistance

# 5

Anil Kumar Sharma, Sachin Kumar, Gajanan M. Chigure,
Nitin D. Jadhav, and M. Sankar

**Abstract**

More than 80% livestock are facing severe problems of ticks and tick-borne diseases (TTBDs), which create remarkable capital loss to animal owners in terms of direct blood feeding and indirectly by transmitting pathogens. Due to the overburden of synthetic chemicals in the management of TTBDs, tick populations have developed acaricide resistance against commonly used chemicals. Laboratory-based monitoring tools have been developed and adopted in different countries for the diagnosis of acaricidal resistance and its monitoring. The Food and Agriculture Organization of the United Nations recommends in vitro tests such as larval packet test (LPT), larval immersion test (LIT), and adult immersion test (AIT). Similarly, resistance diagnosis is developed using a multiplex polymerase chain reaction (PCR), which facilitates the detection of variation in nucleotide substitutions responsible for conferring resistance to synthetic pyrethroids in tick population. PCR diagnostic assays are used to identify the resis-

A. K. Sharma (✉)
School of Agriculture, Uttaranchal University, Dehradun, Uttarakhand, India

S. Kumar
Entomology Laboratory, Division of Parasitology, ICAR-Indian Veterinary Research Institute, Izatnagar, Bareilly, Uttar Pradesh, India

G. M. Chigure
Department of Veterinary Parasitology, College of Veterinary and Animal Sciences (MAFSU, Nagpur), Parbhani, Maharashtra, India

N. D. Jadhav
Department of Veterinary Pharmacology and Toxicology, College of Veterinary and Animal Sciences (MAFSU, Nagpur), Parbhani, Maharashtra, India

M. Sankar
Entomology Laboratory, Division of Parasitology, ICAR-Indian Veterinary Research Institute, Izatnagar, Bareilly, Uttar Pradesh, India



S. Kumar et al. (eds.), *Acaricides Resistance in Ticks*,
https://doi.org/10.1007/978-981-97-7411-1_5

tance-associated mutation in different regions of the targeted gene. To understand the involvement of metabolic enzymes in the development of resistance, biochemical tests using tick larvae are also developed and are commonly used methods. Thus, in this chapter, various in vitro tools for monitoring acaricide resistance in tick populations are discussed.

**Keywords**
Acaricides · Bioassay · Monitoring · Resistance · Ticks

## 5.1 Introduction

Among the major infections of livestock, ticks and diseases transmitted by them rank fourth (Ghosh et al. 2007), and approximately 80% of cattle population in the world is affected either by tick attacks or tick-borne diseases. In addition to causing direct blood loss through hematophagous activity, ticks also serve as vectors for conveying the pathogens responsible for severe diseases such as babesiosis, Crimean-Congo hemorrhagic fever (CCHF), anaplasmosis, theileriosis, and Kyasanur Forest disease (KFD). Ticks in the dairy industry result in economic losses due to their negative impact on the weight increase and milk production of afflicted animals. The presence of tick bite marks significantly contributes to the degradation of hide quality in the leather industry. Ticks also show their presence in cracks and crevices of animal sheds, becoming a major cause of persistent infestation in livestock (Figs. 5.1 and 5.2).

Ticks and tick-borne diseases pose a persistent global concern for livestock owners. The primary approach to managing them is through the use of various classes of chemical acaricides. However, prolonged use of incorrect dilution of acaricides, improper application methods, continuous and frequent use, and wrong dosing have led to the emergence of resistance against routinely employed chemical acaricides. In addition, the overuse of chemical acaricides has inherent disadvantages, such as

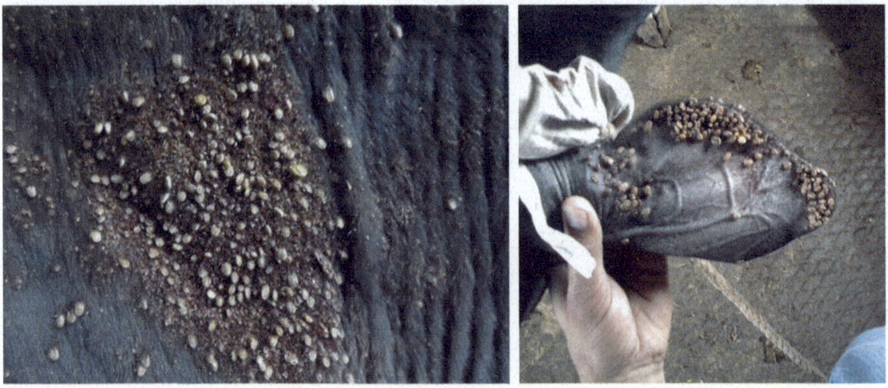

**Fig. 5.1** Tick infestation on animals

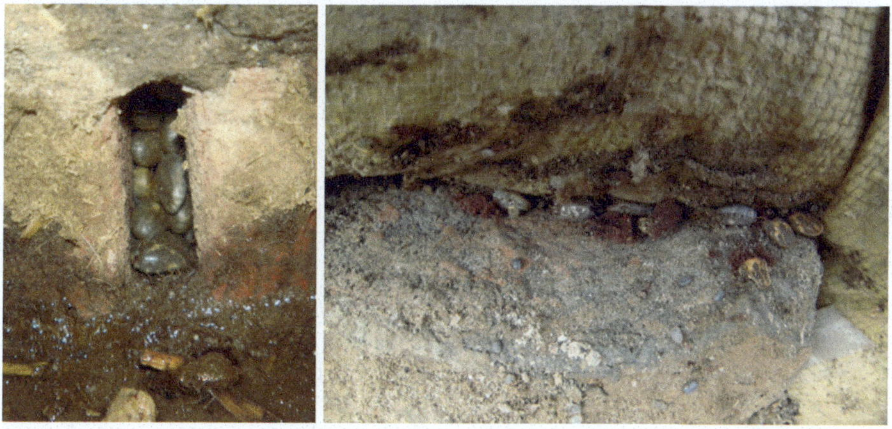

**Fig. 5.2** Tick infestations in cracks and crevices of animal shed

environmental pollution and toxic residues in milk and other dairy products. FAO (2004) projected a picture of development of widespread resistance in ticks from India based on the manner of a questionnaire in a sampled population. Subsequently, reports were released in the literature showing acaricidal resistance and its developmental process in ticks from various countries with emphasis on country-based discriminating concentrations (DC) of commercially used chemical acaricides (Jonsson et al. 2007; Castro-Janer et al. 2010; Kumar et al. 2011; Sharma et al. 2012; Klafke et al. 2017; Chigure et al. 2018; Rinesh Kumar et al. 2020).

Resistance to a specific acaricide can be defined as a decrease in the tick's susceptibility to acaricide when it is applied at the advised concentration. The development of resistance in ticks is a hereditary trait that arises from continuous selection pressure. It occurs when populations of ticks are exposed to chemicals causing problems in their existence and progenies, which show less susceptibility. A decrease in susceptibility may be a consequence of various mechanisms including alteration in target site (amino acid substitutions in receptors or enzymes), development in individual behavior to acaricides, development of detoxification either by metabolic pathway or by ATP transporters, and reduced absorption ability of acaricide into the parasite body (Rosario-Cruz et al. 2009).

Continuous monitoring of commercially used chemicals for tick control is an important step for early detection of resistance to prevent further selection of resistant ticks and their proliferation (FAO 2004). For this purpose, the World Health Organization (1970) recommended a testing procedure to differentiate between resistant and susceptible adult ticks. However, the Food and Agriculture Organization (2004) suggested a need for a uniform and standard testing kit for characterizing acaricide resistance in ticks to be adopted by different laboratories in the world under a Global Acaricide Resistance Monitoring Program. Thus, in this chapter, different methods to diagnose acaricide resistance in different tick populations have been discussed.

## 5.2 Background

In most of the tick research laboratories, acaricide resistance in tick populations has been detected following larval immersion test (LIT), larval packet test (LPT), adult immersion test (AIT), and molecular and biochemical assays. These are the basic tools to characterize field population against various classes of acaricides globally. FAO (1971) suggested a testing method using unfed larvae of ticks in an envelope known as larval packet made from filter paper sprayed with acaricide solution in olive oil. Recently, other resistance-characterizing techniques have been developed and adopted. Shaw (1966) designed a resistance monitoring procedure popularly named "Shaw test" employing tick larvae enclosed in a filter paper bag and dipped in acaricide solution. This technique has been extensively used to determine resistance in ticks in different parts of the world. Fiedler (1968) designed a "tea bag" method employing ticks in tea bag-like packets and dipping in chemical solution. This procedure was adopted to evaluate a number of acaricides for controlling dog tick, *Rhipicephalus sanguineus*. The AIT is also very common to detect resistance in tick population and is adopted by a number of laboratories with minor modifications.

## 5.3 Methods for Detecting Resistance in Ticks

Regular monitoring of resistance emergence in ticks is mandatory for judicious and appropriate use of acaricides, identification of resistance, and surveillance of acaricide-resistant tick species in the world. Acaricide resistance in tick population can be detected through potential and cost-effective tests that are commonly adopted by tick researchers (Sabatini et al. 2001). For any effective pest management program, it is essential to adopt a testing method that is practically applicable, time saving, less expensive, and more reliable to identify even small traces of phenotypic resistance in target organisms. In vitro testing tools are relatively user-friendly, easy to perform, cost-effective, and have minimum specific laboratory setup. In the case of ticks, these testing procedures require nonparasitic engorged females and larvae. The most popular procedures for monitoring phenotypic resistance in cattle tick include the adult immersion test (AIT) (Drummond et al. 1973), larval packet test (LPT) (Stone and Haydock 1962), which is advised by the Food and Agriculture Organization (FAO 1971), and larval immersion test (LIT) (Shaw 1966). In the AIT procedure, engorged females are bathed in technical- or commercial-grade acaricidal solution and the oviposition rate between treated and control ticks is compared.

Currently, these four bioassays are adopted in different laboratories in the world to identify acaricidal tolerance in ticks, where its mode of resistance development is limited or unknown. As reported by Rodriguez-Vivas et al. (2018), LPT is the most popular and widely used testing procedure to detect resistance that might be due to the availability of the larval stage in the field or can be developed in sufficient number from single female ticks. On the other hand, AIT is a highly sensitive procedure for resistance characterization phenotypically in *R. microplus* but it is time-consuming, and engorged female ticks are not generally present in the fields (Kumar et al. 2015). It requires engorged females as a basic test material that is bathed in technical chemical solution with observations on tick mortality and inhibition of egg-laying capacity in treated ticks compared to control ticks (Benavides et al. 2001). LPT is supposed to be a commercially exploitable testing procedure, and comparative studies have revealed its acceptability among various tests (FAO 2004). The two procedures, that is, LPT and AIT, are generally adopted to discriminate resistance in ticks against SP and OP compounds, on the contrary. LIT is popular to detect ivermectin, amitraz, and fipronil resistance providing consistent results (Rodriguez-Vivas et al. 2018). Larval immersion test is currently emerging as one of the common bioassays for tolerance detection against ivermectin. Another larval-based procedure, that is, larval tarsal test (LTT), was first developed in Switzerland in 2011, which is also known for its sensitivity and time-saving test, and is used to characterize resistance in ixodid ticks including *R. microplus* (Lovis et al. 2011).

### 5.3.1 Host Animals

It is difficult to collect a sufficient number of tick stages from fields. Thus, to conduct any in vitro test, a statistically significant number of tick stages, that is, larvae, nymphs, engorged females, and host animals, are the basic requirements for tick feeding and rearing. Ticks collected from fields can be maintained on cross-bred male calves (*Bos taurus* male × *B. indicus* female) to obtain engorged females quantitatively. These animals are maintained according to the rules and regulations of the Indian statutory body, "Committee for the Purpose of Control and Supervision on Animals" (CPCSEA). These guidelines may be different in different countries and must be followed for experimentation. Furthermore, these guidelines are also essential for maintaining reference tick strains on the animals. It must be ensured before releasing ticks on the hosts that animals should be free from any previous infestation so that any contamination in reference or field ticks can be avoided. The animals should be kept in a tick-free condition adopting routine management practices and fed with calf starter, mineral mixture, wheat bran, and water ad libitum for their growth and development. The larvae are released on the ears of animals for feeding according to ear bag tick feeding method as suggested by Ghosh and Azhahianambi (2007) (Fig. 5.3).

### 5.3.2 Chemical Acaricides

It is clear that commercially available chemical products contain so many ingredients as stabilizer, solvent and delivery matrix, preservatives, etc., along with active ingredients. In this situation, it becomes impossible to identify the actual effects of the acaricide on the ticks as these products will show synergistic action of these ingredients. Thus, to study the actual effects on ticks and regular resistance

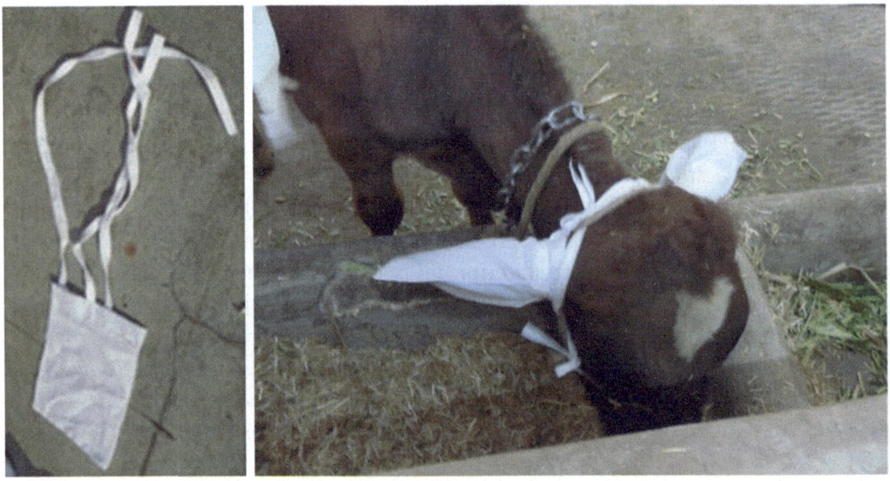

**Fig. 5.3** Ear bag method of tick rearing on animals

monitoring, we should use technical grade acaricide and properly developed concentration in using recommended solvents.

### 5.3.3 Preparation of Concentrations

Technical grade pure chemical acaricides, that is, deltamethrin, cypermethrin, diazinon, amitraz, malathion, etc., should be used in the preparation of mother stock solution in recommended solvents. For resistance characterization, different working concentrations of acaricides (i.e., x/2, x, 2x, 3x, 4x, 5x) are prepared from the mother solution. Here, "x" is the LC95 value of the acaricide against the reference-susceptible strain of *Rhipicephalus microplus* (IVRI-1). The references strain and DCs may be different in different countries. The discriminating concentration (DC = LC95 × 2) of a particular acaricide can be prepared as follows:

$$\text{Working conc.}(\%) = \frac{\text{desired conc.X desired volume}}{\text{Conc.of the stock solution}}$$

### 5.3.4 Reference Tick Strains

Reference susceptible tick strains are another basic and essential material used for determining $LC_{50}$ or $LC_{95}$ concentration of different chemicals. These are used to determine discriminating concentrations (DCs) of various acaricides which may be country-specific. DC is the double of $LC_{95}$ or $LC_{99}$ of a particular chemical against reference strain of a specific country. To determine resistance in tick population, we should have the baseline data of each chemical against reference susceptible tick strains which may vary in different countries due to several factors like frequency, schedule, environmental condition, host species, tick infestation levels, socio-economic status of animal owner etc. Researchers from the world studied resistance using the baseline data against susceptible tick strains of *R. microplus* like Media Joya in Mexico, Yeerongpilly in Australia, Mozo and Porto Alegre in Brazil, IVRI-I in India, Gonzalez, Remireno and Munoz in Texas to study acaricide resistance. The resistance factor (RF) or resistance ratio (RR) is determined on the basis of $LC_{50}$, $LC_{95}$ or $LC_{99}$ values of any field ticks as compared to reference strain.

## 5.4 In Vitro Tests for Resistance Monitoring

The following tests for resistance monitoring in field tick population are commonly adopted in various laboratories globally.

### 5.4.1 Adult Immersion Test (AIT)

For studying acaricide resistance and evaluation of antitick activities of any chemical or herbal compounds, AIT is the most suitable and widely adopted method (Ghosh et al. 2013), especially in countries where animal rearing infrastructure is available to maintain ticks. A dose–response assay is conducted by preparing a series of concentrations of the chemical acaricide as per the following steps:

- Collect the engorged females from animal shed and wash them thoroughly in tap water.
- Separate the ticks into batches of different concentrations.
- The ticks are bathed in the prepared concentrations of acaricide for 2 min while control group ticks should also be run parallel in the respective solvent.
- Transfer the ticks to glass or plastic Petri plates floored with Whatman filter paper no.1 to provide a coarse surface for oviposition.
- After 24 h, ticks are transferred to the glass vials encapped with a cotton cloth and are kept in a BOD incubator maintained at 28 °C and 85 ± 5% RH.
- Four replicas of each experiment are maintained having five ticks in each ($n = 4 \times 5$).
- The experimental observations should be recorded for 10–12 days. If any treated engorged female does not lay eggs till the experiment, it is assumed to be dead.
- The data of any dead ticks should be noted regularly by carefully noticing the lack of pedal movement under light.
- The survived ticks are observed subsequently for generating oviposition data and the efficacy of acaricides (Fig. 5.4).
- The inhibition of oviposition is calculated by the following formula of Bennett (1974):

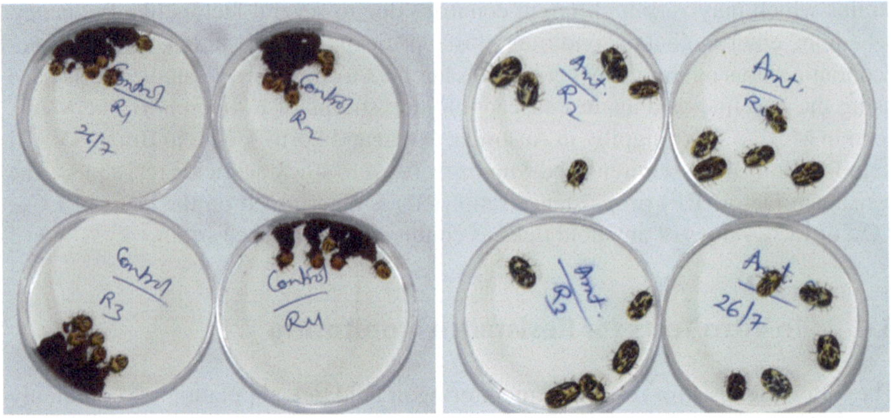

a. Control ticks laying eggs b. Acaricide treated ticks

**Fig. 5.4** AIT bioassay using engorged female *R. microplus* ticks. (**a**) Control ticks laying eggs. (**b**) Acaricide treated ticks

$$RI = EW / IFW$$

$$\%IO = \left[ \left( RI_{control} - RI_{treated} \right) / RI_{control} \right] \times 100$$

where RI is the reproductive index, EW the egg weight, IFW the initial female weight, and %IO the percentage inhibition of oviposition.

### 5.4.2 Larval Immersion Test (LIT)

Shaw (1966) developed a larval-based bioassay known as LIT. Shaw's immersion sandwich approach involves larval immersion in an acaricide solution or suspension, which often enhances toxicity. LIT is a less frequently adopted method for resistance monitoring in field ticks. About 10–14-day-old tick larvae should be used for immersion in different concentrations of acaricides for 10 min. The test is performed as follows:

- To perform the test procedure, approximately more than a hundred tick larvae are transferred to each 1.5 mL Eppendorf tube and then 200 µL of acaricide solution is poured for 10 min immersion.
- After 10 min larval bathing, the test solution is withdrawn from the tube and dried using a filter paper strip.
- Then, the Eppendorf tubes having exposed larvae are sealed with a cotton cloth using rubber bands (Fig. 5.5).
- The control group should be maintained by exposing in respective solvents.
- For each experiment, three replicas are maintained and the treated larvae are placed in a BOD incubator at 28 °C and 85 ± 5% RH (Ajithkumar et al. 2016).

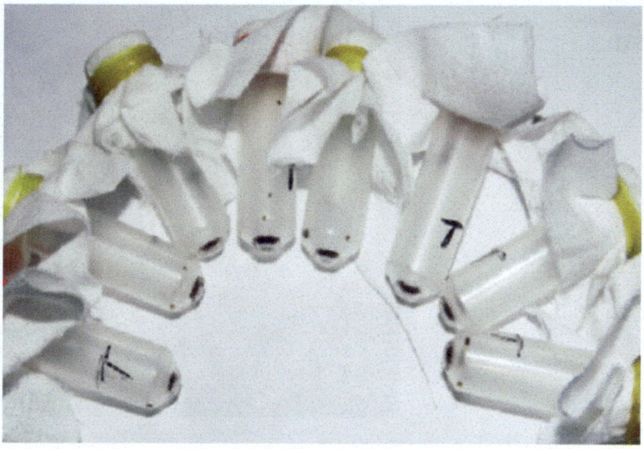

**Fig. 5.5** Larval immersion test in Eppendorf tube capped with cotton cloth

- After 24 h, the tubes are opened under light and larval death is confirmed by loss of active movement in the treated larvae.
- The larvae moving their legs at a place with no crawling are also considered dead and, consequently, larval mortality is determined in different concentrations of acaricides.

### 5.4.3 Larval Packet Test (LPT)

FAO (1971) recommended the LPT for characterization of acaricide resistance using the larval stage. It is the most widely used bioassay as it can be performed with larvae directly procured from the fields. Later many researchers modified it with minor changes and adopted this test (Sharma et al. 2012; Shakya et al. 2020). LPT is performed as follows:

- Parallelogram-shaped packets (5.5 cm × 5.5 cm) are prepared with Whatman filter paper No.1 (Fig. 5.6).
- Briefly, 0.5–0.6 mL of working solution of acaricide is used to impregnate filter paper rectangles.
- The impregnated paper is kept in an incubator at 37 °C for 30 min to evaporate solvent.
- The dried rectangle filter paper is turned in midway and its sides closed using a cellotape, thus a one-side open packet is formed to introduce tick larvae.
- Tests are performed within 30 min of drying of paper.
- Insert approximately 100 larvae of 10–14 days old into the packet with the help of a brush.

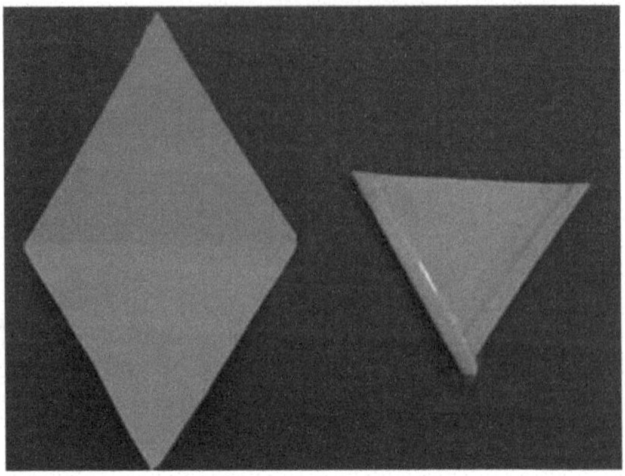

**Fig. 5.6** Larval packets (opened and sealed)

- After inserting the larvae, the remaining side of the packet is also closed with a cellotape and the packets are put in a BOD incubator scheduled at 28 °C and 85 ± 5% RH.
- After 24 h, the packets are opened to record dead and live larvae by observing them on a paper under light exposure; accordingly, the larval mortality is calculated.
- Then, the dose–response data is subjected to probit analysis to determine $LC_{50}$ or $LC_{95}$ values.
- Then, resistance ratio is calculated as.
- Resistance ratio ($RR_{50}$) = $LC_{50}$ value for field ticks/$LC_{50}$ value for reference-susceptible ticks.

### 5.4.4 Larval Tarsal Test (LTT)

The LTT was conducted by Lovis et al. (2013) to characterize field tick population of *R. microplus* from Brazil as follows:

- For the assay, the eggs are placed into the wells of 96-well microtiter plates pre-applied with a serial dilution of acaricides, and control wells are exposed to the vehicle.
- These egg-bearing plates are then closed and spotted at 28–29 °C and 70–85% RH to facilitate hatching.
- After 3 weeks of egg placement in the plate, larvae are also exposed to acaricide in the plate and death of the larvae is observed in each well based on their movement and physical appearance.
- The test is repeated four times to subject probit analysis, and lethal doses of particular acaricide are estimated.
- The resistance was measured by calculating the resistance ratios (RR) of field ticks.

### 5.4.5 Statistical Analysis

The dose-mortality data obtained from various test procedures are analyzed by probit analysis (Finney 1962). All the analyses can be performed using any statistical software program. The analysis includes log-transformed dose of acaricide and plotting it against probit-transformed mortality data. Linear regression analysis may be done to obtain the regression equation, and the $LC_{50}$ and $LC_{95}$ values are estimated from the regression equation. The significant difference in mean values among different groups is calculated using one-way ANOVA while mean the difference between two different groups is analyzed by performing *t*-test. However, standard error of the raw data on mortality, oviposition, and egg weight is also determined.

## 5.5 Biochemical Assays

The biochemical tool for resistance detection was initiated in the pests of agricultural importance and mosquitoes even before the establishment of veterinary parasites (Hemingway 1998). To date, protocols used in the tick system were mainly developed from mosquitoes and agriculture insects. The biochemical assays were subsequently adopted with minor changes to work out the probable process of acaricide resistance development in ticks without any standardization (Jamroz et al. 2000; Miller et al. 2001; Enayati et al. 2010; Ghosh et al. 2015). In ticks, various enzymes like esterases, monooxygenases, and glutathione S- transferases (GSTs) have been supposed to be associated with metabolic detoxification in conferring resistance (Bellgard et al. 2012; Gupta et al. 2016; Fular et al. 2020). These enzymes are quantified using pooled larvae of each field tick isolate as per the standardized and validated methods.

### 5.5.1 Esterase Assay

The larvae ($n = 40$, 10–15 days old) of each tick isolate are homogenized in 150 μL homogenization buffer and centrifuged. The fresh working solution of α-naphthyl and β-naphthyl acetate is developed with 100 μL of 30 mM α- and β-naphthyl acetate (prepared in acetone in 9.9 mL of 0.02 M phosphate buffer, pH 7.2). The fast-blue stain solution (15 mg fast-blue mixed with 1.5 mL distilled water and 3.5 mL 5% SDS in 0.1 M sodium phosphate buffer, pH 7.0) is freshly prepared. A homogenate (20 μL) in multiple replicates is loaded in each well of the 96-well microtiter plate and 200 μL α- or β-naphthyl acetate is added in each well. Control wells are filled with 20 μL homogenization buffer only. The plate is incubated at room temperature for 15 min and then 50 μL fast-blue solution is added and reincubated for 5 min for reaction and absorbance taken at 570 nm (Fig. 5.7). To determine the mean protein concentration in each isolate, a standard curve of protein is developed. The quantity of naphthol per minute is obtained as above and is divided by the

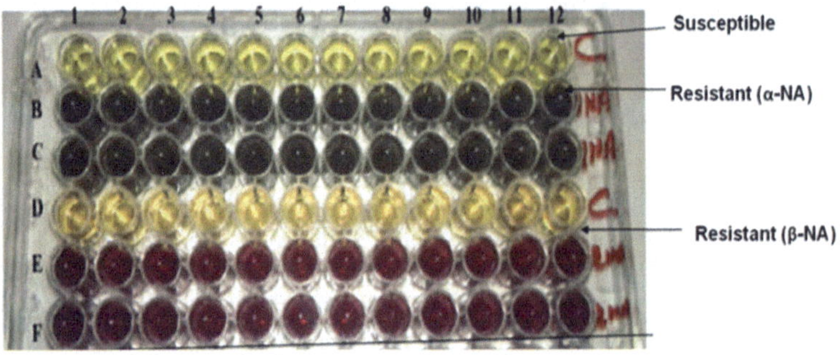


**Fig. 5.7** ELISA plate showing esterase activity in resistant ticks

protein value. Esterase activities are estimated in μmoles of product formed/min/mg protein (Habig et al. 1974).

### 5.5.2 Glutathione S-Transferase (GST) Assay

The homogenate is prepared from 40 tick larvae of 15–20 days old. The assay mixtures of 10 μL of larval homogenate (four replications) with 200 μL working solution containing 10 mM reduced glutathione in phosphate buffer (2.5 mL, pH 6.5) and 63 mM chlorodinitrobenzene (125 μL, CDNB) are incubated at room temperature in a dark area and absorbance at 340 nm is recorded. GST estimation is determined following Lambert–Beer's eq. ($A = \varepsilon CL$), where A represents absorbance at 340 nm; ε denotes the extinction coefficient of product 3-(2-chloro-4-nitrophenyl)-glutathione, which is 4.39 $mM^{-1}$; L denotes path length, which is 6 mm; and C denotes concentration. To estimate specific activity, GST concentration in homogenate is divided by total protein concentration. The activity in the sample is measured as GST (mM/mg/min) = O.D/4.39 $mM^{-1}$ × 6 mm × total protein in 10 mL homogenate ×reaction time in min × 1000. GST activity is compared with the $RR_{50}$ value determined from dose-mortality test using larvae.

### 5.5.3 Monooxygenase Assay

The monooxygenase activity (cytochrome P450) is quantified on the basis of the quantity of heme substance in the homogenate. The homogenate of 80 larvae of 10–15 days old is prepared in 150 μL homogenization buffer and 20 μL of the same is loaded in various wells. Potassium phosphate buffer (0.625 M, pH 7.2) and 3,3′,5,5′-tetramethylbenzidine (0.008 M) are mixed together to form working solution. Potassium phosphate buffer (80 μL), TMBZ (200 μL), and 3% hydrogen peroxide (25 μL) are transferred to each well. The microtiter plates are kept at room temperature (5 min) in a dark area to take absorbance at 650 nm. The control wells are filled with homogenization buffer (20 μL) without larval homogenate (Fig. 5.8).

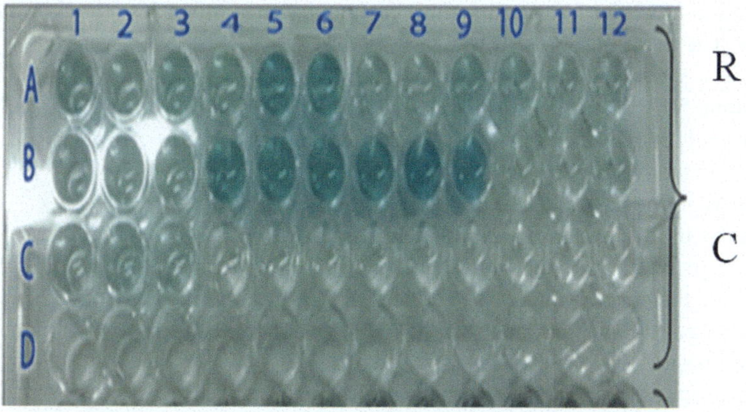


**Fig. 5.8** ELISA plate showing monooxygenase content in resistant ticks

To determine the concentration of monooxygenase per mg of protein, the resulting optical densities (OD) are rectified to the total protein substance in the larval homogenate. The values are compared with the standard curve of purified cytochrome C and are represented as nanomoles equivalent of cytochrome P450/mg protein.

## 5.6 Molecular Bioassay

Overdependency on synthetic pyrethroids for managing insects/pests has resulted in the worldwide problem of resistance emergence in pest populations. Studies showed that sodium channel is the primary target site of pyrethroids. Various reports on the presence of point mutations in sodium channel gene causing knockdown resistance have been published in different arthropods. In ticks, the detection of mutations at different sites of sodium channel gene was also reported in different reference and field tick populations (Morgan et al. 2009; Stone et al. 2014). In India, C190A mutation in domain II of S4–5 linker region of sodium channel gene has been reported (Kumar et al. 2013; Nagar et al. 2018; Fular et al. 2021). The following sections describe the protocol for the identification of sodium channel mutation for monitoring of resistance.

### 5.6.1 Genomic DNA Extraction

The protocol described below has been adapted from *Molecular Cloning: A Laboratory Manual* (fourth edn.) by Green and Sambrook et al. (2001) with some modifications. The method for genomic DNA extraction does not require extraction with phenol:chloroform and is based on the precipitation of DNA by isopropanol.

The method is suited for small sample size, consumes much less time, and is user friendly. The procedure is as follows:

- Triturate 50–100 frozen or fresh larvae in a pestle and mortar.
- Add 1 mL of lysis buffer.
- Incubate the homogenate at 37 °C for an hour.
- Centrifuge the homogenate at 10,000 rpm for 10 min.
- Transfer the supernatant to another Eppendorf tube.
- Add 5 μL (final concentration 100 μg/mL) of Proteinase-K (20 mg/mL) and incubate the suspension at 55 °C overnight with vortexing every 2–3 h.
- Centrifuge the homogenate at 10,000 rpm for 10 min to sediment undigested tissue.
- Transfer the supernatant to another 2 mL Eppendorf tube.
- Add 1 mL of isopropanol at room temperature and mix the contents by inversion multiple times.
- When the stringy DNA precipitate becomes visible, centrifuge at 10,000 rpm for 10 min at 4 °C to collect the DNA pellet.
- If no visible or very little DNA precipitate is seen, mark the outside of the tube before centrifugation to allow the pellet to be located.
- The supernatant is carefully removed without disturbing the pellet.
- Wash the DNA pellet with freshly prepared 70% ethanol (1 mL).
- Centrifugation is done at 10,000 rpm for 10 min at 4 °C.
- The supernatant is removed carefully to allow the DNA pellet to air drying at room temperature.
- Dissolve the DNA in 50–100 μL of TE buffer. If required, incubate it at 55 °C for 15 min to dissolve the DNA pellet.
- The DNA can be stored at 4 °C for 1–2 days and at −20 °C for long term.

### 5.6.2 Amplification of S4–5 Linker Region of Sodium Channel Gene

- The C190A point mutation site in the domain II S4–5 linker region is amplified using primer pair, Fwd: 5′-TACGTGTGTTCAAGCCTA-3′ and Rev.: 5′-ACTTTCTTCGTAGTTCTTG-3′.
- For 25 μL PCR setup, add DNA (1.0 μL), 10X buffer (2.5 μL), dNTP (0.5 μL of 10 mM), forward primer (0.5 μL), reverse primer (0.5 μL), DreamTaq DNA polymerase (0.3 μL of 5 IU/μL) (Thermo Scientific, USA).
- The PCR conditions include an initial denaturation step at 95 °C for 3 min, followed by 35 cycles of 95 °C for 30 sec, 50 °C for 30 s, and 72 °C for 30 s with a final extension step at 72 °C for 10 min.
- The 167 bp PCR product is visualized in agarose gel (1.5%) stained with ethidium bromide or similar dyes.

**Lysis buffer:** 50 mM Tris (pH 8.5), 0.1 M EDTA, 1% SDS.
**TE buffer:** 10 mM Tris, 1 mM EDTA (pH 8.0).

### 5.6.3 Sequence Analysis and Identification of C190A Mutation

- The PCR product can be cloned into a TA cloning vector and sent for double-stranded sequencing. Alternatively, PCR product can be gel extracted using any commercial gel extraction kit and directly sent for sequencing.
- The sequences are analyzed using multiple sequence alignment on a DNA analysis software like GeneTool or DNA Star with published sequences from GenBank and screen for C190A mutation.

  A C C A T C G G T G C C **C** T C G G G A A C T T G A C Australian susceptible

  A C C A T C G G T G C C **A** T C G G G A A C T T G A C Australian resistant

  A C C A T C G G T G C C **C** T C G G G A A C T T G A C IVRI-I (HM579820) (susceptible)

  A C C A T C G G T G C C **A** T C G G G A A C T T G A C IVRI-IV (JQ693154) (resistant)
- Partial alignment of nucleotide sequence in the domain II S4–5 linker region of sodium channel gene shows C to A mutation in deltamethrin-resistant IVRI-IV strain of *R. microplus*. This position is located at 190 in the reference sequence.

## 5.7 Factors that Influence the Efficacy of Acaricides

Tick management is mainly focused on the large-scale consumption of synthetic chemicals, and there are many factors that can affect the effectiveness of these acaricides. These factors include the following.

**Variation in Tick Species and Strain** The potency of acaricide varies in different tick species. Some tick species may be susceptible at varying levels to acaricides. For instance, some acaricides are highly toxic to one species but comparatively less toxic to another species. Moreover, there may be intra-specific genetic variations or strains that are responsible for the inefficacy of acaricides in tick management. Thus, it is essential to understand targeted tick species and its biological characteristics for selecting the most effective acaricide.

**Emergence of Acaricide-Resistant Populations** Indiscriminate application and continuous exposure of ticks to acaricides are responsible for the growth of multiacaricide-resistant tick species in the field. Certain genetic mutations in ticks conferring acaricide resistance are responsible for effective survival and reproduction and transferring the resistant genes to the next generations. After a certain period, these factors contribute to a complete diminishing of the efficacy of acaricides. It is believed that resistance can develop against both synthetic and natural acaricides, but proper rotation or combination of different acaricides should be used to manage resistant populations in a very effective manner.

**Mechanism of Action** Acaricides have various mechanisms to kill or repel ticks such as disrupting neurotransmission, interfering with metabolic pathways, or causing physical damage to the tick's cuticle, which causes death in the exposed ticks. The mechanism of action can also influence the knockdown efficacy of acaricides.

Ticks may show different levels of susceptibility to different mechanisms of action, and therefore, combining acaricides with such modes of action can enhance efficacy and delay resistance development.

**Acaricidal Formulation and Delivery System** A number of commercial acaricides are sold in the market in various formulations such as sprays, dips, spot-ons, pour-on, powders, collars, injectable, and ear tags. Each formulation provides some specific advantages and limitations in terms of ease of application, duration of efficacy, and distribution over the animal body. The choice of acaricidal formulation depends on factors like tick species, host animal characteristics, animal breed, and environmental conditions. For effective tick management, it is essential to adopt proper application techniques to ensure uniform coverage and maximize efficacy.

**Dosage and Concentration** The dosage and concentration of the active ingredient(s) in the acaricide formulation determine its effectiveness. Improper dose schedule with incorrect acaricide concentration is a major contributing factor in the failure of effective tick control. However, excessive dosage can increase the risk of adverse effects on the host animal, residual toxicity in milk and dairy products, and the environment. It is important to apply appropriate dosage based on certain factors such as the size and species of the animal through which we can optimize efficacy and minimize potential risks.

**Environmental Factors** Different climatic conditions prevail in different parts of the world like temperature, humidity, rainfall, altitude, and sunlight that can affect acaricidal activity toward different tick species. Some acaricides may degrade easily and rapidly under certain environmental conditions, reducing their effectiveness. Besides, environmental factors can affect tick behavior and biology, activity patterns, and population dynamics, impacting the timing and frequency of acaricide applications.

**Host Factors** Characteristics of the host animals, such as skin thickness, hair coat density, grooming behavior, and immune response, can influence the distribution and absorption of acaricides. For instance, animals with thick fur may require higher doses or specialized application methods to ensure proper drug penetration to the skin. Thus, while selecting the suitable acaricidal formulation and application method, the characteristics of the host animals should be kept in mind.

**Interaction with Other Chemicals** Concurrent use of multiple chemicals, such as shampoos, conditioners, pesticides, or medications, may interact with acaricides and affect their efficacy. Some chemicals may enhance or inhibit the absorption, metabolism, or excretion of acaricides, altering their pharmacokinetics and efficacy. Compatibility testing should be conducted while using multiple products simultaneously to avoid adverse interactions and ensure optimal efficacy.

**Frequency and Timing of Application** The timing and frequency of acaricide application are critical key factors for efficacy testing. Applying acaricides at the right time relative to the tick life cycle and peak activity periods maximizes their efficacy. Based on the level of tick infestation on animals, repeat application of the acaricides especially in areas with high tick burdens or during tick active season may be effective to maintain adequate tick control.

**Product Quality and Storage** The quality and storage conditions of acaricide products can impact their efficacy. Improper storage, exposure to extreme temperatures, or prolonged shelf life can degrade the active ingredients, reducing their potency and effectiveness. Such products are strictly prohibited for application in tick management. It is necessary to promote fresh, properly stored antitick products and adhere to manufacturer's recommendations for handling and storage for optimal tick control efficacy.

**Monitoring and Surveillance of Ticks** Regular monitoring and surveillance for efficacy, acaricide resistance, and changes in tick populations are essential for effective formulation of tick management strategy in particular regions. It can help identify heterogeneity in tick populations and a list of ineffective chemicals. These factors may be essential for adapting control measures, maintaining long-term effectiveness, and minimizing the risk of resistance development.

## 5.8 Strategies for Monitoring Resistance over Time

Monitoring acaricide resistance in tick populations over time is a continuous process and is very important for sustainable tick management programs. It is country-specific and helps prevent the spread of resistance and preserve the effectiveness of acaricides. The particular tick control strategy of a country or region cannot be adopted effectively in other countries or regions due to the vast variations in the environmental and host–parasite factors. The following strategies can be adopted for monitoring acaricide resistance.

**Baseline Surveys** Baseline data on susceptibility/resistance status of tick populations in a particular region is an essential tool prior to implementing tick control programs and also provides a clue for monitoring changes in resistance levels over time. Baseline data can be collected through field surveys, tick collection from various locations, and characterization of resistance status using standardized laboratory bioassays and concentrations of acaricides (Garcia et al. 2022). The baseline information can help tick researchers and animal owners identify susceptible or resistant tick populations for the selection of effective tick control measures.

**Regular Surveillance Programs** Surveillance studies are an important component of integrated tick management program to monitor the development of acaricide resistance in tick populations, and variations in resistance patterns and trends. Surveillance can be accomplished by sampling of tick population from different regions, and testing their susceptibility/resistant status to commonly used acaricides using established testing tools (Abbas et al. 2014). The surveillance data can be used to identify hotspots of emerging resistance, effectiveness of control measures, assess the spread of resistance genes, and guide targeted interventions for tick management strategies in the region.

**Laboratory Bioassays** In vitro bioassays involve testing laboratory-reared ticks or reference tick strains, and field-collected ticks against country-specific discriminating concentrations (DCs) of commonly used acaricides in a laboratory setup

(Kumar et al. 2015). These in vitro assays can be conducted using different life stages of ticks (larvae, nymphs, adults) to evaluate mortality, reproductive inhibition, and molting inhibition and resistance status of the collected population. The laboratory-generated research provides quantitative data on resistance level, development of resistance map of the region or country, and also can help track any variation in resistance patterns over time.

**Resistance Phenotyping** Phenotypic characterization provides various resistance levels and mechanism of acaricide resistance in field ticks. Phenotypic traits of field-collected ticks can be characterized in terms of the resistance ratio (RR) or resistance factor (RF), which compares the mortality of treated field ticks with susceptible reference strain. Resistance phenotyping can also help identify cross-resistance to different acaricides and explore in-depth knowledge of the underlying genetic mechanisms of resistance.

**Field Trials** Field trials are an important factor in determining the actual efficacy of acaricide by applying a known or recommended concentration of acaricide on the infested animals. It provides valuable insights into the practical effectiveness of acaricides against the susceptibility status of ticks on naturally infested animals and also helps identify emerging resistance issues in a particular region or area where the field trials are conducted (George 2006). Monitoring tick populations before and after field trials reveals actual variation in susceptibility and, if necessary, guides for suitable modifications to control better strategies for tick management. This approach helps evaluate and compare the results of laboratory-based bioassays and natural field trials. It was observed that the efficacy of antitick products was reduced when applied in field conditions (Sharma et al. 2022).

**Molecular Techniques** Molecular tools are generally adopted in different tick research laboratories to study the role of specific gene sequence responsible for resistance to a particular class of acaricide. In the approach, polymerase chain reaction (PCR) and DNA sequencing can be used to detect genetic markers associated with resistance development in field ticks (Ghosh and Nagar 2014). These markers may include mutations in target sites (e.g., acetylcholinesterase, sodium channels) or increased expression of metabolic detoxification enzymes (e.g., cytochrome P450s), which also help the mechanism of development of resistance. Molecular tools allow for a rapid and sensitive detection of resistance mechanisms and can complement traditional bioassays for resistance monitoring.

**Dose–Response Studies** Dose–response studies involve testing ticks against a series of concentrations of acaricides to determine the minimum effective concentration required to achieve a specific level of mortality in treated ticks. These studies provide significant information on the efficacy of acaricides against resistant tick populations and can help establish appropriate dose regime for effective control.

**Cross-Resistance and Synergistic Studies** Cross-resistance studies involve testing ticks resistant to one acaricide for their susceptibility to other acaricides with different modes of action. Synergism studies assess the effect of combining acaricides with synergists or inhibitors of detoxification enzymes to overcome resistance and improve the control strategies for ticks and tick-borne diseases. Synergists can be used to decrease the concentration of active ingredients of acaricide and increase the efficacy of the product when combined with a low concentration of acaricide (Shakya et al. 2022). These studies provide a deep understanding of resistance mechanisms and clues for selecting alternative tick control strategies.

**Resistance Management Programs** Developing and implementing tick resistance management plans integrating multiple control practices of TTBDs is essential for mitigating the development of multiacaricide-resistant populations. Resistance management programs may suggest rotational use of acaricides belonging to different classes, using synergists to overcome resistance problem, and implementing ecofriendly tick control measures, that is, biological control agents, herbal acaricide, or habitat modification. Regular review and updating of resistance management strategies based on surveillance data and emerging resistance trends can play an important role in maintaining the efficacy of acaricidal formulation.

**Collaboration and Data Sharing** Establishing collaborative networks among researchers, government agencies, veterinarians, extension agents, and industry stakeholders is essential for effective resistance monitoring and management. Collaboration between research institutions, government agencies, veterinary professionals, and industry stakeholders can facilitate the establishment of surveillance networks for monitoring acaricide resistance through multi-institutional research project proposals. These networks help in sharing data and resources, thereby enhancing the effectiveness of monitoring efforts (Madder et al. 2011).

**Integrated Tick Management (ITM) Program** Incorporating resistance monitoring into integrated tick management programs ensures resistance data, decision-making, and management strategies. ITM approaches consist of multiple control tactics, including chemical, biological, cultural, and mechanical methods, to mitigate the global problem of multiacaricide-resistant ticks and provide sustainable management of ticks and tick-borne diseases. For this purpose, continuous monitoring and surveillance studies are basic tools for proactive management of acaricide resistance and minimizing the excessive burden of chemicals in the environment.

## 5.9 Conclusion

For monitoring acaricide resistance in field populations, in vitro bioassays like AIT, LPT, LIT, and LTT can be performed with engorged females and larvae collected directly from the fields. Further, biochemical and molecular assays can be performed to study the acaricide resistance. The abovementioned resistance monitoring tools will definitely be helpful for tick researchers.

**Acknowledgments** The authors are grateful to the Indian Council of Agriculture Research and Indian Council of Medical Research (ICMR), New Delhi.

## References


Abbas RZ, Zaman MA, Colwell DD, Gilleard J, Iqbal Z (2014) Acaricide resistance in cattle ticks and approaches to its management: the state of play. Vet Parasitol 203(1–2):6–20. https://doi.org/10.1016/j.vetpar.2014.03.014

Ajithkumar KG, Tayade AB, Kumar R, Gupta S, Sharma AK, Nagar G, Tewari SS, Kumar B, Rawat AKS, Srivastava S, Kumar S (2016) Chemo-profiling and bioassay of phytoextracts from *Ageratum conyzoides* for acaricidal properties against *Rhipicephalus* (*Boophilus*) *microplus* (Acari: Ixodidae) infesting cattle and buffaloes in India. Ticks Tick Borne Dis 7(2):342–349

Bellgard MI, Moolhuijzen PM, Guerrero FD, Schibeci D, Rodriguez-Valle M, Peterson DG, Dowd SE, Barrero R, Hunter A, Miller RJ, Lew-Tabor AE (2012) Cattle Tick Base: an integrated internet-based bioinformatics resource for *Rhipicephalus microplus*. Int J Parasitol 42(2):161–169

Benavides OE, Hernandez MG, Castro AH (2001) Preliminary evaluation of neem *(Azadirachta indica)* extract as alternative for cattle ticks *Boophilus microplus*. Rev Colomb Entomol 27:1–8

Bennett GF (1974) Oviposition of *Boophilus microplus* (Canestrini)(Acarida: Ixodidae). I. Influence of tick size on egg production. Acarologia 16(1):52–61

Castro-Janer E, Martins JR, Mendes MC, Namindome A, Klafke GM, Schumacher TTS (2010) Diagnoses of fipronil resistance in Brazilian cattle ticks (*Rhipicephalus* (*Boophilus*) *microplus*) using in vitro larval bioassays. Vet Parasitol 173(3–4):300–306

Chigure GM, Sharma AK, Kumar S, Fular A, Sagar SV, Nagar G, Upadhaya D, Saravanan BC, Kumar R, Ghosh S (2018) Role of metabolic enzymes in conferring resistance to synthetic pyrethroids, organophosphates, and phenylpyrazole compounds in *Rhipicephalus microplus*. Int J Acarol 44:28–34

Drummond RO, Ernst SE, Trevino JL, Gladney WJ, Graham OH (1973) *Boophilus annulatus* and *Boophilus microplus*: laboratory test of insecticides. J Econ Entomol 66:130–133

Enayati AA, Asgarian F, Amouei A, Sharif M, Mortazavi H, Boujhmehrani H, Hemingway J (2010) Parathyroid insecticide resistance in *Rhipicephalus bursa*. Pestic Biochem Physiol 97:243–248

FAO (1971) Recommended methods for the detection and measurement of resistance of agricultural pests to pesticides—tentative method for larvae of cattle tick, *Boophilus microplus* spp. FAO method no. 7. Plant Prot Bull 19:15–18

FAO (2004) Resistance management and integrated parasite control in ruminants-guidelines, module I-ticks: acaricide resistance: diagnosis. Management and Prevention. Food and Agriculture Organization, Animal Production and Health Division, FAO, Rome, pp 25–77

Fiedler OGH (1968) A new biological method for evaluating the efficiency of acaricides against ticks. J South Afr Med Assoc 39:84–87

Finney DJ (1962) Probit analysis—a statistical treatment of the response curve. Cambridge University Press, Cambridge, pp 1–318

Fular A, Gupta S, Sharma AK, Kumar S, Upadhaya D, Shakya M, Nagar G, Ghosh S (2020) Standardization of tick specific biochemical tools for estimation of esterases, monooxygenases and glutathione S-transferase for characterization of acaricide resistance. Pestici Biochem Physiol 164:130–139

Fular A, Sharma AK, Upadhaya D, Nandi A, Nagar G, Bisht N, Shakya M, Kumar S, Kumar S, Kumar R, Ghosh S (2021) Evaluation of acaricidal resistance status of *Rhipicephalus microplus* ticks from the hilly state (Uttarakhand) of India and evaluation of efficacy of a natural formulation for the management of resistant ticks. Exp Appl Acarol 85(2):355–377

Garcia K, Weakley M, Do T, Mir S (2022) Current and future molecular diagnostics of tick-borne diseases in cattle. Vet Sci 9(5):241. https://doi.org/10.3390/vetsci9050241

George JE (2006) Present and future technologies for tick control. Ann N Y Acad Sci 916:583–588. https://doi.org/10.1111/j.1749-6632.2000.tb05394.x

Ghosh S, Azhahianambi P (2007) Laboratory rearing of *Theileria annulata*-free *Hyalomma anatolicum anatolicum* ticks. Exp Appl Acarol 43(2):137–146

Ghosh S, Nagar G (2014) Problem of ticks and tick-borne diseases in India with special emphasis on progress in tick control research: a review. J Vector Borne Dis 51(4):259–270

Ghosh S, Bansal GC, Gupta SC, Ray DD, Khan MQ, Irshad H, Shahiduzzaman M, Seitzer U, Ahmed JS (2007) Status of tick distribution in Bangladesh, India and Pakistan. Parasitol Res 101:207–216

Ghosh S, Tiwari SS, Srivastava S, Sharma AK, Kumar S, Ray DD, Rawat AKS (2013) Acaricidal properties of *Ricinus communis* leaf extracts against organophosphate and pyrethroids resistant *Rhipicephalus microplus*. Vet Parasitol 192(1–3):259–267

Ghosh S, Tiwari SS, Kumar B, Srivastava S, Sharma AK, Kumar S, Bandyopadhyay A, Julliet S, Kumar R, Rawat AKS (2015) Identification of potential plant extracts for anti-tick activity against acaricide resistant cattle ticks, *Rhipicephalus microplus* (Acari: Ixodidae). Exp Appl Acarol 66(1):59–171

Gupta S, Ajithkumar KG, Sharma AK, Nagar G, Kumar S, Saravanan BC, Ravikumar G, Ghosh S (2016) Esterase mediated resistance in deltamethrin resistant reference tick colony of *Rhipicephalus microplus*. Exp Appl Acarol 69(2):239–248

Habig WH, Pabst MJ, Jako WB (1974) Glutathione S-transferasesthe first enzymatic step in mercapturic acid formation. J Biochem 249:7130–7139

Hemingway J (1998) Techniques to detect insecticide resistance mechanisms (field and laboratory manual). Document WHO/CDS/CPC/MAL/98.6. World Health Organization, Geneva

Jamroz RC, Guerrero FD, Pruett JH, Oehler DD, Miller RJ (2000) Molecular and biochemical survey of acaricide resistance mechanisms in larvae from Mexican strains of the southern cattle tick, *Boophilus microplus*. J Insect Physiol 46:685–695

Jonsson NN, Miller RJ, Robertson JL (2007) Critical evaluation of the modified-adult immersion test with discriminating dose bioassay for *Boophilus microplus* using American and Australian isolates. Vet Parasitol 146:307–315

Klafke G, Webster A, Agnol BD, Pradel E, Silva J, de La Canal LH, Becker M, Osório MF, Mansson M, Barreto R, Scheffer R (2017) Multiple resistance to acaricides in field populations of *Rhipicephalus microplus* from Rio Grande do Sul state, Southern Brazil. Ticks Tick Borne Dis 8(1):73–80

Kumar S, Paul S, Sharma AK, Kumar R, Tewari SS, Chaudhuri P, Ray DD, Rawat AKS, Ghosh S (2011) Diazinon resistant status in *Rhipicephalus microplus* collected from different agro-climatic regions of India. Vet Parasitol 181(2–4):274–281

Kumar R, Nagar G, Sharma AK, Kumar S, Ray DD, Chaudhuri P, Ghosh S (2013) Survey of pyrethroids resistance in Indian isolates of *Rhipicephalus (Boophilus) microplus*:Identification of C190A mutation in the domain II of the para-sodium channel gene. Acta Trop 125:237–245

Kumar S, Sharma AK, Nagar G, Ghosh S (2015) Determination and establishment of discriminating concentrations of malathion, coumaphos, fenvalerate and fipronil for monitoring acaricide resistance in ticks infesting animals. Ticks Tick Borne Dis 6:383–387

Kumar R, Sharma AK, Ghosh S (2020) Menace of acaricide resistance in cattle tick, *Rhipicephalus microplus* in India: status and possible mitigation strategies. Vet Parasitol 278:108993. https://doi.org/10.1016/j.vetpar.2019.108993

Lovis L, Perret JL, Bouvier J, Fellay JM, Kaminsky R, Betschart B, Sager H (2011) A new in vitro test to evaluate the resistance level against acaricides of the cattle tick *Rhipicephalus* (*Boophilus*) *microplus* Vet Parasitol 182(2-4):269–280. https://doi.org/10.1016/j.vetpar.2011.06.004

Lovis L, Mendes MC, Perret JL, Martins JR, Bouvier J, Betschart B, Sager H (2013) Use of the larval tarsal test to determine acaricide resistance in *Rhipicephalus microplus* Brazilian field populations. Vet Parasitol 191(3–4):323–331

Madder M, Thys E, Achi L, Touré A, De Deken R (2011) *Rhipicephalus (Boophilus) microplus*: a most successful invasive tick species in West-Africa. Exp Appl Acarol 53(2):139–145. https://doi.org/10.1007/s10493-010-9390-8

Miller RJ, George JE, Guerrero FD, Carpenter, Welch JB (2001) Characterization of acaricide resistance in *Rhipicephalus sanguineus*, collected from Corozol army veterinary quarantine Centre, Panama. J Med Entomol 38:298–302

Morgan JAT, Corley SW, Jackson LA, Lew-Tabor AE, Moolhuijzen PM, Jonsson NN (2009) Identification of point mutation in the Para-sodium channel gene of the cattle *Rhipicephalus microplus* associated with resistance to synthetic pyrethroids acaricides. Int J Parasitol 39:775–779

Nagar G, Sharma AK, Kumar S, Sarvanan BC, Kumar R, Gupta S, Kumar S, Ghosh S (2018) Molecular mechanism of synthetic pyrethroid and organophosphate resistance in field isolates of *Rhipicephalus microplus* tick collected from a northern state of India. Exp Appl Acarol 75:319–331

Rodriguez-Vivas RI, Jonsson NN, Bhusan C (2018) Strategies for the control of *Rhipicephalus microplus* ticks in a world of conventional acaricide and macrocyclic lactone resistance. Parasitol Res 117:3–29

Rosario-Cruz R, Almazan C, Miller RJ, Dominguez-Gracia DI, Hernandez-Ortiz R, De la Fuente J (2009) Genetic basis and impact of tick acaricide resistance. Front Biosci 14:2657–2665

Sabatini GA, Kemp DH, Hughes S, Nari A, Hansen J (2001) Test to determine LC50 and discriminating doses for macrocyclic lactones against the cattle tick *Boophilus microplus*. Vet Parasitol 95:53–62

Sambrook J, Russell DW, Irwin N, Janseen KA (2001) Molecular cloning—a laboratory manual, 3rd edn. Cold SpringHarbor Laboratory Press, Cold spring harbor, New York, p 6.1–6.62

Shakya M, Kumar S, Fular A, Upadhaya D, Sharma AK, Bisht N, Nandi A, Ghosh S (2020) Emergence of fipronil resistant *Rhipicephalus microplus* populations in Indian states. Exp App Acarol 80:591–602

Shakya M, Nandi A, Fular A, Kumar S, Bisht N, Sharma AK, Singh K, Kumar R, Kumar S, Juliet S, Ghosh S (2022) Synergistic property of piperonyl butoxide, diethyl maleate, triphenyl phosphate and verapamil hydrochloride with deltamethrin and ivermectin against *Rhipicephalus microplus* ticks. Ticks Tick-borne Dis 13:102006. https://doi.org/10.1016/j.ttbdis.2022.102006

Sharma AK, Kumar R, Kumar S, Nagar G, Singh NK, Rawat SS, Dhakad ML, Rawat AKS, Ray DD, Ghosh S (2012) Deltamethrin and cypermethrin resistance status of *Rhipicephalus* (*Boophilus*) *microplus* collected from six agro-climatic regions of India. Vet Parasitol 188(3–4):337–345

Sharma AK, Tiwari SS, Kumar S, Rawat AKS, Srivastava S, Ray DD, Singh NK, Rawat SS, Sangwan AK, Ghosh S (2022) Establishment of antitick efficacy of a phytopharmaceutical formulation prepared from *Annona squamosa* leaf extracts for the management of acaricide resistant tick infestations on cattle. Acta Trop 233:106463. https://doi.org/10.1016/j.actatropica.2022.106463

Shaw RD (1966) Culture of an organophosphate resistance strain of *Boophilus microplus* (canestrini.) and assessment of its resistance spectrum. Bull Entomol Res 56:398–405

Stone BF, Haydock P (1962) A method for measuring the acaricides susceptibility of the cattle tick *Boophilus microplus* (Can.). Bull Entomol Res 53:563–578

Stone NE, Olafson PO, Davey RB, Buckmeier G, Bodine D, Sidak-Loftis LC, Giles JR, Duhaime R, Miller RJ, Mosqueda J, Scoles GA, Wagner DM, Busch JD (2014) Multiple mutations in the Para sodium channel gene are associated with pyrethroid resistance in *Rhipicephalus microplus* from the United States and Mexico. Parasit Vectors 7:456. https://doi.org/10.1186/s13071-014-0456-z

World Health Organization (1970) Health aspects of chemical and biological weapons: report of a WHO group of consultants. WHO, Geneva

# Managing Acaricide Resistance in the Cattle Tick, *Rhipicephalus microplus* (Acari: Ixodidae) 6

Roger I. Rodríguez-Vivas, José A. Rosado Aguilar, and Gabriela J. Flota-Burgos

**Abstract**

Ticks and tick-borne diseases are widely distributed worldwide, mainly in tropical and subtropical areas. Acaricides and macrocyclic lactones (MLs) are pivotal in controlling the cattle tick *Rhipicephalus microplus*. However, intensive exposure to acaricides and MLs has resulted in selecting resistant tick populations and negatively affects the livelihoods of millions of cattle producers worldwide. To reduce the impact of acaricide resistance, integrated tick management (ITM) is needed using chemical and nonchemical strategies. This ITM consists of the association of the environment and the monthly fluctuation of tick species using a combination of sustainable tools that are compatible and that maintain low levels of parasite populations that cause economic losses. The objective of this chapter is to highlight the main chemical and nonchemical strategies comprehensively for the control of the cattle tick (*R. microplus*) and minimize the impact of acaricide resistance on global cattle farming.

**Keywords**

*Rhipicephalus microplus* · Integrated tick management · Acaricides · Nonchemical methods · Strategies

---

R. I. Rodríguez-Vivas (✉) · J. A. Rosado Aguilar · G. J. Flota-Burgos
Campus de Ciencias Biológicas y Agropecuarias, Facultad de Medicina Veterinaria y Zootecnia, Universidad Autónoma de Yucatán, Mérida, Yucatán, Mexico
e-mail: rvivas@correo.uady.mx


S. Kumar et al. (eds.), *Acaricides Resistance in Ticks*,
https://doi.org/10.1007/978-981-97-7411-1_6

## 6.1 Introduction

Ticks and the pathogens they transmit to cattle are widely distributed worldwide, especially in tropical and subtropical areas (Rodriguez-Vivas et al. 2018a). The FAO (2004) mentioned that 80% of the bovine population worldwide is exposed to tick infestation.

The cattle tick *Rhipicephalus microplus* (Canestrini) (Acari: Ixodidae) is responsible for many losses caused by the direct effect of blood consumption (i.e., injection of toxins and production of anemia) or due to the negative clinical aspects and death caused by tick-borne pathogens (i.e., *Babesia bovis*, *B. bigemina*, and *Anaplasma marginale*). Ticks also cause stress in animals that affects their behavior and welfare, which compromises the immune response (Abbas et al. 2014), as well as the loss of energy due to the constant movement to counteract the effects of tick blood-sucking (Fig. 6.1) (Betancur-Hurtado and Giraldo-Ríos 2018).

The potential annual cost associated with ticks and tick-transmitted pathogens worldwide is US$ 22–30 billion (Lew-Tabor and Rodriguez Valle 2016). In Mexico and Brazil, the infestation of *R. microplus* results in losses in milk and meat, thus incurring an annual economic loss of US$ 0.573 and 3.24 billion, respectively. In Colombia, the annual losses associated with ticks and tick-borne diseases are estimated to be US$168 million (Rodriguez-Vivas et al. 2017).

Acaricides and macrocyclic lactones continue to be the best alternatives in controlling *R. microplus* ticks worldwide, and the frequent use of these drugs has led to the development of several resistant tick populations (Rodriguez-Vivas et al. 2018a, 2021).

Several populations of *R. microplus* have been found resistant to almost all commercially available acaricides that have been used for their control, including arsenics, organochlorides, carbamates, organophosphates (OPs), synthetic pyrethroids (SPs), macrocyclic lactones (MLs), formamidines, fipronil, and fluazuron

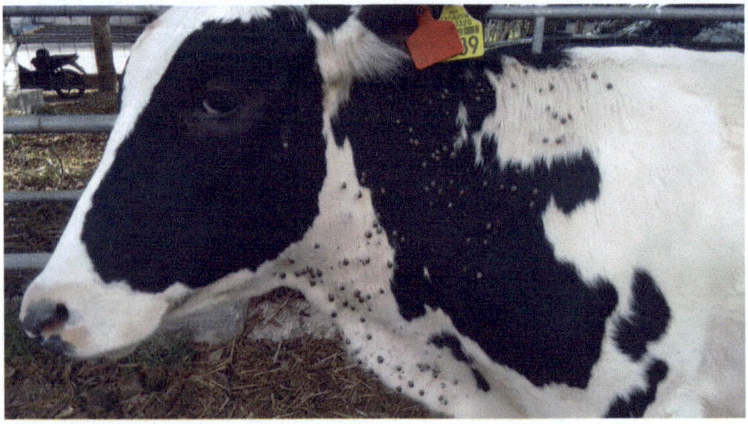

**Fig. 6.1** Cattle heavily infested with *R. microplus* ticks

(Perez-Cogollo et al. 2010a, b; Ghosh et al. 2015; Klafke et al. 2017; Rodriguez-Vivas et al. 2006, 2007, 2018a, 2022).

Resistance to acaricides is a natural selection in response to selection pressure and the frequent use of different classes of acaricides for tick control (Rodriguez-Vivas et al. 2018a).

The distribution of this resistance makes efficient control of ticks impossible; for this reason, it is prudent to administer these acaricides wisely. In this chapter, we will describe the use of integrated tick management to minimize the impact of acaricide resistance on livestock production worldwide.

## 6.2 Chemical Control of Cattle Ticks

The use of acaricides and MLs has been the main tool for controlling ticks in cattle. The main classes of these chemicals used in cattle for tick control are described below.

### 6.2.1 Acaricides and Macrocyclic Lactones

The acaricides and LM available on the market to control ticks act systemically or through direct contact with the ectoparasite. All commercial acaricides are neurotoxic and have their action on the nervous system of ticks (Taylor 2001). The main application methods for the delivery of an acaricide for control in livestock require different formulations such as emulsifiable concentrates, wettable powders, or flowable products that could be diluted in water and applied to animals by immersion in a dipping vat, spray race, and hand sprayer (Fig. 6.2). In developing countries, hand-dressing is another procedure (apply acaricide according to the sites where the tick preferentially attaches to the host, according to the species of the tick to be treated) (De Meneghi et al. 2016). More recently, other methods have been used such as pour-on products, acaricide-impregnated ear tags, pheromone acaricide-impregnated devices attached in different ways to cattle, and injectables (Rodríguez-Vivas et al. 2022).

The drug classes, arsenicals, and organochlorides were used to control cattle ticks, and nowadays safer drug classes are used as acaricides to treat cattle ticks; this includes carbamates, OPs, SPs, phenylpyrazoles, amidines, insect growth regulators, MLs, and recently, isoxazolines (Aguilar-Tipacamu and Rodriguez-Vivas 2003; Rodriguez-Vivas et al. 2014; da Costa et al. 2023).

In this chapter, the main acaricides and LMs used to control ticks in cattle farming will be presented in two tables that include the families to which they belong, modes and sites of action, as well as the main characteristics for their use in cattle.

The site and mode of action of currently used acaricides and MLs to control cattle ticks are presented in Table 6.1.

Although acaricides and LMs have been effective in controlling ticks in cattle, they have negative aspects such as the high direct cost of drugs, the selection of resistant populations, and the risk of losing the stability of enzootic diseases and

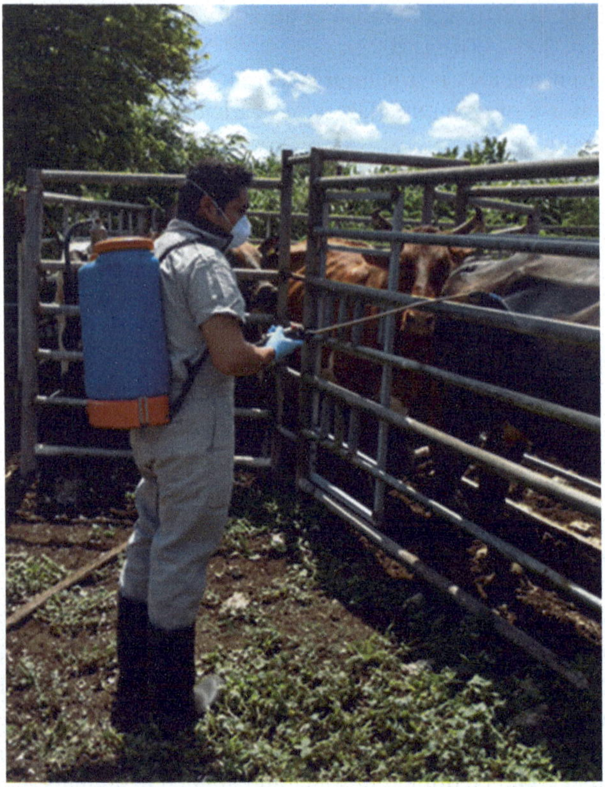

**Fig. 6.2** Spraying method for acaricide treatment in cattle

causing production losses during animal handling. Additionally, they produce an environmental impact and can be toxic to public health (De Meneghi et al. 2016).

### 6.2.2 Acaricide Mixture Formulations

Mixtures of acaricides are used to reduce the rate of evolution of acaricide resistance. It is based on the assumptions that one individual tick will not have resistant alleles to two chemical classes with different modes of action, the resistance to each acaricide is monogenic, there is no potential for cross-resistance, each acaricide has a similar persistent effect, resistant individuals in the population are rare, and some individuals in the population remain untreated (Tabashnik 1990; Githaka et al. 2022). It is worth clarifying that acaricide mixtures for tick control must be used before the resistance phenomenon to one acaricide occurs, and each acaricide must have similar treatment rates and different modes of action, sites of action, or different resistance mechanisms.

**Table 6.1** Site and mode of action of currently used acaricides, macrocyclic lactones, and isoxazolines to control cattle ticks

| Antiparasitic drug | Site of action | Mode of action |
|---|---|---|
| *Acaricides* | | |
| Organophosphates | Acetylcholinesterase | Inhibit the action of acetylcholinesterase at cholinergic synapses and at muscle end plates |
| Pyrethroids | Voltage-gated $Na^+$-channel | Prolonged opening of Na+-channels in nerve, muscle, and other excitable cells |
| Formamidines | Octopamine tyramine receptors | Act as agonists by stimulating the octopamine receptors, the consequence is a decrease in intracellular $Ca2^+$ and activation of $K^+$ efflux, leading to interruption of the nerve impulse and death. Inhibit the activity of monoamine oxidase enzymes |
| Phenylpyrazoles | GABA receptor | Block transmission of signals by the inhibitory neurotransmitter, GABA. The compound binds within the chloride channel and consequently inhibits the flux of $cl^-$ ions into the nerve cell |
| Benzoylphenyl urea | Chitin formation | Chitin synthesis inhibitors |
| Isoxazolines | γ-Aminobutyric acid chloride channels and glutamate-gated chloride channels | Inhibit γ-aminobutyric acid chloride channels and glutamate-gated chloride channels |
| *Macrocyclic lactones* | | |
| Milbemycins | Glutamate-gated chloride channel | High affinity for the glutamate-gated ion channels near GABA-gated Cl-channels |
| Avermectins | Glutamate-gated chloride channel | Block nerve signals by interfering with the glutamate-gated chloride channel receptors |
| Spinosyns | Nicotinic acetylcholine receptors | Disruption of nicotinic acetylcholine receptors. Spinosyn A may have another mode of action |

Adapted from Rodriguez-Vivas et al. (2014, 2018a, b)

The mixture of different groups of acaricides/insecticides has been synergistically effective, and this has been used for several years in many countries to control ticks (Lovis et al. 2013; Rodriguez-Vivas et al. 2018a). The following synergist effects of acaricide have been demonstrated to control ticks: amitraz + permethrin (Li et al. 2007), amitraz + fipronil (Prullage et al. 2011), and amitraz + deltamethrin (Barré et al. 2008). The combination of OPs (chlorfenvinphos + ethion) with SPs (cypermethrin + deltamethrin) has been successfully applied for the control of *R. microplus* (George et al. 2004). The combination of OPs (i.e., dichlorvos) with tetrachlorvinphos was successfully used to control OPs-resistant populations of *R. microplus* (Davey et al. 2013).

### 6.2.3 Synergized Acaricide Formulation

The use of synergists helps eliminate resistant tick populations and prolong the use of acaricides with low efficacy due to metabolic resistance (Rodriguez-Vivas et al. 2018a). Enzyme activity inhibitors such as diethyl maleate (an inhibitor of glutathione-S-transferases), triphenyl phosphate (an esterase inhibitor), verbutin (an inhibitor of certain cytochrome P450 isoforms), and piperonyl butoxide (PBO) (an inhibitor of cytochrome P450 monooxygenase) (Li et al. 2007) should be appropriately added to pesticides to mitigate metabolic resistances (Showler et al. 2020). Li et al. (2010) showed the potentiation effect of reduced verbutin and PBO concentrations on the efficacy of permethrin, amitraz, and coumaphos on a resistant strain of *R. microplus*.

In the Mexican tropics, Rodriguez-Vivas et al. (2013) demonstrated under in vitro (laboratory bioassays) and in vivo (field efficacy trials in cattle) conditions that the mixture of cypermethrin, amitraz, and PBO caused high mortality of SP-resistant ticks.

### 6.2.4 Rotation of Acaricides

Alternating acaricides in tick treatment reduce the selection pressure from any acaricide, but this assumes that resistance no longer exists and that the resistant frequency of individuals to each acaricide used will decline during the application of the alternate product (Rodriguez-Vivas et al. 2018a).

Some studies have demonstrated the benefits of rotating acaricides in terms of delaying the development of strong resistance in a population of ticks that initially presented a low level of resistance to an acaricide. It has been shown that amitraz can be used effectively in a rotation program because there is some evidence of loss of resistance to amitraz in populations of ticks on farms where cattle were treated with other alternatives. This may be due to the recessive mode of inheriting resistance to amitraz (Jonsson et al. 2010a). Conversely, in *R. microplus* resistant to SPs and OPs, reversion to susceptibility is difficult because it has been demonstrated that resistance persists for several years (Rodriguez-Vivas et al. 2011). In addition, Aguilar-Tipacamú et al. (2008) determined that the main mode of inheritance of SPs in *R. microplus* is through a partially dominant trait.

In a field study in Australia, cattle with *R. microplus* amitraz resistance were treated with spinosad alone, amitraz alone, or a rotation between amitraz and spinosad every 2 months over 4 years. The application of spinosad alone and the application of spinosad in rotation with amitraz treatments produced the loss of amitraz resistance and a return to total or almost total susceptibility to amitraz (Jonsson et al. 2010b).

Another method of using rotation is the use of "generational treatment," in which each tick generation is treated with a different class of acaricide (Centenaro et al. 2022). For generational treatment to be efficient, the tick population must be susceptible to at least three acaricides classes. In Argentina, Nava et al. (2020) showed the efficacy of rotating treatments for the control of *R. microplus* using three classes of acaricides over 1 year. Although generational treatment was originally designed for areas with three generations of ticks per year, this concept might be used in areas where there are 4–5 generations per year by performing additional treatments (Centenaro et al. 2022).

### 6.2.5 Selective Treatments

Selective treatment is based on the preservation of a subpopulation not treated with an acaricide, that is, refugia (Molento et al. 2013). In selective treatment, only cattle that have a parasite load greater than a predetermined threshold should be treated with acaricides (i.e., ≥30 standard engorged female ticks/animal).

Centenaro et al. (2022) evaluated two schemes to control a multiresistant *R. microplus* population on cattle under field conditions: (a) a rotation treatment with six treatments per year (spring–spring period) where four different classes of acaricide are used, and (b) a selective (partial) and rotation treatment, where only half of the cattle with the highest tick loads were treated. The author found that the two schemes were lower ticks loads than the nontreated group, but no significant differences between them.

## 6.3 Nonchemical Control of Cattle Ticks

It is imperative to develop and implement nonchemical techniques to minimize selection for acaricide resistance in cattle tick. Furthermore, the frequent use of acaricides due to the resistance phenomenon produces negative impacts on the environment, animal health, and animal-derived products. For these reasons, it is necessary to implement nonchemical alternatives that are environmentally friendly and important for the mitigation of acaricide resistance.

The main nonchemical control alternatives that have been used to control ticks in cattle are described below.

### 6.3.1 Manual Removal of Ticks

The manual removal of ticks is a practice used on farms where there are a small number of animals and generally in developing countries (Rodriguez-Vivas et al. 2018a). Engorged ticks, ranging from 5 to 10 mm in length, are removed from cattle in the morning.

In a study carried out in Nigeria, it was found that the lowest prevalence of *A. variegatum* (6.3%) was due to the manual collection of ticks, carried out up to three times a week during the wet season of the year (Pullan 1980). In central Nigeria, combining manual removal of ticks with conventional acaricides during the wet season when the parasite load is high, efficient tick control was achieved (Lorusso et al. 2013).

WingChing-Jones (2015) demonstrated the benefit of manual removal of *R. microplus* ticks on Jersey dairy cows in Costa Rica. The technique reduced the tick population by 21%. During the hand-picking of ticks, care is required. Cattle ticks can transmit pathogens to humans (i.e., Crimean–Congo hemorrhagic fever virus) (Muhammad et al. 2008).

The efficacy of hand removal is conditional on the number of animals in the herd and personnel availability. This practice is only used on small farms where the number of tick loads on cattle is low.

### 6.3.2 Host Resistance

Cattle exhibit contrasting, heritable phenotypes for infestation with *R. microplus* and related tick species due to the co-evolution of resistant cattle with ticks and many years of selective breeding. *Bos taurus taurus* cattle breeds have a lower resistance (~90% resistance) to *R. microplus* ticks than *Bos taurus indicus* cattle (~98–99% resistance), which is highly resistant (Fig. 6.3) (Jonsson et al. 2014; Tabor et al. 2017). The heritability of tick resistance in cattle is high. In *Bos indicus*–cross cattle, for example, the heritability estimate for the burden of *R. microplus* is moderate ($h^2 = 0.34$, Mackinnon et al. 1991).

Physical barriers, immunological response, and behavior that affect tick resistance include immune response, density of the fur coat, skin pigmentation, skin vibration, skin thickness, and/or self-cleaning ability, tongue papillae, and odor (Gasparin et al. 2007).

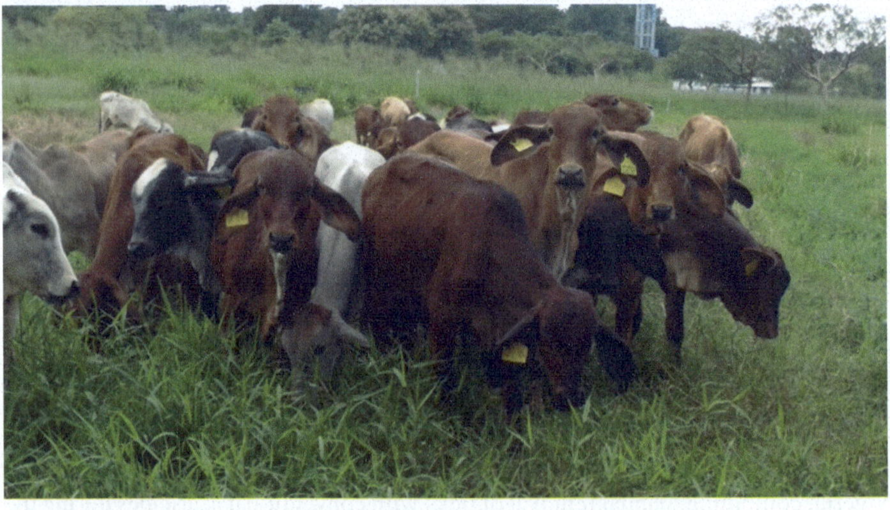

**Fig. 6.3** *Bos indicus* cattle identify as resistant to ticks

The difference in tick resistance between breeds is attributed to differences in immunological and cellular responses. Tick resistance generally occurs against attaching immature stages (i.e., larvae). The greatest larval mortality occurs mostly within 24 h of finding a host. There is evidence of innate and adaptive immune response to tick infestation, and it appears that the relative importance of each differs between *Bos taurus taurus* and *Bos taurus indicus* cattle. There are conflicting results regarding the role of humoral immunity in tick resistance, and some studies indicate that strong IgG responses to tick antigens are not protective. A strong T-cell-mediated response directed against larval stages, as mounted by *Bos taurus indicus* cattle, might be protective (Jonsson et al. 2014). The skin of resistant breeds also contained higher numbers of mast cells, eosinophils, and basophils with upregulated proteases, collagens, cathepsins, keratins, and extracellular matrix proteins in response to feeding ticks (Tabor et al. 2017).

Susceptible breeds are commonly found to be associated with the increased expression of toll-like receptors, calcium-binding proteins, MHC class II, and complement factors with an increased presence of neutrophils in the skin following tick feeding. *B. taurus indicus* breeds had higher levels of T cells present in the skin before tick infestation and thus seemed to respond to ticks more efficiently (Tabor et al. 2017). For more information on the resistance mechanisms of cattle to tick infestation, we recommend Jonsson et al. (2014) and Tabor et al. (2017).

The potential reduction in acaricide requirement arising from the concerted selection and breeding of cattle for increased host resistance is very substantial (Rodriguez-Vivas et al. 2018a). In Holstein cattle, out of 100 *R. microplus* larvae they rejected 85 and in Brahman out of 100 larvae, they rejected 99, and as *Bos taurus taurus* is crossed with *Bos taurus indicus* the natural resistance of *Bos taurus taurus* increases noticeably (Rodriguez-Vivas et al. 2018b). Given that resistance to ticks is a polygenic trait, which is heritable (Mapholi et al. 2014), the genetic selection of resistant cattle is an important tool to reduce dependence on the use of acaricides. The use of genomic technologies can help improve the accuracy of genetic selection by identifying markers or genes associated with the resistance of cattle breeds to ticks (Marima et al. 2020).

### 6.3.3 Plant Species that Are Unfavorable to Ticks

The identification and application of some types of leguminous or grass plants with acaricidal activity or repellent effects still need greater validation at the field level for possible inclusion in integrated tick management schemes (FAO 2004). Some plants have been shown to act as attractants for ticks, that is, *Stylosanthes scabra* (tropical legume) can trap between 12 and 27% of larvae in the sticky exudate of glandular trichomes found on stems and leaves (Wilson et al. 1989). Another example is the African shrub *Acalypha fruticosa*, which attracts larvae of *R. appendiculatus*, which lie quiescent on the underside of the leaf plant (Hassan et al. 1994).

In Mexico, the effect of the forage grasses *Melinis minutiflora* and *Andropogon gayanus* has been evaluated, which can trap ticks through their stylozating secretions and adherent villi, the first being more capable of control. This type of plant, grown in strategically used pastures, can decrease the risk of tick–cattle encounters, and thus contribute to reducing the use of acaricides (Rodriguez-Vivas et al. 2018b).

### 6.3.4 Pasture Alternation and/or Rotation

The survival time of the nonparasitic phase of ticks in pastures depends directly on the climate condition and the type of vegetation, which determines the abundance of the populations (Nava et al. 2013). Pasture spelling was implemented to produce the death of tick larvae by rotating cattle into "clean" paddocks at given time intervals. Rotational grazing with a short rest period (20 days) showed higher tick infestations on host than did those in continuous grazing. When pastures are grazed with longer rest times, it is a promising nonpharmacological tool to control cattle ticks (Cruz-González et al. 2023).

Generations of new populations of *R. microplus* increase throughout the year, a phenomenon linked with global warming, leading to the need for studies of the monthly fluctuation of this tick species. A successful tick-control strategy will also depend on the interaction of biotic and abiotic factors that lead to seasonal population abundance that, in turn, determines the behavior of ticks in each area (Cruz-González et al. 2023).

Depending on the weather, under tropical field conditions, the average pre-hatching time is 30–35 days. In tropical climates, larvae have better activity adhering to the potential host when they have 3–5 days of hatching, indicating that the adequate time for the presence of viable and vigorous larvae in the pasture could be between 33 and 40 days after the detachment of engorged ticks (Rodriguez-Vivas et al. 2014). In Venezuela, the use of computer modeling made it possible to predict that using a pasture rotation of 36 days of rest in dry seasons and 24 days in rainy seasons allows a substantial reduction in tick infestations (FAO 2004).

Recently, in the humid tropics of Mexico, Cruz-González et al. (2023) found that a 30-day rest period for pastures (without the presence of cattle) did not reduce the presence of ticks on animals but a 45-day rest period does reduce the presence of *R. microplus* ticks on cattle.

### 6.3.5 Pasture Burning

In many farms in different countries, burning pasture is a widely used practice for tick control (Abbas et al. 2014). Fire directly affects ticks due to the physical exposure of larvae, adult females, and eggs to high temperatures. Indirectly, pasture burning affects the vegetation layer that serves as protection against ticks (Rodriguez-Vivas et al. 2014).

In Zambia, cattle on land that was annually burnt had fewer ticks than those on land that was not annually burnt (Baars 1999), and the tick species involved were

*A. variegatum*, *H. truncatum*, *R. e. evertsi*, *B. decoloratus*, and *R. sanguineus*. A South African study of pasture burning also showed a reduction in tick populations (*A. hebraeum*, *B. decoloratus*, *R. appendiculatus*, *R. e. evertsi*, *R. zambeziensis*) after burning (Spickett et al. 1992). Studies in the United States with *A. americanum* have shown that annual burning reduces the density of all life stages but only temporarily as ticks recolonize burnt areas (Cully Jr 1999). Most published studies demonstrated that in the time immediately following a prescribed burn there is a considerable reduction in the number of ticks at the burn site. Fulk et al. (2022) showed the effects of prescribed fire on ticks (*Ixodes* spp. vectors of Lyme disease) spread and propagation in a spatial setting. It was found that while ticks can recover relatively quickly following a burn, annual and high-intensity-prescribed burns could reduce the incidence of ticks in and around the area that is burned. In another study, Polito et al. (2013) studied the tick abundance and tick loading on cattle in response to patch burning. The authors found significant reductions in tick infestation on cattle in burning-treated pastures, indicating that pasture burning could be used to help control ticks in pastures.

Only when pastures have a very high infestation of tick larvae, multiple tick resistance to acaricide is present in a farm, and other nonpharmacological methods are not available, burning of some pastures is recommended. However, fire removes the ground cover, increases the risk of erosion, and generally reduces the quality of pasture. In some countries or specific areas, pasture burning is illegal.

### 6.3.6 Nutritional Management

Strategic feed supplementation with protein and energy is important in mediating acquired resistance to ticks. In a field study conducted in eastern Queensland, Australia, feeding cattle with poor-quality pastures resulted in a significant loss of resistance in the *Bos taurus* and *B. indicus* × *B. taurus* heifers and steers to *R. microplus* (Maryam et al. 2012).

### 6.3.7 Plant Products and Secondary Metabolites with Acaricide Properties against Ticks

Medicinal plants have been demonstrated to be an alternative tool for the control of ticks by the secondary metabolites produced as a defense mechanism against conditions of biotic and abiotic stress. Such secondary metabolites can inhibit the synthesis of chitin or feeding and can decrease development, growth, or reproduction. Many species of plants have been evaluated for acaricidal activity, with the species studied mainly being members of the families Lamiaceae, Asteraceae, Fabaceae, Piperaceae, Poaceae, and Verbenaceae. Several studies have identified secondary metabolites (terpenes, coumarins, alcohols, stilbenes, acids, sulfureted compounds, and aldehydes) of essential oils and plant extracts, associated with acaricidal activities against different species of ticks (Rosado-Aguilar et al. 2017). Plant extracts and essential oils against different species of ticks have proven mortalities of 5–100% (larvae) and 60–100% (adults), as well as inhibition of egg hatching of 60–100%. Only a few secondary metabolites have confirmed acaricidal effects. For the essential oils, the plant compounds with confirmed activity are carvacrol, thymol, 1,8-cineol, and n-hexanal (Daemon et al. 2009; De Oliveira-Cruz et al. 2013). Meanwhile, for the plant extracts the active secondary metabolites are dibenzyldisulfide, dibenzyltrisulfide, and nicotine (Arceo-Medina et al. 2016). Currently, plumbagin, a naphthoquinone from *Diospyros*, was evaluated on *R. microplus* resistant to acaricides obtaining mortalities of 100 to 36.26%, and LC50% and LC99% of 0.011% and 0.019%, respectively (Gutiérrez-Wong et al. 2023). Only carvacrol, thymol, and 1,8-cineol have been evaluated for acaricidal activity under in vivo conditions (Borges et al. 2011; Rosado-Aguilar et al. 2017). *Eucalyptus* spp. leaf extracts demonstrated 6% efficacy against female *R. microplus* ticks (Costa et al. 2008).

In some countries, plants based on commercially available formulations such as MyggA Natural® from Sweden (*Corymbia citriodora* oil with a minimum of 50% *p*-menthane-3,8-diol (PMD), Citriodiol® from the United Kingdom [64% PMD (a mixture of the *cis* and *trans* isomers of *p*-menthane-3,8-diol), and Ixodes® from Mexico (neem extract) are being used for controlling ticks.

Several plant extracts and essential oils have shown good efficacies in in vitro conditions; however, only a few of them have also been evaluated on *R. microplus* naturally infested cattle to validate the results obtained.

For more information on the use of plant extracts, essential oils, and secondary metabolites with acaricidal properties against ticks, we recommend consulting the article by Rosado-Aguilar et al. (2017).

### 6.3.8 Vaccination

Vaccination is one of the alternatives for the control of *R. microplus*. Several tick vaccines were introduced to the market that are based on the use of the Bm86 antigen. The tick vaccines available on the market are based on hidden antigens from the gut of the tick that once inoculated into cattle induce the production of antibodies, which, when ingested by the tick, result in lysis of intestinal cells, reduced egg production, and reduced hatchability of eggs. Consequently, tick populations decline over time, although there is a little direct effect on tick mortality.

Two vaccines were placed on the market in the 1990s, TickGARD® (Australian origin) and Gavac® (Cuban origin) (Pereira et al. 2022), and one in 2017 Bovimune Ixovac® (Mexico) (https://lapisa.com/productos/bovimune-ixovac). The Tick Vac® vaccine was launched in Colombia and marketed in 2005 (polyprotein antigen from *R. microplus* larvae) and in Brazil (2010), with the sale restricted to farms that adhere to the cattle tick strategic control program. In 2018, the Go-Tick® vaccine (with the same formulation as Tick Vac®) was placed in the Colombian market without success.

There are some field challenge studies of current commercial vaccines, all of which show a trend of effective reduction in dependence on conventional acaricides for the control of *R. microplus*, up to 87% in the case of Gavac® in Cuba (Rodriguez-Valle et al. 2004). Go-Tick® in Colombia has presented satisfactory results in controlling up to 74.6% of the reproduction of *R. microplus* in cattle (Betancourt et al. 2005), and the use of this vaccine reduced the use of acaricides in 50% (from every 21 days to 5–72 days) (Betancourt 2017).

Currently, only two vaccines are on the market, Gavac® is used in Cuba, Brazil, Nicaragua, Panama, Bolivia, and Ecuador; meanwhile, Bovimune Ixovac® is in Mexico.

Vaccination is a safe tool because it does not generate residues that can contaminate milk, meat, and the environment, or otherwise pose a risk to animal health and humans (Willadsen 2006). The vaccines against ticks reduce tick loads but do not eliminate exposure to tick-borne diseases (TBDs) (Fragoso et al. 1998). Homologs of the BM86 antigen are present across species of the genus *Rhipicephalus* and in *Hyalomma* ticks and cross-protection using TickGARD® against *R. decoloratus* and *R. annulatus* (Pipano et al. 2003; Odongo et al. 2007) has been demonstrated. Additionally, an effect of a recombinant version of the Ra86 homolog encoded by *R. appendiculatus*, a three-host tick, on molting from larvae to adults has also been demonstrated (Olds et al. 2012).

In addition to the Bm86 antigen and its variants, different antigens have recently been characterized that are in the experimental phase as vaccine candidates; extracts and proteins from salivary glands (serpinas), ribosomal proteins, intracellular proteins (subolesin), aquaporins, ferritin 2, vitellogenin, among others. These antigens, when inoculated into animals, produce antibodies that, upon contact with ticks, cause lysis of intestinal cells and consequently a reduction in the survival of the arthropod, reducing reproductive parameters, and causing death (Rodriguez-Vivas et al. 2018b).

### 6.3.9 Biological Control

Biological control of ticks is the use of live organisms to reduce tick populations. It includes pathogens, nematodes, predators, and resistant plants. Research on predators has been conducted on nematodes, ants, beetles, and many bird species (Samish et al. 2004; Ojeda-Chi et al. 2011). African oxpeckers (*Buphagus africanus* and *B. erythrorhynchus*) are birds that feed on ticks (Samish et al. 2004).

### 6.3.10 Predators

In Guadeloupe, French West Indies, the common predators of parasitic or free stages of *Amblyomma variegatum* include birds, free-ranging chickens, grackles (*Quiscalus lugubris*), and cattle egrets (*Bubulcus ibis*) and tropical fire ants, *Solenopsis*

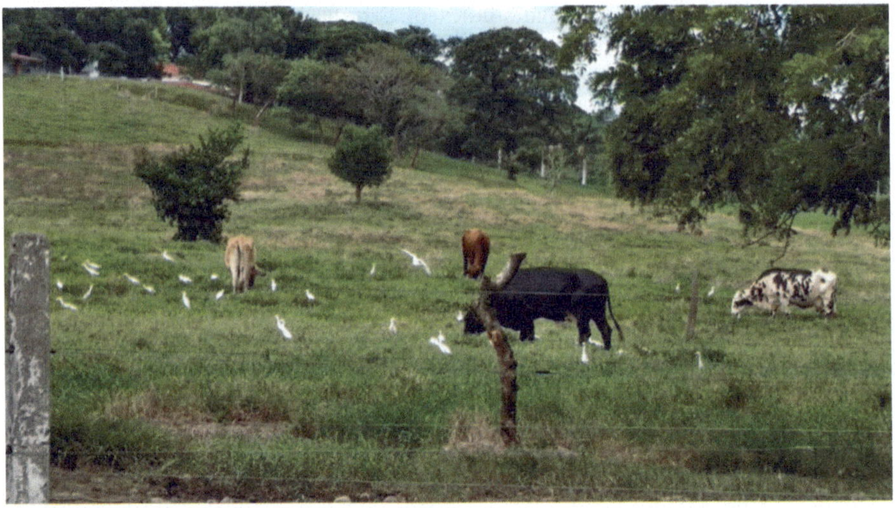

**Fig. 6.4** Birds (*Bubulcus ibis*) are common predators of ticks in the Mexican tropics

*geminate* (Barré et al. 1991). Wild birds and domestic fowl can be efficient predators of ticks. Oxpeckers (*B. erythrorhynchus* and *Buphagus africanus*), guinea fowl (*Numida meleagris*), domestic fowl (*Gallus domesticus*), and cattle egrets (*Bubulculus ibis*) are the species generally considered to have the most significant effects on tick populations (Fig. 6.4).

Although releases of the genus *Ixodiphagus* show potential value in controlling ticks, parasitoids and most predators have limited potential in integrated tick management because parasitoid wasps are not natural enemies of ticks and most predators of ticks are generalists (Samish et al. 2004).

### 6.3.11 Entomopathogenic Fungi

Entomopathogenic fungi (EPF), or arthropod pathogenic fungi, can naturally cause enzootic and epidemic infections against arthropod host populations (Fernandes et al. 2012). A plethora of laboratory and field studies have demonstrated that arthropod pathogenic fungi can induce high mortalities and reduce fecundity and egg viability in experimentally infected ticks (Kaaya et al. 1996; Fernandes et al. 2012). So far, most studies on the anti-tick activities of EPF have mainly used isolates of three fungal genera *Beauveria* (Hypocreales: Cordycipitaceae), *Metarhizium* (Hypocreales: Clavicipitaceae), and *Akanthomyces* (formerly, *Lecanicillium*, Cordycipitaceae, Hypocreales) (Alonso-Díaz and Fernández-Salas 2021).

In the Mexican tropics, *M. anisopliae* were evaluated to control *R. microplus*. The efficacies in laboratory conditions for larvae and adult stages were 45–100 and

100%, respectively. Meanwhile, the efficacy of controlling *R. microplus* larvae on vegetation varied from 68% to 100%. Global efficacy to control *R. microplus* in laboratory and field conditions (on cattle and vegetation) are 50–100 and 36–90% (Ojeda-Chi et al. 2010).

In Kenya, Kaaya and Hassan (2000) sprayed *R. decoloratus* with aqueous suspensions of *M. anisopliae* and *B. bassiana* feeding on Zebu cattle in farms, and the mortality and egg viability of the engorged ticks were recorded after 6 weeks. They also conducted field experiments by spraying paddocks infested with larvae of *R. appendiculatus* and containing Zebu cattle with aqueous suspensions and then counting the number of ticks on all cattle. The aqueous formulations of both fungi induced 30–40% higher mortality and reduced *R. decoloratus* egg hatchability by 48–68% relative to the control treatment. Moreover, after 6 months of spraying the paddocks, the mean numbers of adult *R. appendiculatus* on cattle had been reduced by 80–92% compared to controls. In Brazil, the efficacy after spraying *R. microplus*-infested cattle with an oil-based formulation of Metarril SPs Organic (an *M. anisopliae*-based commercial pesticide) with a backpack pump sprayer system increased in the second week after treatment, reaching 90.5% over the control group, corresponding to a substantial reduction in the number of ticks observed with the control (Camargo et al. 2016). The use of entomopathogenic fungal formulations (based on conidia, blastospores, or microsclerotia) against the nonparasitic phases of *R. microplus* (i.e., applied to the infested pasture) in Brazil under field and semi-field conditions has also been reported with successful results (Mesquita et al. 2020; Marciano et al. 2021).

In Brazil, Marciano et al. (2021) tested granular formulations based on microsclerotia and blastospores of *M. robertsii* against *R. microplus* in a semi-field experiment and recorded a significantly reduced number of tick larvae, with 64.8% relative efficacy.

Although many studies have demonstrated that entomopathogenic fungi can infect and kill all developmental stages of tick species, their efficacies in the field are often weak and inconsistent with the laboratory results (Fernandes et al. 2012). Low relative humidity, high UV radiation, and high temperature can negatively affect entomopathogenic fungal virulence (Scheepmaker and Butt 2010). Formulations and delivery methods are actively being enhanced to optimize the infectivity and virulence of entomopathogenic fungi under field conditions (Maniania et al. 2007; Jackson et al. 2010).

One of the main limitations of entomopathogenic fungi is their stability, which is why their large-scale production can be expensive. Most manufacturers would recommend the same application method for entomopathogenic fungi as used for other chemical pesticides (Shelton and Roush 2000).

Despite these limitations, entomopathogenic fungi can become established in the field and continue to constantly act on ticks when there are adequate humidity and temperature conditions (Rodriguez-Vivas et al. 2018b).

### 6.3.12 Entomopathogenic Nematodes

Several studies have demonstrated that entomopathogenic nematodes (EPN) are potential tick control agents (Singh et al. 2018; Goolsby et al. 2019). Some species such as *Rhipicephalus annulatus* are far more susceptible to EPN than *Hyalomma excavatum*, *R. sanguineus*, or *R. bursa*, which may be due to the thickness of their cuticle (Samish et al. 2000). In laboratory studies that looked at the virulence of entomopathogenic nematodes to the larval, nymphal, and adult stages of *H. excavatum*, *R. bursa*, *R. microplus*, and *R. sanguineus* to two strains of *Steinernema riobravae*, *Steinernema carpocapsae*, and three strains of *Heterorhabditis bacteriophora*, adult ticks were more susceptible (80–100% mortality) in a dish containing 5000 infective juveniles of *H. bacteriophora* IS-3 or IS-5 strains, isolated in Israel, compared to preimaginal stages (Samish et al. 1999; Singh et al. 2018).

In Brazil, a study reported the efficacy of *H. bacteriophora* for tick control under field conditions (Filgueiras et al. 2023). This study used insect cadavers (*Tenebrio molitor*) fully colonized with *H. bacteriophora*. After placing the insect cadavers, *R. microplus* engorged females were distributed on the soil. On days 42 and 63, the apical portion of the grasses with *R. microplus* larvae was collected and quantified. The larval population of *R. microplus* was reduced up to 73.1% in plots treated with *H. bacteriophora* at day 63 after treatment (Filgueiras et al. 2023).

Remotely operated sprayers have been designed to apply *H. bacteriophora* in a water solution to control tick-infested deer and nilgai antelope in South Texas (Goolsby et al. 2019). Entomopathogenic nematodes have no mammalian toxicity and are therefore viable alternatives to conventional or organic acaricides, especially in environmentally sensitive areas (Shapiro-Ilan et al. 2017).

## 6.4 Integrated Tick Management (ITM)

Integrated tick management (ITM) consists of the association of the population dynamics of tick species and the environment using a combination of sustainable methods and techniques that are compatible and that maintain low levels of tick populations that cause economic losses (Rodriguez-Vivas et al. 2018b).

The ITM involves the systematic application of two or more techniques to control tick populations, which adversely affect cattle. The principal aim is to obtain tick control in a more sustainable, environmentally compatible, and cost-effective manner than is achievable with a single technology (Willadsen 2006).

In the development of approaches that allow effective management of tick populations, minimize nontarget effects, and preserve the availability of our existing acaricides, it is essential to develop more fully the use of ITM. In such approaches, cascades of management tactics may be deployed as and when necessary, with acaricide available as just one component, to be used in appropriate circumstances (Rodriguez-Vivas et al. 2022). The consensus in the ITM is to reduce the frequency of acaricide application, but this is not always easy in some animal production in the tropics and subtropics (Kunz and Kemp 1994).

### 6.4.1 Basic Knowledge before ITM Implementation

Before the implementation of ITM, basic knowledge of the region is required. It is important to understand the biology of the cattle tick in the region, its epidemiology, and climatic conditions during the year, as well as knowledge of the pharmacological and nonpharmacological control, government policies in each country, the effectiveness of the acaricides applied over time, and establish the best application strategies.

### 6.4.2 Barriers to Their Availability and Implementation

Besides the advantages of the ITM, there is poor adoption, mainly in developing countries. Parsa et al. (2014) studied the obstacles to ITM adoption in developing countries and found that the main obstacles are insufficient technical support and training for producers (53%), lack of policies and government support for tick control (39%), and producers having low levels of education (22%). Other barriers are ITM being too difficult to implement (18%), the powerful influence of the pharmaceutical industry (16%), and lack of financing to implement ITM, especially long-term funding (16%), among others.

### 6.4.3 Role of Technical Support

Trained technical personnel play an important role in the implementation of ITM. Personnel must be in direct contact with farmers, field workers, and extension veterinarians. They must be trained to identify tick species present on animals, calculate an average number of standard ticks per animal, indicate when to apply acaricide treatments to tick-infested cattle, practical use of different acaricide application methods, establish acaricide rotation program, determine the capacity in liters of the immersion dip, etc. (Rodriguez-Vivas et al. 2022).

### 6.4.4 Economic Threshold

Economic threshold levels of tick load rather than a calendar date should indicate when animals are treated. Cattle should be inspected for ticks, and the number of standard females (>4 mm) must be calculated on one side of the animal and then multiplied by 2. In the tropics when cattle have ≥50 standard ticks, acaricide treatment is recommended (Rodriguez-Vivas et al. 2022). If the tick infestation is below economic thresholds, then acaricide treatments should not be made. This will decrease the environmental and safety concerns for the cattle, the livestock producers, and the consumers (FAO 2004).

### 6.4.5 ITM Success Stories

Several studies have been conducted to evaluate the ITM in different countries to control cattle ticks. Some success histories in the use of ITM are presented below.

***Antitick Vaccine and Acaricides*** In Mexico, Redondo et al. (1999, 2004), using an ITM employing vaccination with Gavac® and amidine treatments, under field conditions achieved nearly 100% control of *R. microplus* populations resistant to OPs and SPs. This technique effectively controls tick infestations while reducing the number of acaricide treatments and consequently the rise of *R. microplus* populations resistant to acaricides. Additionally, after 10 years of using this ITM in a Mexican farm, a substantial reduction in acaricide treatments has been achieved (from 24 to 7–8 per year) with a consequent reduction in tick infestation from 100 to 20 adult ticks per animal (De la Fuente et al. 2007). In Uruguay, Solari et al. (2007) carried out an ITM using ivermectin, acaricides, and hemoparasite vaccine. In this study, the benefit achieved with the use of integrated control was proven by reducing the number of ticks, clinical cases of hemoparasites, and blood-sucking flies.

***Entomopathogenic Fungus and Acaricides*** In Brazil, Bahiense et al. (2006) evaluated the association of deltamethrin and the entomopathogenic fungus *M. anisopliae* against *R. microplus* larvae resistant to SPs. High mortality rates were observed when deltamethrin was associated with the entomopathogen. The authors concluded that this association could be used as a method for integrated control of *R. microplus*. Bahiense et al. (2008) evaluated the combination of deltamethrin and *M. anisopliae* in calves artificially infested with *R. microplus* ticks and reported a 30.2% effectiveness in controlling this tick species and a 60% reduction in their oviposition.

***Acaricides and Synergists*** In the United States, Li et al. (2010) evaluated the synergistic effects of verbutin (a member of alkynyl synergists that act as a specific inhibitor of certain P450 isoforms that are involved in the metabolic detoxification of certain pesticides) on three commonly used acaricides against larvae of both susceptible and resistant strains of *R. microplus*. The use of verbutin/permethrin increased the synergism ratio from 2.4 to 4.4, verbutin/coumaphos from 1.5 to 6.0, and verbutin/amitraz from 1.8 to 15.

Rodriguez-Vivas et al. (2013) determined the efficacy of cypermethrin, amitraz, and piperonylbutoxide (PBO, a potent inhibitor of the P450) mixtures, through laboratory bioassays and on-animal efficacy studies, for the control of SP-resistant *R. microplus* on cattle in the Mexican tropics. Excellent synergism was observed with the mixture of cypermethrin + amitraz + PBO, and this mixture was the most effective in killing resistant tick larvae in laboratory conditions (96.7–100% of larval mortality). In the field study, the mixtures containing cypermethrin + PBO (80.6–97.3%) and cypermethrin + amitraz (87.0–89.7%) showed higher efficacies than cypermethrin alone (76.3–80.5%). The highest level of efficacy was obtained with the mixture of cypermethrin + amitraz + PBO, which yielded >95% control that persisted for 28 days after treatment against naturally infested cattle with *R. microplus* in the Mexican tropics.

***Acaricides and Pheromones*** Nchu et al. (2009) evaluated the use of attraction–aggregation–attachment pheromone to enhance exposure to *Amblyomma variegatum*. The emulsifiable formulation gave the highest relative tick reduction in both seasons: 46.5% and 54.7% and in dry and rainy seasons, respectively. This association could be used to control *R. microplus* on cattle.

***Acaricides, Pasture Burning, Fungi, Selected Cattle Treatment, and Paddock Rotation*** In a farm with cattle and red deer (with 15% mortality due to tick infestation) in the sub-humid tropics of Mexico, both animal species were treated with acaricides 11–12 times per year. An ITM program was established with six acaricides treatments (fluazuron and coumaphos) a year, paddock rotation (every 42 days in the dry season, every 28 days in the rainy season), annual burning of 20% of grasslands, selective treatment in cattle in months of lower incidence of ticks (2 times/year), and application of two treatments with *M. anisopliae* to 20% of pastures. In the cattle herd, the ITM effectively controls tick infestations while reducing the number of chemical acaricide treatments (50%), and tick reduction burden by 30% (ticks/animal did not exceed 70), tick larvae were reduced by 40–80% in paddocks treated with *M. anisopliae*. In the red deer herd, the mortality due to tick infestations was reduced from 15% to 0%.

ITM in cattle has been successful in certain circumstances, but it is necessary to emphasize comprehensive parasite control and transfer this technology to the field level. The main challenge for veterinarians, the veterinary pharmaceutical industry, governments, and farmers is to integrate the chemical and nonchemical technologies available for sustainable tick control.

## References

Abbas RZ, Zaman MA, Colwell DD, Gilleard J, Iqbal Z (2014) Acaricide resistance in cattle ticks and approaches to its management: the state of play. Vet Parasitol 203(1–2):6–20. https://doi.org/10.1016/j.vetpar.2014.03.006

Aguilar-Tipacamu G, Rodriguez-Vivas RI (2003) Effect of moxidectin against natural infestation of the cattle tick *Boophilus microplus* (Acari: Ixodidae) in the Mexican tropics. Vet Parasitol 111:211–216. https://doi.org/10.1016/s0304-4017(02)00355-2

Aguilar-Tipacamú G, Miller RJ, Hernández-Ortiz R, Rodriguez-Vivas RI, Vásquez-Peláez C, García-Vázquez Z, Olvera VF, Rosario-Cruz R (2008) Inheritance of pyrethroid resistance and a sodium channel gene mutation in the cattle tick *Boophilus microplus*. Parasitol Res 103(3):633–639. https://doi.org/10.1007/s00436-008-1024-2

Alonso-Díaz MA, Fernández-Salas A (2021) Entomopathogenic fungi for tick control in cattle livestock from Mexico. Front Fungal Biol 2:657694. https://doi.org/10.3389/ffunb.2021.657694

Arceo-Medina GN, Rosado-Aguilar JA, Rodríguez-Vivas RI, Borges-Argaez R (2016) Synergistic and antagonistic action of fatty acids: sulphides and stilbene against acaricide-resistant *Rhipicephalus microplus* ticks. Vet Parasitol 228:121–125. https://doi.org/10.1016/j.vetpar.2016.08.023

Baars RMT (1999) The effect of rangeland fires cattle tick infestation in Western Zambia. Trop Anim Health Prod 31:275–278. https://doi.org/10.1023/A:1005299605959

Bahiense TC, Fernandes EKK, Bittencourt VR (2006) Compatibility of the fungus *Metarhizium anisopliae* and deltamethrin to control a resistant strain of *Boophilus microplus* tick. Vet Parasitol 141(3–4):319–324. https://doi.org/10.1016/j.vetpar.2006.05.011

Bahiense TC, Fernandes EKK, Angelo Ida C, Perinotto WM, Bittencourt VR (2008) Performance of *Metarhizium anisopliae* and its combination with deltamethrin against a pyrethroid-resistant strain of *Boophilus microplus* in a stall test. Ann NY Acad Sci 1149:242–245. https://doi.org/10.1196/annals.1428.031

Barré N, Mauléon H, Garris G, Kermarrec A (1991) Predators of the tick *Amblyomma variegatum* (Acari: Ixodidae) in Guadeloupe, French West Indies. Exp Appl Acarol 12(3–4):163–170. https://doi.org/10.1007/bf01193464

Barré N, Li AY, Miller RJ, Gaia H, Delathiere JM, Davey RB, George JE (2008) *In vitro* and *in vivo* evaluation of deltamethrin and amitraz mixtures for the control of *Rhipicephalus* (*Boophilus*) *microplus* (Acari,Ixodidae) in New Caledonia. Vet Parasitol 155:110–119. https://doi.org/10.1016/j.vetpar.2008.04.016

Betancourt A (2017) Las vacunas contra la garrapata común del ganado: componente fundamental para el control integrado del parásito. Acovez 46(3):15–20

Betancourt A, Patiño F, Torres O, Eugenio B (2005) Prueba de establo para evaluar la efectividad de la vacuna Tick Vac®, contra la garrapata *Boophilus microplus*. Acovez 34(3):18–25

Betancur-Hurtado OJ, Giraldo-Ríos C (2018) Ticks and tick-borne pathogens. In: Economic and health impact of the ticks in production animals. IntechOpen, pp 1–19. https://doi.org/10.5772/intechopen.81167

Borges LMF, Sousa LAD, Barbosa CS (2011) Perspectives for the use of plant extracts to control the cattle tick *Rhipicephalus* (*Boophilus*) *microplus*. Revista Brasileria de Parasitología Veterinaria 20(2):89–96. https://doi.org/10.1590/s1984-29612011000200001

Camargo MG, Nogueira MRS, Marciano AF, Wendell MSP, Coutinho-Rodrigues CJB, Scott FB, Angelo IC, Prata MCA, Bittencourt VREP (2016) *Metarhizium anisopliae* for controlling *Rhipicephalus microplus* ticks. Vet Parasitol 223:38–42. https://doi.org/10.1016/j.vetpar.2016.04.014

Centenaro FC, Barbieri A, Rico IB, Gonchoroski GZ, Jardim FT, Doyle RL, Dall'Agnol B, Reck J, Webster A (2022) Rotational and selective protocols using acaricides to control a multi-resistant strain of *Rhipicephalus microplus* under field conditions in Southern Brazil. Ticks and Tick-borne Diseases 13(5):101987. https://doi.org/10.1016/j.ttbdis.2022.101987

Costa FB, Vasconcelos PSDS, Silva AMM, Brandão VM, Silva IA, Teixeira WC, Guerra RDMSN, Santos ACG (2008) Eficácia de fitoterápicos em fêmeas ingurgitadas de *Boophilus microplus*, provenientes da mesorregião oeste do Maranhão, Brasil. Revista Brasileria de Parasitologia Veterinária 17(1):83–86

Cruz-González G, Pinos-Rodríguez JM, Alonso-Díaz MA, Romero-Salas D, Vicente-Martínez JG, Fernández-Salas A, Jarillo-Rodríguez J, Castillo Gallegos E (2023) Rotational grazing modifies *Rhipicephalus microplus* infestation in cattle in the humid tropics. Animals 13:915. https://doi.org/10.3390/ani13050915

Cully JF Jr (1999) Lone star tick abundance, fire and bison grazing in tallgrass prairie. J Range Manag 52:139–144

da Costa AJ, de Souza Martins JR, de Almeida Borges F, Vettorato LF, Barufi FB, Arreiro Amaral HO, Abujamra LC, Castro Rodrigues D, Zanetti LWD (2023) First report of the efficacy of a fluralaner-based pour-on product (Exzolt® 5%) against ectoparasites infesting cattle in Brazil. Parasit Vectors 16:336. https://doi.org/10.1186/s13071-023-05934-7

Daemon E, Monteiro CMO, Rosa LS, Clemente MA, Arcoverde A (2009) Evaluation of the acaricide activity of thymol on engorged and unengorged larvae of *Rhipicephalus sanguineus* (Latreille, 1808) (Acari: ixodidae). Parasitol Res 105(2):495–497. https://doi.org/10.1007/s00436-009-1426-9

Davey RB, Thomas DB, Pound JM, Lohmeyer KH, Miller RJ (2013) Efficacy of an organophosphate mixture against an organophosphate-resistant strain of *Rhipicephalus* (*Boophilus*) *microplus* (Acari: Ixodidae). J Entomol Sci 48(4):306–316. https://doi.org/10.18474/0749-8004-48.4.306

De la Fuente J, Almazán C, Canales M, Pérez de la Lastra JM, Kocan KM, Willadsen P (2007) A ten-year review of commercial vaccine performance for control of tick infestations on cattle. Anim Health Res Rev 8(1):23–28. https://doi.org/10.1017/s1466252307001193

De Meneghi D, Stachurski F, Adakal H (2016) Experiences in tick control by acaricide in the traditional cattle sector in Zambia and Burkina Faso: possible environmental and public health implications. Front Public Health 4:239. https://doi.org/10.3389/fpubh.2016.00239

De Oliveira-Cruz EM, Costa-Junior LM, Oliveira-Pinto JA, Santos DA, Alves S, Arrigoni-Blank MF, Bacci L, Barreto-Alves P, Cavalcanti SCH, Fitzgerald Blank A (2013) Acaricidal activity of *Lippia gracilis* essential oil and its major constituents on the tick *Rhipicephalus* (*Boophilus*) *microplus*. Vet Parasitol 195(1–2):198–202. https://doi.org/10.1016/j.vetpar.2012.12.046

FAO (Food and Agriculture Organization) (2004) Module 1. Ticks: Acaricide resistance: diagnosis, management and prevention. In: FAO (ed) Guidelines resistance management and integrated parasite control in ruminants. FAO Animal Production and Health Division, pp 25–77

Fernandes ÉKK, Bittencourt VREP, Roberts DW (2012) Perspectives on the potential of entomopathogenic fungi in biological control of ticks. Exp Parasitol 130(3):300–305. https://doi.org/10.1016/j.exppara.2011.11.004

Filgueiras MDG, Matos RS, Barreto LP, Mascarin GM, Rizzo PV, Freitas FMC, de Azevedo Prata MC, Monteiro C, Fernandes ÉKK (2023) From the laboratory to the field: efficacy of entomopathogenic nematodes to control the cattle tick. Pest Manag Sci 79(1):216–225. https://doi.org/10.1002/ps.7190

Fragoso H, Rad PH, Ortiz M, Rodriguez M, Redondo M, Herrera L, de la Fuente J (1998) Protection against *Boophilus annulatus* infestations in cattle vaccinated with the *B. microplus* Bm86-containing vaccine Gavac. off. *Vaccine* 16(20):1990–1992. https://doi.org/10.1016/s0264-410x(98)00116-9

Fulk A, Huang W, Agusto F (2022) Exploring the effects of prescribed fire on tick spread and propagation in a spatial setting. Comput Math Methods Med 5031806. https://doi.org/10.1155/2022/5031806

Gasparin G, Miyata M, Coutinho LL, Martinez ML, Teodoro RL, Furlong J, Machado LA, Silva MVGB, Sonstegard TS, Regitano LCA (2007) Mapping of quantitative trait loci controlling tick *Riphicephalus* (*Boophilus*) *microplus* resistance on bovine chromosomes 5, 7 and 14. Anim Genet 38:453–459. https://doi.org/10.1111/j.1365-2052.2007.01634.x

George JE, Pound JM, Davey RB (2004) Chemical control of ticks on cattle and the resistance of these parasites to acaricides. Parasitology 129(Suppl S1):S353–S366. https://doi.org/10.1017/s0031182003004682

Ghosh S, Kumar R, Nagar G, Kumar S, Sharma AK, Srivastava A, Kumar S, Kumar KA, Saravanan B (2015) Survey of acaricides resistance status of *Rhipiciphalus* (*Boophilus*) *microplus* collected from selected places of Bihar, an eastern state of India. Ticks Tick Borne Dis 6(5):668–675. https://doi.org/10.1016/j.ttbdis.2015.05.013

Githaka NW, Kanduma EG, Wieland B, Darghouth MA, Bishop RP (2022) Acaricide resistance in livestock ticks infesting cattle in Africa: current status and potential mitigation strategies. Curr Res Parasitol Vector-Borne Dis 2:100090. https://doi.org/10.1016/j.crpvbd.2022.100090

Goolsby JA, Cantu D, Vasquez A, Racelis A (2019) Development of a remotely activated field sprayer and evaluation of temperature and aeration on the longevity of *Steinernema riobrave* entomopathogenic nematodes for treatment of cattle fever tick-infested Nilgai. Subtropical Agric Environ 70:1–5

Gutiérrez-Wong JR, Rosado-Aguilar JA, Rodríguez-Vivas RI (2023) First report of acaricidal efficacy from plumbagin on larvae of *Rhipicephalus microplus* and *Rhipicephalus sanguineus* resistant to conventional acaricides. Exp Parasitol 255:108632. https://doi.org/10.1016/j.exppara.2023.108632

Hassan SM, Dipeolu OO, Malonza MM (1994) Natural attraction of livestock ticks by the leaves of a shrub. Trop Anim Health Prod 26:87–91. https://doi.org/10.1007/BF02239905

Jackson MA, Dunlap CA, Jaronski ST (2010) Ecological considerations in producing and formulating fungal entomopathogens for use in insect biocontrol. BioControl 55:129–145. https://doi.org/10.1007/s10526-009-9240-y

Jonsson NN, Cutullè C, Corley SW, Seddon JM (2010a) Identification of a mutation in the para-sodium channel gene of the cattle tick *Rhipicephalus microplus* associated with resistance to flumethrin but not to cypermethrin. Int J Parasitol 40(14):1659–1664. https://doi.org/10.1016/j.ijpara.2010.07.006

Jonsson NN, Miller RJ, Kemp DH, Knowles A, Ardila AE, Verrall RG, Rothwel JT (2010b) Rotation of treatments between spinosad and amitraz for the control of *Rhipicephalus (Boophilus) microplus* populations with amitraz resistance. Vet Parasitol 169(1–2):157–164. https://doi.org/10.1016/j.vetpar.2009.12.026

Jonsson NN, Piper EK, Constantinoiu CC (2014) Host resistance in cattle to infestation with the cattle tick *Rhipicephalus microplus*. Parasite Immunol 36(11):553–559. https://doi.org/10.1111/pim.12140

Kaaya GP, Hassan S (2000) Entomogenous fungi as promising biopesticides for tick control. Exp Appl Acarol 24:913–926. https://doi.org/10.1023/A:1010722914299

Kaaya GP, Mwangi EN, Ouna EA (1996) Prospects for biological control of livestock ticks, *Rhipicephalus appendiculatus* and *Amblyomma variegatum* using the entomogenous fungi *Beauveria bassiana* and *Metarhizium anisopliae*. J Invertebr Pathol 67(1):15–20. https://doi.org/10.1006/jipa.1996.0003

Klafke G, Webster A, Dall Agnol B, Pradel E, Silva J, de La Canal LH, Becker M, Osório MF, Mansson M, Barreto R, Scheffer R, Souza UA, Corassini VB, Dos Santos J, Reck J, Martins JR (2017) Multiple resistance to acaricides in field populations of *Rhipicephalus microplus* from Rio Grande do Sul state, Southern Brazil. Ticks Tick Borne Dis 8(1):73–80. https://doi.org/10.1016/j.ttbdis.2016.09.019

Kunz SE, Kemp DH (1994) Insecticides and acaricides: resistance and environmental impact. Rev Sci Tech 13(4):1249–1286. https://doi.org/10.20506/rst.13.4.816

Lew-Tabor AE, Rodriguez Valle M (2016) A review of reverse vaccinology approaches for the development of vaccines against ticks and tick borne diseases. Ticks Tick Borne Dis 7(4):573–585. https://doi.org/10.1016/j.ttbdis.2015.12.012

Li AY, Chen AC, Davey RB, Miller RJ, George JE (2007) Acaricide resistance and synergism between permethrin and amitraz against susceptible and resistant strains of *Boophilus microplus* (Acari, Ixodidae). Pest Manag Sci 63(9):882–889. https://doi.org/10.1002/ps.1417

Li AY, Davey RB, Miller RJ (2010) Laboratory evaluation of verbutin as a synergist of acaricides against larvae of *Rhipicephalus* (*Boophilus*) *microplus* (Acari: Ixodidae). J Econ Entomol 103(4):1360–1364. https://doi.org/10.1603/ec09329

Lorusso V, Picozzi K, de Bronsvoort BM, Majekodunmi A, Dongkum C, Balak G, Igweh A, Welburn SC (2013) Ixodid ticks of traditionally managed cattle in Central Nigeria: where *Rhipicephalus* (*Boophilus*) *microplus* does not dare (yet?). Parasit Vectors 6:171. https://doi.org/10.1186/1756-3305-6-171

Lovis L, Reggi J, Berggoetz M, Betschart B, Sager H (2013) Determination of acaricide resistance in *Rhipicephalus (Boophilus) microplus* (Acari: Ixodidae) field populations of Argentina, South Africa, and Australia with the larval tarsal test. J Med Entomol 50(2):326–335. https://doi.org/10.1603/me12127

Mackinnon MJ, Meyer K, Hetzel DJS (1991) Genetic variation and correlation for growth, parasite resistance and heat tolerance in tropical cattle. Livest Prod Sci 27(2–3):105–122. https://doi.org/10.1016/0301-6226(91)90090-D

Maniania NK, Nchu F, Ekesi S (2007) Fungal pathogen for biocontrol of ticks. In: Ekesi S, Maniania NK (eds) Use of entomopathogenic fungi in biological Pest management. Research Signpost, pp 295–392

Mapholi NO, Marufu MC, Maiwashe A, Banga CB, Muchenje V, MacNeil MD, Chimonyo M, Dzama K (2014) Towards a genomics approach to tick (Acari: Ixodidae) control in cattle: a review. Ticks Tick Borne Dis 5(5):475–483. https://doi.org/10.1016/j.ttbdis.2014.04.006

Marciano AF, Mascarin GM, Franco RFF, Golo PS, Jaronski ST, Kamp Fernandes ÉK, Pinheiro Bittencourt VR (2021) Innovative granular formulation of *Metarhizium robertsii* microsclerotia and blastospores for cattle tick control. Sci Rep 11:4972. https://doi.org/10.1038/s41598-021-84142-8

Marima JK, Nel CL, Marufu MC, Jonsson NN, Dube B, Dzama K (2020) A genetic and immunological comparison of tick-resistance in beef cattle following artificial infestation with *Rhipicephalus* ticks. Exp Appl Acarol 80:569–590. https://doi.org/10.1007/s10493-020-00480-8

Maryam J, Babar ME, Nadeem A, Hussain T (2012) Genetic variants in interferon gamma (IFN-gamma) gene are associated with resistance against ticks in *Bos taurus* and *Bos indicus*. Mol Biol Rep 39(4):4565–4570. https://doi.org/10.1007/s11033-011-1246-8

Mesquita E, Marciano AF, Corval ARC, Fiorotti J, Corrêa TA, Quinelato S, Bittencourt VREP, Golo PS (2020) Efficacy of a native isolate of the entomopathogenic fungus *Metarhizium anisopliae* against larval tick outbreaks under semifield conditions. BioControl 65:353–362. https://doi.org/10.1007/s10526-020-10006-1

Molento MB, Fortes FS, Buzatti A, Kloster FS, Sprenger LK, Coimbra E, Soares LD (2013) Partial selective treatment of *Rhipicephalus microplus* and breed resistance variation in beef cows in Rio Grande do Sul, Brazil. Vet Parasitol 192(1–3):234–239. https://doi.org/10.1016/j.vetpar.2012.10.021

Muhammad G, Naureen A, Firyal S, Saqib M (2008) Tick control strategies in dairy production medicine. Pak Vet J 28(1):43–50

Nava S, Mastropaolo M, Guglielmone AA, Mangold AJ (2013) Effect of deforestation and introduction of exotic grasses as livestock forage on the population dynamics of the cattle tick *Rhipicephalus* (*Boophilus*) *microplus* (Acari: Ixodidae) in northern Argentina. Res Vet Sci 95(3):1046–1054. https://doi.org/10.1016/j.rvsc.2013.09.013

Nava S, Rossner MV, Torrents J, Morel N, Martinez NC, Mangold AJ, Guglielmone AA (2020) Management strategies to minimize the use of synthetic chemical acaricides in the control of the cattle tick *Rhipicephalus* (*Boophilus*) *microplus* (Canestrini, 1888) in an area highly favorable for its development in Argentina. Med Vet Entomol 34(3):264–278. https://doi.org/10.1111/mve.12432

Nchu F, Maniania NK, Touré A, Hassanali A, Eloff JN (2009) The use of a semiochemical bait to enhance exposure of *Amblyomma variegatum* (Acari: Ixodidae) to *Metarhizium anisopliae* (Ascomycota: Hypocreales). Vet Parasitol 160(3–4):179–284. https://doi.org/10.1016/j.vetpar.2008.11.005

Odongo D, Kamau L, Skilton R, Mwaura S, Nitsch C, Musoke A, Taracha E, Daubenberger C, Bishop R (2007) Vaccination of cattle with TickGARD induces cross-reactive antibodies binding to conserved linear peptides of Bm86 homologues in *Boophilus decoloratus*. Vaccine 25(7):1287–1296. https://doi.org/10.1016/j.vaccine.2006.09.085

Ojeda-Chi MM, Rodriguez-Vivas RI, Galindo-Velasco E, Lezama-Gutiérrrez R (2010) Laboratory and field evaluation of *Metarhizium anisopliae* (Deuteromycotina: Hyphomycetes) for the control of *Rhipicephalus microplus* (Acari: Ixodidae) in the Mexican tropics. Vet Parasitol 170(3–4):348–354. https://doi.org/10.1016/j.vetpar.2010.02.022

Ojeda-Chi MM, Rodriguez-Vivas RI, Galindo-Velasco E, Lezama-Gutiérrrez R, Cruz-Vazquez C (2011) Control de *Rhipicephalus microplus* (Acari: ixodidae) mediante el uso del hongo entomopatógeno *Metarhizium anisopliae* (Hipocreales: Clavicipitaceae). Revista Mexicana de Ciencias Pecuarias 2(2):177–192

Olds C, Mwaura S, Crowder D, Odongo D, Van Oers M, Owen J, Bishop R, Daubenberger C (2012) Immunization of cattle with Ra86 impedes *Rhipicephalus appendiculatus* nymphal-to adult molting. Ticks Tick Borne Dis 3(3):170–178. https://doi.org/10.1016/j.ttbdis.2012.03.003

Parsa S, Morse S, Bonifacio A, Chancellor TC, Condori B, Crespo-Pérez V, Hobbs SL, Kroschel J, Ba MN, Rebaudo F, Sherwood SG, Vanek SJ, Faye E, Herrera MA, Dangles O (2014) Obstacles to integrated pest management adoption in developing countries. Proc Natl Acad Sci USA 111(10):3889–3894. https://doi.org/10.1073/pnas.1312693111

Pereira DFS, Ribeiro HS, Gonçalves AAM, da Silva AV, Lair DF, de Oliveira DS, Boas DFV, Conrado IDSS, Leite JC, Barata LM, Reis PCC, Mariano RMDS, Santos TAP, Coutinho DCO, Gontijo NF, Araujo RN, Galdino AS, Paes PRO, Melo MM, Nagem RAP, Dutra WO, Silveira-Lemos DD, Rodrigues DS, Giunchetti RC (2022) *Rhipicephalus microplus*: an overview of vaccine antigens against the cattle tick. Ticks Tick Borne Dis 13(1):101828. https://doi.org/10.1016/j.ttbdis.2021.101828

Perez-Cogollo LC, Rodriguez-Vivas RI, Ramirez-Cruz GT, Miller RJ (2010a) First report of the cattle tick *Rhipicephalus microplus* resistant to ivermectin in Mexico. Vet Parasitol 168(1–2):165–169. https://doi.org/10.1016/j.vetpar.2009.10.021

Perez-Cogollo LC, Rodriguez-Vivas RI, Ramirez-Cruz GT, Rosado-Aguilar JA (2010b) Survey of *Rhipicephalus microplus* resistance to ivermectin at cattle farms with history of macrocyclic lactones use in Yucatan, Mexico. Vet Parasitol 172(1–2):109–113. https://doi.org/10.1016/j.vetpar.2010.04.030

Pipano E, Alekceev E, Galker F, Fish L, Samish M, Shkap V (2003) Immunity against *Boophilus annulatus* induced by the Bm86 (Tick-GARD) vaccine. Exp Appl Acarol 29(1–2):141–149. https://doi.org/10.1023/a:1024246903197

Polito VJ, Baum KA, Payton ME, Little SE, Fuhlendorf SD, Reichard MV (2013) Tick abundance and levels of infestation on cattle in response to patch burning. Rangel Ecol Manag 66(5):545–552. https://doi.org/10.2111/REM-D-12-00172.1

Prullage JB, Cawthorne WG, Hir L, de Fallois LP, Timmons PR (2011) Synergy between fipronil and amitraz in a *Rhipicephalus sanguineus* tick residual contact test. Exp Appl Acarol 54(2):173–176. https://doi.org/10.1007/s10493-011-9424-x

Pullan NB (1980) Productivity of White Fulani cattle on the Jos Plateau, Nigeria. III. Disease and management factors. Trop Anim Health Prod 12(2):77–84. https://doi.org/10.1007/bf02242612

Redondo M, Fragoso H, Ortíz M, Montero C, Lona J, Medellín JA, Fría R, Hernández V, Franco R, Machado H, Rodríguez M, de la Fuente J (1999) Control of chemically resistant *Boophilus microplus* populations on grazing cattle vaccinated with Gavac® in Mexico. Exp Appl Acarol 23:841–849. https://doi.org/10.1023/A:1015925616490

Redondo M, Fragoso H, Montero C, Lona J, Medellin JA, Fria R, Hernandez V, Franco R, Machado H, Rodriguez M, de la Fuente J (2004) Integrated control of acaricide-resistant *Boophilus microplus* populations on grazing cattle in Mexico using vaccination with Gavac and amidine treatments. Exp Appl Acarol 23(10):841–849. https://doi.org/10.1023/a:1015925616490

Rodriguez-Valle M, Méndez L, Valdez M, Redondo M, Espinosa CM, Vargas M, Cruz RL, Barrios HP, Seoane G, Ramirez ES, Boue O, Vigil JL, Machado H, Nordelo CB, Piñeiro MJ (2004) Integrated control of *Boophilus microplus* ticks in Cuba based on vaccination with the anti-tick vaccine Gavac. Exp Appl Acarol 34(3–4):375–382. https://doi.org/10.1007/s10493-004-1389-6

Rodriguez-Vivas RI, Alonso-Dıaz MA, Rodrıguez-Arevalo F, Fragoso-Sanchez H, Santamaria VM, Rosario-Cruz R (2006) Prevalence and potential risk factors for organophosphate and pyrethroid resistance in *Boophilus microplus* ticks on cattle ranches from the state of Yucatan, Mexico. Vet Parasitol 136(3–4):335–342. https://doi.org/10.1016/j.vetpar.2005.05.069

Rodriguez-Vivas RI, Rivas AL, Chowell G, Fragoso SH, Rosario CR, Garcia Z, Smith SD, Williams JJ, Schwager SJ (2007) Spatial distribution of acaricide profiles (*Boophilus microplus* strains susceptible or resistant to acaricides) in southeastern Mexico. Vet Parasitol 146(1–2):158–169. https://doi.org/10.1016/j.vetpar.2007.01.016

Rodriguez-Vivas RI, Trees AJ, Rosado-Aguilar JA, Villegas-Perez SL, Hodgkinson JE (2011) Evolution of acaricide resistance: phenotypic and genotypic changes in field populations of *Rhipicephalus* (*Boophilus*) *microplus* in response to pyrethroid selection pressure. Int J Parasitol 41(8):895–903. https://doi.org/10.1016/j.ijpara.2011.03.012

Rodriguez-Vivas RI, Li AY, Ojeda-Chi MM, Trinidad-Martinez I, Rosado-Aguilar JA, Miller RJ, Pérez de León AA (2013) *In vitro* and *in vivo* evaluation of cypermethrin, amitraz, and piperonyl butoxide mixture s for the control of resistant *Rhipicephalus* (*Boophilus*) *microplus* (Acari: Ixodidae) in the Mexican tropics. Vet Parasitol 197(1–2):288–296. https://doi.org/10.1016/j.vetpar.2013.07.018

Rodriguez-Vivas RI, Rosado-Aguilar JA, Ojeda-Chi MM, Pérez-Cogollo LC, Trinidad-Martínez I, Bolio-González ME (2014) Control integrado de garrapatas en la ganadería bovina. Ecosistemas y Recursos Agropecuarios 1(3):295–308

Rodriguez-Vivas R, Grisi L, Pérez A, Silva H, Torres-Acosta J, Fragoso H, Romero D, Rosario R, Saldierna F, García D (2017) Potential economic impact assessment for cattle parasites in Mexico. Review. Revista Mexicana de Ciencias Pecuarias 8(1):61–74. https://doi.org/10.22319/rmcp.v8i1.4305

Rodriguez-Vivas RI, Jonsson NN, Bhushan C (2018a) Strategies for the control of *Rhipicephalus microplus* ticks in a world of conventional acaricide and macrocyclic lactone resistance. Parasitol Res 117(1):3–29. https://doi.org/10.1007/s00436-017-5677-6

Rodriguez-Vivas RI, Torres Acosta JFJ, Cruz Vázquez C, Almazán García C, Alcalá Canto T, Alonso Díaz MA, Chan Pérez JI, Domínguez García DI, Fernández Salas A, Figueroa Castillo JA, Galindo Velasco E, Lagunes Quintanilla RE, López Arellano ME, Martínez Ibáñez F, Martínez Ortíz de Montellano C, Mendoza de Gives P, Ojeda Robertos NF, Ortega Pacheco A, Rosario Cruz R, Rosado Aguilar JA, Torres Rodríguez L, Vitela Mendoza I (2018b) Epidemiología y control de garrapatas, moscas y nematodos gastrointestinales que afectan a los bovinos en México. In: Rodriguez Rivera O (ed) Estado del Arte Sobre Investigación e Innovación Tecnológica en Ganadería Bovina Tropical, 2nd edn. Red de Investigación e Innovación Tecnológica para la Ganadería Bovina Tropical, pp 255–308. https://redgatro.fmvz.unam.mx/docs/Estado_arte.pdf

Rodriguez-Vivas RI, Ramirez España E, Lozano Blanco I, Ojeda-Chi MM, Trinidad-Martinez I, Torres Islas JA, Bhushan C (2021) Monitoring the resistance of *Rhipicephalus microplus* to amitraz, flumethrin, coumaphos, and ivermectin on cattle farms in Mexico. Vet Parasitol Reg Stud Reports 26(1):100644. https://doi.org/10.1016/j.vprsr.2021.100644

Rodriguez-Vivas RI, Almazán GC, Castellanos HJL, Cortés GB, Domínguez GDI, Figueroa CJA, Jasso VCE, Hernández OR, Martínez IF, Mendoza GP, Ojeda RNF, Martínez OC, Rosado AJA, Rosario CR, Soberanes CN, Torres AJF, Vega MC, Zárate RJJ (2022) Manual para el control de garrapatas que afectan al ganado bovino. Servet Editorial Grupo Asís

Rosado-Aguilar JA, Arjona-Cambranes K, Torres-Acosta JF, Rodríguez-Vivas RI, Bolio-González ME, Ortega-Pacheco A, Alzina-López A, Gutiérrez-Ruiz EJ, Gutiérrez-Blanco E, Aguilar-Caballero AJ (2017) Plant products and secondary metabolites with acaricide activity against ticks. Vet Parasitol 238:66–76. https://doi.org/10.1016/j.vetpar.2017.03.023

Samish M, Alekseev E, Glazer I (1999) Interaction between ticks (Acari: Ixodidae) and pathogenic nematodes (Nematoda): susceptibility of tick species at various developmental stages. J Med Entomol 36(6):733–740. https://doi.org/10.1093/jmedent/36.6.733

Samish M, Alekseev E, Glazer I (2000) Biocontrol of ticks by entomopathogenic nematodes. Research update. Ann N Y Acad Sci 916:589–594. https://doi.org/10.1111/j.1749-6632.2000.tb05341.x

Samish M, Ginsberg H, Glazer I (2004) Biological control of ticks. Parasitology 129(S1):S389–S403. https://doi.org/10.1017/s0031182004005219

Scheepmaker JWA, Butt TM (2010) Natural and released inoculum levels of entomopathogenic fungal biocontrol agents in soil in relation to risk assessment and in accordance with EU regulations. Biocontrol Sci Tech 20(5):503–552. https://doi.org/10.1080/09583150903545035

Shapiro-Ilan DI, Hazir S, Glazer I (2017) Basic and applied research: entomopathogenic nematodes. In: Lacey LA (ed) Microbial agents for control of insect pests: from discovery to commercial development and use. Academic Press, pp 91–105

Shelton AM, Roush RT (2000) Resistance to insect pathogens and strategies to manage resistance. In: Lacey LA, Kaya HK (eds) Field manual of techniques in invertebrate pathology. Springer, pp 829–845

Showler AT, Garcia AR, Caesar RM (2020) Lethal effects of a silica gel + pyrethrins (Drione) on *Amblyomma americanum* (Ixodida: Ixodidae) larvae and nymphs. J Med Entomol 57(6):1864–1867. https://doi.org/10.1093/jme/tjaa119

Singh NK, Goolsby JA, Shapiro-Ilan DI, Miller RJ, Setamou M, Perez De Leon AA (2018) Effect of immersion time on efficacy of entomopathogenic nematodes against engorged females of cattle fever tick, *Rhipicephalus* (=*Boophilus*) *microplus*. Southwest Entomol 43:19–28. https://doi.org/10.3958/059.043.0120

Solari MA, Cuore U, Sanchis J, Gayo V, Trelles A, Bermudez F, Rizzo E (2007) Aplicación del control integrado de parásitos (CIP) a la garrapata *Boophilus microplus* en Uruguay. Aplicación del control integrado de parásitos (CIP) en un establecimiento comercial [Conference presentation]. Seminario Regional FAO, Montevideo, Uruguay

Spickett AM, Horack IG, Van Niekerk A, Braack LE (1992) The effect of veld-burning on the seasonal abundance of free-living ixodid ticks as determined by drag-sampling. Onderstepoort J Vet Res 59(4):285–292

Tabashnik BE (1990) Modeling and evaluation of resistance management tactics. In: Roush RT, Tabashnik BE (eds) Pesticide resistance in arthropods. Chapman Hall, pp 153–182

Tabor AE, Ali A, Rehman G, Rocha Garcia G, Zangirolamo AF, Malardo T, Jonsson NN (2017) Cattle tick *Rhipicephalus microplus*-host interface: a review of resistant and susceptible host responses. Front Cell Infect Microbiol 7:506. https://doi.org/10.3389/fcimb.2017.00506

Taylor MA (2001) Recent developments in ectoparasiticides. Vet J 161(3):253–268

Willadsen P (2006) Tick control: thoughts on a research agenda. Vet Parasitol 138(1–2):161–168. https://doi.org/10.1016/j.vetpar.2006.01.050

Wilson LJ, Sutherst RW, Kerr JD (1989) Trapping of the cattle tick *Boophilus microplus* by *Stylosanthes scabra* under grazing conditions. Aust J Agric Res 40(6):1301–1308. https://doi.org/10.1071/AR9891301

WingChing-Jones R (2015) Extracción manual de garrapatas *Riphicephalus* (*Boophilus*) *microplus* en ganado bovino como estrategia de control. Nutrición Animal Tropical 9(1):88–101. https://doi.org/10.15517/nat.v9i1.19393

# Tick-Borne Diseases

# 7

Hira Muqaddas, Naunain Mehmood, Madiha Rasool,
Farhana Yousaf, and Furhan Iqbal

**Abstract**

Ticks are important arthropod vectors, distinguished by their ability to transfer a wide range of disease-causing agents (bacteria, virus, and protozoa), thereby having socioeconomic significance, particularly in countries with low income. Transmission of tick-borne diseases (TBDs) occurs during tick feeding, although in some instances, infection can also happen through inhalation of the pathogen or ingestion of infected food products, without the direct involvement of ticks. Many TBDs are zoonotic, and in this regard, our understanding of the interactions between pathogens, hosts, host population dynamics, and vectors is still lacking. Tick and TBD research has been overlooked in comparison to studies on mosquito-borne diseases such as malaria, dengue, and Zika. Drug-based treatments and vaccinations are available for certain TBDs but not for all. There is no denying that prevalence and distribution of ticks have been increased in the environment since the beginning of the twentieth century due to human activities.

---

H. Muqaddas · F. Yousaf
Department of Zoology, The Women University Multan, Multan, Pakistan

N. Mehmood
Department of Zoology, University of Sargodha, Sargodha, Pakistan

Department of Veterinary Medicine, University of Sassari, Sassari, Italy

M. Rasool
Department of Zoology, The Women University Multan, Multan, Pakistan

Institute of Zoology, Bahauddin Zakariya University, Multan, Pakistan

F. Iqbal (✉)
Institute of Zoology, Bahauddin Zakariya University, Multan, Pakistan
e-mail: furhan.iqbal@bzu.edu.pk


S. Kumar et al. (eds.), *Acaricides Resistance in Ticks*,
https://doi.org/10.1007/978-981-97-7411-1_7

Therefore, it is important to control TBDs, for which it is necessary to enhance the knowledge of health professionals and the general community so as to reduce the current burden of TBDs, "One Health approach" is necessary for improved multidisciplinary management of disease. This chapter specifically addresses the various TBDs that impact both humans and animals globally with a note on their vectors and treatments.

**Keywords**

Tick-borne diseases · TBD · Bacterial · Viral · Protozoan

## 7.1 Introduction

Ticks are among the most common vectors that are found globally, inhabiting diverse environments ranging from extremely dry to exceptionally humid conditions (Brites-Neto et al. 2015). Ticks are known to transmit huge varieties of pathogens and tick-borne illnesses and are frequently encountered in medical and veterinary clinical settings. Livestock is the main source of income for farmers in developing nations and serves as a means of livelihood in many parts of the world and for livestock, ticks pose a hazard to economic prospects (Karim et al. 2017). It has been estimated that ticks and tick-borne diseases (TBDs) cause production economic losses (Singh et al. 2022). The ratio of these economic losses is higher in tropical and subtropical regions as the geoclimatic conditions of these areas are conducive to tick growth and reproduction (Eisen et al. 2016). The process of a tick bite is remarkably sophisticated. Once they locate a warm and moist area on the skin, ticks use their sharp chelicerae (blades) to pierce through the epidermis and secure themselves with their serrated harpoon-like structure called the hypostome (John et al. 2017). They then secrete a cement-like substance to firmly attach themselves to the skin, preventing premature detachment. This action creates an inoculation compartment around their feeding apparatus, which is followed by hemorrhaging (Bonnet and Boulanger 2017). Ticks play a crucial role in transmitting various infectious agents, including bacteria, viruses, and protozoan parasites, and several of the TBDs are primarily zoonotic where humans are incidental hosts and sometimes represent a dead end for the infectious agent (Dantas-Torres et al. 2012; Piesman and Eisen 2008). The control and prevention of these diseases are frequently challenging due to the limitations associated with their diagnosis and clinical management. It is necessary to disrupt the complex transmission chain that involves ticks and vertebrate hosts that interact in a constantly changing environment. Few TBDs have vaccines or treatments available but many of them do not have and these diseases are considered neglected in many parts of the world (Boulanger et al. 2019). Here, we have discussed some of the common tick-transmitted bacteria, viruses, and protozoan-borne diseases that have been reported from various parts of the world (Fig. 7.1).

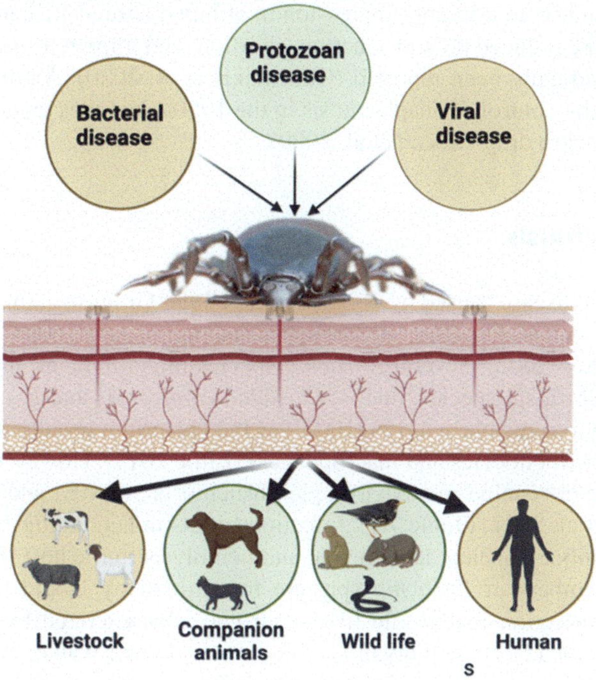


**Fig. 7.1** Ticks transmit a variety of bacteria, viruses, and protozoa to livestock, wild animals, as well as humans, resulting in their morbidity and mortality under acute infection conditions. (Image created with BioRender.com)

## 7.2 Tick-Transmitted Bacterial Diseases

### 7.2.1 Anaplasmosis

Anaplasmosis is a disease that is caused by a variety of small, obligate intracellular Gram-negative bacteria that are included in the family Anaplasmataceae that is placed in the order Rickettsiales (Atif 2015). A member of the family Anaplasmataceae, including *Anaplasma marginale, A. centrale, A. platys, A. phagocytophilum, A. bovis*, and *A. ovis* infects humans as well as a large number of livestock, pets, and wild animals (Rjeibi et al. 2018). The disease caused by this bacterium in humans is referred to as the "human granulocytic anaplasmosis" (Bakken and Dumler 2015), while in animals, it is known as "bovine anaplasmosis" in cattle, "ovine anaplasmosis" in sheep, and "canine anaplasmosis" in dogs (Carrade et al. 2009). The disease is mainly transmitted by tick's bite but can also spread accidentally during medical procedures. The bacterium causes leukocyte infection, indicated by the presence of bacterial merulae in infected granulocytes on peripheral blood smears. Cattle fever occurs when body temperature exceeds 40 °C (normal is 38.5 °C). Leukocyte destruction causes granulocytopenia and neutropenia, leading to immunosuppression in afflicted animals (Ziam et al. 2020). Other factors like reduced milk production, abortion, and impaired spermatogenesis have also sporadically been reported (Chochlakis et al. 2020). Antibiotic therapy, first tested for the control of anaplasmosis in the 1950s, includes the use of tetracycline and imidocarb drug (Kocan et al. 2000).

### 7.2.2 Ehrlichiosis

Ehrlichiosis is a disease caused by obligate intracellular Gram-negative bacteria that belong to the genus *Ehrlichia* in Ehrlichiaceae family and order Rickettsiales (Blanco and Oteo 2002). Several *Ehrlichia* species infect humans and animals. In humans, two *Ehrlichia* species, that is, *Ehrlichia chaffeensis* and *E. ewingii*, cause human monocytotropic ehrlichiosis (HME) as the bacterium usually infects human monocytic cells (monocytes and macrophages) (Little 2017). However, in dogs, the disease is termed "canine monocytotropic ehrlichiosis" (CME) and is caused by *E. canis* (Bai et al. 2017) (Table 7.1). Infection results in hematological alterations, including thrombocytopenia, leukopenia, and hemolysis in the host (Fonseca et al. 2017). The members of *Ehrlichia* spp. are transmitted by ixodid ticks, and the symptoms of infection include flu-like syndrome, characterized by fever, chills, cough, malaise, headache, and myalgia (Thirumalapura and Walker 2015). In dogs, if canine ehrlichiosis occurs, infection can result in an acute multisystemic illness characterized by the presence of petechiae (red patches caused by leaking of blood vessels) and/or cutaneous ecchymosis (bruising) (Laferl et al. 1999). Dogs may exhibit ocular illness because of anterior uveitis and retinal detachment, leading to blindness (Sainz et al. 2015). Treatment for ehrlichiosis includes the use of doxycycline; sometimes tetracycline is another option. The treatment must start promptly as soon as the infection is noticed (Horowitz et al. 2001).

### 7.2.3 Borreliosis (Lyme Disease)

Borreliosis is a bacterial disease caused by Gram-negative *Borrelia* species that belongs to the order Spirochaetales and the family Spirochaetaceae (Madison-Antenucci et al. 2020). It is a highly mobile, spiral-shaped bacteria and is characterized by having two membranes, two flagella, and outer surface protein (OSP role in virulence) (Trevisan et al. 2021). There are two main bacterial groups in this genus: *Borrelia burgdorferi sensu lato* (Bbsl) complex (which is responsible for causing Lyme disease) and *Borrelia* species that causes relapsing fever (Cutler et al. 2017) (Table 7.1). Lyme borreliosis is the predominant tick-borne illness affecting humans. Transmission of the pathogen from animals to humans primarily occurs through the bites of hard-shell ticks belonging to the genus *Ixodes* (Stone and Brissette 2017). The first sign of Lyme disease is often the appearance of a characteristic circular rash at the site of the tick bite, known as erythema migrans (Biesiada et al. 2012). Although Lyme disease is typically not fatal, it can lead to various manifestations

**Table 7.1** A brief overview of the principal bacterial pathogens, the tick vectors, and the diseases they cause

| Pathogen | Tick vector[a] | Disease caused | References |
|---|---|---|---|
| **Bacteria: *Anaplasma* spp.** | | | |
| *Anaplasma phagocytophilum* | *Ixodes scapularis, Ixodes ricinus, Haemaphysalis punctata, Ixodes pacificus, Rhipicephalus bursa, Haemaphysalis concinna* | Human granulocytic anaplasmosis Tick-borne fever | Burri et al. (2011), Dumler et al. (2005) |
| *A. marginale* | *Ixodes ricinus, Rhipicephalus sanguineus* | Bovine anaplasmosis | Kocan et al. (2003) |
| *A. centrale* | *Rhipicephalus bursa, R. annulatus* | | Ouedraogo et al. (2021), Jongejan and Uilenberg 2004 |
| *A. bovis* | *Hyalomma excavatum, Rhipicephalus sanguineus, R. turanicus* | Bovine mononuclear | Piesman and Eisen (2008), Aktas et al. 2010 |
| *A. ovis* | *Rhipicephalus bursa* | Ovine anaplasmosis | Aktas et al. (2011), Chochlakis et al. 2010 |
| *A. platys* | *Rhipicephalus bursa, R. Turanicus* | Canine infectious cyclic thrombocytopenia | Renneker et al. (2013), Chochlakis et al. (2010) |
| **Bacteria: *Borrelia* spp.** | | | |
| *Borrelia burgdorferi* sensu lato [b] | *Ixodes hexagonus, I. pacificus, I. persulcatus, I. ricinus, I. scapularis* | Lyme borreliosis | Jongejan and Uilenberg (2004), Piesman and Eisen (2008), Eisen and Lane (2002), Wang et al. (1999) |
| *B. hermsii* | *Ornithodoros hermsi* | | Schwan et al. (2009), Fritz et al. (2013) |
| *B. turicatae* | *Ornithodoros turicata* | | Schwan et al. (2005), Boyle et al. (2014) |
| *B. parkeri* | *Ambyloma maculatum* | | Schott et al. (2010), Schwan et al. (2005) |
| *B. garinii*[b] | *Ixodes ricinus, I. persulcatus* | | Tveten (2013) |
| *B. lusitaniae*[b] | *Ixodes ricinus* | | Skotarczak and Wodecka (2005), Ragagli et al. (2011) |
| *B. valaisiana*[b] | *Ixodes ricinus* | | Tveten (2013), Leal et al. (2020), Quessada et al. 2003 |

(continued)

**Table 7.1** (continued)

| Pathogen | Tick vector[a] | Disease caused | References |
|---|---|---|---|
| **Bacteria: *Anaplasma* spp.** | | | |
| *B. persica* | *Ornithodoros tholozani* | | Verdiere-de et al. (2011), Barmaki et al. (2010), Safdie et al. (2010) |
| *B. afzelli*[b] | *Ixodes ricinus*, *I. Persulcatus* | | Tonetti et al. ((2015), Crippa et al. (2002) |
| *B. miyamotoi*[b] | *I. Ricinus* | | Wagemakers et al. (2015), Kubiak et al. (2021) |
| *Borrelia* spp. [b] | *Ornithodoros* spp. | Relapsing fever | Yagupsky and Moses (1985), Trevisan et al. (2022) |
| **Bacteria: *Ehrlichia* spp.** | | | |
| *Ehrlichia canis* | *Rhipicephalus sanguineus* | Ehrlichiosis | Stich et al. (2008), Aguiar et al. (2007) |
| *E. chaffeensis* [b] | *Amblyomma americanum* | Human monocytic ehrlichiosis | Dawson et al. (1996), Cohen et al. (2010), Beall et al. (2022) |
| *E. ewingii* [b] | *Amblyomma americanum* | Granulocytic ehrlichiosis | Paddock et al. (2001) |
| *E. ruminantium* | *Amblyomma variegatum*, *Rhipicephalus microplus* | Heartwater/ Cowdriosis | Allsopp (2010), Biguezoton et al. (2016) |
| **Bacteria: *Francisella* spp.** | | | |
| *Francisella tularensis*[b] | *Dermacentor* spp. *Lxodes ricinus* | Tularemia | Jongejan and Uilenberg (2004), Piesman and Eisen (2008), Milutinović et al. (2008), Petersen et al. 2009 Gyuranecz et al. (2011) |
| **Bacteria: *Rickettsia* spp.** | | | |
| *Rickettsia rickettsia* [b] | *Amblyomma americanum*, *A. aureolatum*, *A. cajennense*, *Dermacentor andersoni*, *D. variabilis*, *Rhipicephalus sanguineus* | Rocky Mountain spotted fever | Jongejan and Uilenberg (2004), Piesman and Eisen (2008) Breitschwerdt et al. (2011), Labruna et al. (2009) |
| *R. africae*[b] | *Amblyomma hebraeum*, *A. variegatum* | African tick bite fever | Kelly et al. 1996, Raoult et al. 2001, Silva-Ramos et al. 2021 |

(continued)

**Table 7.1** (continued)

| Pathogen | Tick vector[a] | Disease caused | References |
|---|---|---|---|
| **Bacteria: *Anaplasma* spp.** | | | |
| *R. conorii*[b] | *Rhipicephalus sanguineus*, *R. turanicus* | Mediterranean spotted fever | Socolovschi et al. 2012, Levin et al. 2012 |
| *R. japonica* | *Haemaphysalis flava* | | Jongejan and Uilenberg 2004, Qin et al. 2019 |

[a] Associated vector list may be longer
[b] Pathogenicity for humans

affecting the skin, musculoskeletal system, nervous system, and cardiovascular system (Steere et al. 2016). Lyme disease is usually treated with doxycycline, amoxicillin, cefuroxime, and azithromycin. Intravenous ceftriaxone is sometimes needed for refractory arthritis or neurological disease (Cutler et al. 2017).

The other clinical manifestation of *Borrelia* spp. is tick-borne relapsing fever (TBRF), prevalent in various regions of Africa, Asia, and America, which can be transmitted to humans usually through the bite of Argasid ticks belonging to the *Ornithodoros* genus (Ogden et al. 2011). The most common symptoms include severe joint pain (arthralgias), dizziness, nausea, and vomiting. In some cases, fever exceeds 40 °C (104 °F), with an irregular pattern, and may be accompanied by delirium (Bratton and Corey 2005). TBRF can be treated using doxycycline and tetracycline (Jakab et al. 2022).

### 7.2.4 Tularemia

Tularemia is a potentially serious illness that is commonly called rabbit fever that results from infection with Gram-negative coccobacillus bacterium, *Francisella tularensis* (Busch et al. 2018) (Table 7.1). These bacteria are nonmotile, encapsulated facultative intracellular pathogens of humans and many animals (Celli and Zahrt 2013). Although observed worldwide, it is more common in the Northern Hemisphere and typically appears as sporadic cases. Tularemia primarily affects animals and humans, with rodents and lagomorphs being the most susceptible species (Feldman 2003). This disease is highly contagious and can easily be transmitted through direct contact with infected animals, scratches, bites, undercooked meat consumption, and inhalation (Hestvik et al. 2015). In addition to these modes of transmission, *Dermacentor* and *Ixodes* ticks can also transmit the disease (Steiner et al. 2014). Tularemia can progress from the initial infection site to the lungs, resulting in respiratory tularemia, which represents the most severe form of the illness (Ranjbar et al. 2016). Moreover, the potential for intentional release or weaponization of tularemia, particularly through aerosols, adds to its significance as a bioterrorism threat (Barel and Charbit 2019).

Tularemia's clinical presentations can be categorized into several syndromes: ulceroglandular (the most prevalent), glandular, oculoglandular, oropharyngeal/

gastrointestinal, pulmonary typhoidal, and cervical or occipital adenopathy tularemia (Maurin 2020). Fever, chills, headache, malaise, fatigue, and muscle aches appear after a few days of bites. Roughly one-third of the patients may experience a cough. Additional symptoms may encompass skin ulcers, sore throat, pleural effusions, pneumonia, acute respiratory distress syndrome, and pericarditis (Yeom et al. 2015). Streptomycin is the preferred treatment for tularemia, with gentamicin also proving effective. Although chloramphenicol or tetracycline has been utilized, relapses occasionally occur with these medications, and they may not fully prevent lymph node suppuration (Yeni et al. 2021).

### 7.2.5 Rickettsiosis

Rickettsiosis refers to a collection of diseases that are caused by a large number of intracellular obligatory Gram-negative bacteria that belong to the family Rickettsiaceae (Vaca et al. 2022). Rickettsial bacteria are divided into three groups based on the disease they usually cause: spotted fever, typhus, and scrub typhus. These bacteria are transmitted by ticks lice, mites, chiggers, and fleas (Thomas et al. 2016). One of the common diseases is Rocky Mountain spotted fever (RMSF). It is caused by intracellular bacterium *Rickettsia rickettsia* and is transmitted to humans by ticks (Masters et al. 2003) (Table 7.1). Despite being described clinically over a century ago, RMSF remains one of the most aggressive infections in humans, capable of causing fatalities even in young individuals (Anstead 2020; Jay and Armstrong 2020). As the name of the disease indicates, papular skin rash at first develops on wrists and ankles and later spreads to the palms, soles, and other areas of the body. Patients with these illnesses typically display feverish rashes with nausea, vomiting, and loss of appetite. Chloramphenicol and tetracycline are the recommended drugs for treating rickettsial illnesses, but they are known for their side effects. Conversely, sulfonamides stimulate the proliferation of rickettsia and should be avoided for therapeutic purposes (Jain 2018).

## 7.3 Tick-Transmitted Protozoa Diseases

### 7.3.1 Babesiosis

Babesiosis is a tick-borne intra-erythrocytic disease caused by several species that are included in the genera *Babesia* and are closely related to malarial parasites and included in the phylum Apicomplexan (Lempereur et al. 2017). A number of species of this genera including *Babesia bovis, B. ovis, B. canis, B. microti, B. gibsoni, B. vodeli*, and *B. divergens* infect both humans and animals (Bajer et al. 2022). Several hard tick genera including *Rhipicephalus, Dermacentor, Ixodes, Hyalomma*, and *Haemaphysalis* (Table 7.2) are involved in the transmission of *Babesia* species

**Table 7.2** Tick-borne protozoal disease and their associated tick vectors

| Pathogen | Tick vector[a] | References |
|---|---|---|
| ***Babesia* spp. (Babesiosis)** | | |
| *Babesia orientalis* | *Rhipicephalus haemaphysaloides* | Liu et al. (2005), He et al. (2017) |
| *B. divergens* | *Ixodes ricinus, I. scapularis* | Fanelli (2021), Zintl et al. (2003), Springer et al. (2020) |
| *B. microti*[b] | *Ixodes ricinus, I. scapularis* | Bullard et al. (2014), Bloch et al. (2019) |
| *B. trautmanni* | *Rhipicephalus* spp. | Dipeolu et al. (1983) |
| *B. perroncitoi* | *Rhipicephalus* spp. | Vercruysse and Parent (1981) |
| *B. caballi* | *Dermacentor reticulatus, Ixodes ricinus, Hyalomma* spp. | Battsetseg et al. (2001), Jongejan et al. (2015) |
| *B. felis* | *Ixodes, Dermacentor* spp. | Ayoob et al. (2010) |
| *B. gibsoni* | *Rhipicephalus longicornis* | Teodorowski et al. (2022), Chao et al. (2017) |
| *B. vogeli* | *Rhipicephalus sanguinaus* | René et al. (2012); Passos et al. (2005) |
| *B. rossi* | *Rhipicephalus elliptica* | Shabangu et al. (2021), Morters et al. (2020) |
| *B. canis* | *Dermacentor reticulatus* | Schoeman (2009), De Marco et al. (2017) |
| *B. motasi* | *Rhipicephalus punctata* | Hong et al. (2019), Niu et al. (2016) |
| *B. ovata* | *Haemaphysalis longicornis* | Sivakumar et al. (2016), Maeda et al. (2016) |
| *B. ovis* | *Rhipicephalus bursa* | Aouadi et al. (2017), Altay et al. (2008) |
| *B. major* | *Rhipicephalus punctata* | Hornok et al. (2014), Brocklesby and Sellwood (1973) |
| *B. bovis* | *Rhipicephalus annulata* | Simuunza (2009), Scoles et al. (2021) |
| *B. divergens*[b] | *Ixodes ricinus* | Fanelli (2021), Zintl et al. (2003) |
| *B. bigemina* | *Rhipicephalus microplus* | Simuunza (2009), Ola-Fadunsin et al. (2021) |
| ***Theileria* spp. (Theileriosis)** | | |
| *Theileria annulata* | *Hyalomma detritum* | Larcombe et al. (2019) |
| *T. parva* | *Rhipicephalus appendiculatus, R. zambeziensis* | Norval et al. (1985), Konnai et al. (2006) |
| *T. mutans* | *Amblyomma* spp. | Young et al. (1978) |
| *T. velifera* | *Amblyomma* spp. | Ouedraogo et al. (2021) |
| *T. orientalis* | *Haemaphysalis longicornis* | Watts et al. (2016), Lakew et al. (2023) |
| *T. taurotragi* | *Rhipicephalus appendiculatus* | Pienaar et al. (2018) |
| *T. ovis* | *Rhipicephalus turanicus, R. bursa* | Aktas et al. (2006), Zakkyeh et al. (2012), Zaeemi et al. (2011) |

(continued)

**Table 7.2** (continued)

| Pathogen | Tick vector[a] | References |
|---|---|---|
| *T. luwenshuni* | *Haemaphyalis qinghaiensis* | Phipps et al. (2016), Bawm et al. (2018) |
| *T. uilenbergi* | *Haemaphyalis qinghaiensis* | Li et al. (2009) |
| *T. lestoquardi* | *Hyalomma* spp. | Riaz et al. (2019), Tajeri et al. (2016) |
| *T. sergenti* | *Rhipicephalus* spp. | Baek et al. (2003) |

[a] Associated vector list may be longer
[b] Pathogenicity for humans

to a variety of vertebrate hosts including humans, wild and domestic animals like horses, sheep, goats, pigs, and dogs (Shabangu et al. 2021; Morters et al. 2020). *Babesia* spp. are picked up by ticks during their blood meal from sick animals. It has two modes of transmission; parasites can then be transmitted from a female tick to the next generation by passing through eggs called trans-ovarial transmission. However, the parasite is transmitted from the larvae to the nymphs and then to the adults; this mode is termed trans-stadial transmission (Mustafa 2017).

The clinical manifestations caused by babesiosis are similar to those of malaria. Fever, sweating, muscle aches, and headaches are common, along with anemia, hemoglobinuria, jaundice, and sometimes kidney and cardiac failure (Bloch et al. 2019). For mild cases, only symptomatic treatment is necessary. However, for severe cases, patients should receive treatment with either quinine with clindamycin or with atovaquone combined with azithromycin (Rajapakse and Bakirhan 2021).

### 7.3.2 Theileriosis

Theileriosis is a tick-borne protozoan disease that is caused by a number of parasites belonging to the *Theileria* genus in the phylum Apicomplexa and infects small and large ruminants as well as equids and felids (Demessie and Derso 2015). Members of the genus *Theileria*, including *Theileria annulata, T. ovis, T. luwenshuni, T. parva*, and *T. sergenti*, have a huge impact on the global economy as they mainly cause ovine and bovine theileriosis among the dairy animals (Ouedraogo et al. 2021; Lakew et al. 2023) (Table 7.2). Members of the *Theileria* spp. infect red blood cells and lymphocytes of the host animals and mainly two stages of these pathogens can be detected in the blood of infected animals: piroplasm stage in red blood cells and schizonts stage inside lymphocytes (Sojka et al. 2022). These parasites are transmitted from infected animals to others through ticks (*Ixodes* ticks) (Erdemir et al. 2012) and via trans-stadial transmission (Bekloo et al. 2017). The primary clinical signs of tropical theileriosis are fever, mild nasal and ocular discharge, loss of appetite, excessive salivation, swelling of superficial lymph nodes, breathing difficulties, sudden onset of anemia, jaundice, and potentially death caused by asphyxiation (Qayyum et al. 2010). This disease can be treated with imidocarb, oxytetracyclines, and halofuginone drugs (Goud et al. 2020).

## 7.4 Tick-Transmitted Viral Diseases

### 7.4.1 Alkhurma Hemorrhagic Fever

The recently emerged disease Alkhurma hemorrhagic fever (AHF) is an uncommon and possibly fatal viral illness caused by the Alkhurma hemorrhagic fever virus (AHFV), which is a member of the *Flavivirus* genus in the Flaviviridae family (Madani and Abuelzein 2021; Horton et al. 2016). The first detection of AHFV case occurred in 1995 in Alkhurma city, Saudi Arabia (Madani et al. 2014), and is therefore named after it. However, there is an increasing amount of evidence indicating that the virus exists outside of its initial boundaries (Saudi Arabia). The primary mode of transmission of AHFV to humans is through the bite of infected ticks (Table 7.3; *Ornithodoros savignyi* and *Hyalomma dromadarii*) (Bhatia et al. 2020). AHFV is a genetically similar variant (90% similarity) of the Kyasanur Forest disease virus (KFDV) that is responsible for generating viral hemorrhagic fever in specific regions of India (Shah et al. 2018) shedding light on the possible evolutionary divergence. Across the Arabian Peninsula, these ticks have been linked to camels and the locations where they rest and reside (Abdally et al. 2020). The disease initially manifests with nonspecific flu-like symptoms, fever, anorexia, lethargy, diarrhea, and vomiting. A second phase with severe neurological and hemorrhagic symptoms was developed in some individuals (Madani and Abuelzein 2021). There is currently no specific antiviral treatment for AHF. The best approach to combat ALKV involves basic tick bite prevention strategies (Abdulhaq et al. 2022).

### 7.4.2 Colorado Tick Fever

Colorado tick fever (CTF), commonly known as mountain tick fever and American mountain tick fever, is caused by double-stranded RNA virus that belongs to the genus *Coltivirus* and family Reoviridae (Owen et al. 2021). CTF virus (CTFV) is transmitted by the bite of infected ticks, such as *Dermacentor andersoni* (Table 7.3), which transmit the illness to the humans (Padgett et al. 2022) residing in the western United States and western Canada (Williamson et al. 2019). CTFV usually infects the bone marrow and red blood cells of the host, leading to symptoms such as fever, chills, headache, body aches, and fatigue. Around half of the patients get a "biphasic" fever during which individuals experience multiple days (3 days) of elevated body temperature, experience temporary relief for several days (1–3 days), and subsequently encounter a second brief spell of fever and illness (Farooq and Moriarty 2021). In severe instances, encephalitis can develop. Treatment primarily involves supportive measures to facilitate recovery (Bowen 2019).

**Table 7.3** Major tick-borne viral diseases along with their possible tick vectors

| Pathogen | Tick vector[a] | Disease caused | References |
|---|---|---|---|
| Alkhurma hemorrhagic Fever virus[b] | *Ornithodoros savigny* | Alkhurma hemorrhagic fever | Charrel et al. (2001), (2007) |
| Colorado tick fever virus[b] | *Dermacentor andersoni* | Colorado tick fever | Geissler et al. (2014) |
| Crimeane Congo hemorrhagic fever virus[b] | *Hyalomma* spp. | Crimean–Congo hemorrhagic fever | Gargili et al. (2017), Vatansever et al. (2007) |
| Eyach virus[b] | *Ixodes ricinus* | Neuropathy | Moutailler et al. (2016) |
| Kyasanur Forest disease virus[b] | *Haemaphysalis* spp. | Kyasanur Forrest disease | Trapido et al. (1959), Dobler (2010) |
| Omsk hemorrhagic fever virus[b] | *Dermacentor reticulatus* | Omsk hemorrhagic fever | Růžek et al. (2010) |
| Powassan virus[b] | *Ixodes scapularis* | Powassan encephalitis | Anderson and Armstrong (2012) |
| Severe fever thrombocytopenia syndrome virus[b] | *Haemaphysalis* spp. | Severe fever with thrombocytopenia syndrome | Liu et al. 2014 |
| Tick-borne encephalitis virus[b] | *Ixodes ricinus, I. persulcatus* | Tick-borne encephalitis | Jääskeläinen et al. (2006), Michelitsch et al. (2019) |
| Nairobi sheep disease virus | *Rhipicephalus appendiculatus* | Nairobi sheep disease | Lewis (1946), Baron and Holzer (2015) |
| African swine fever virus | *Ornithodoros* spp. | African swine fever | Penrith and Vosloo (2009) |
| LSD virus | *Rhipicephalus decoloratus, R. Appendiculatus, Amblyomma hebraem* | Lumpy skin disease | Inci et al. (2016) |
| Louping ill virus [b] | *Ixodes ricinus* | Louping-ill disease | Clark et al. (2020) |

[a] Associated vector list may be longer
[b] Pathogenicity for humans

### 7.4.3 Crimean–Congo Hemorrhagic Fever

Crimean–Congo hemorrhagic fever (CCHF) was first identified in the Crimea region during an outbreak in 1944, where over 200 cases were reported (Bente et al. 2013). CCHF is prevalent in Africa, the Balkans, the Middle East, and Asia. This is usually caused by the tick-borne virus, Nairo virus, which belongs to the

Bunyaviridae family. The virus causing CCHF (CCHFV) has been reported in a wide range of wild and domestic animals such as sheep, goat, and cattle but the host remained asymptomatic with no pathogenic effects. On the other hand, the virus is particularly virulent for humans (Hawman and Feldmann 2023). Livestock becomes infected by the bites of the infected ticks, leaving the virus in their bloodstream for about 1 week after infection. Humans can get infected by the bites of infected ticks (Vatansever et al. 2007). Human-to-human transmission can also occur as a result of close contact with body fluids such as blood, secretion, and organs of an infected person (Hawman and Feldmann 2023). Hospital-acquired infection may occur as a result of improper sterilization of medical equipment, contamination of medical supplies, and reuse of needles (Kalal 2019). Symptoms of CCHF are sudden fever, dizziness, neck pain, sensitivity to light, sore eyes, headache, nausea, vomiting, diarrhea, enlarged lymph node, fast heart rate, and a rash caused by bleeding into the skin. The antiviral drug ribavirin has been used in the treatment of CCHF (Negredo et al. 2017).

### 7.4.4 Nairobi Sheep Disease

Nairobi sheep disease (NSD) affects small ruminants like sheep and goats, and it is caused by the RNA virus that belongs to the *Orthonairovirus* genus of the Nairoviridae family (Kuhn et al. 2016). Nairobi sheep disease virus (NSDV) shares close similarities to the human pathogenic CCHFV (Kuhn et al. 2016). Similarly, the virus found in India has been designated as the Ganjam virus, which is genetically identical to NSDV (Lasecka et al. 2015). Human infections due to NSDV are very rare. Therefore, it is primarily regarded as a livestock disease that poses a significant threat to the economies of low-income countries (Krasteva et al. 2020). When animals get bitten by infected ticks (*Rhipicephalus appendiculatus*; Table 7.3), they can get a high fever, severe diarrhea with bleeding in the gut, and sometimes miscarriages. Mortality rates within herds might exceed 90% (Tarif et al. 2012). This illness is notifiable by the World Organisation for Animal Health (OIE); therefore, it creates trade barriers, which can have a significant impact on small ruminant farmers around the world (Krasteva et al. 2020). There is no precise medication for NSD; however, providing supportive care, adequate shelter, and high-quality nutrition may enhance the chances of survival.

### 7.4.5 African Swine Fever

African swine fever (ASF) is a highly contagious and deadly viral disease that affects domestic pigs and wild boars, but this disease is not zoonotic (Luskin et al. 2021). ASF is caused by a double-stranded DNA virus that replicates in the cell cytoplasm and is the only member of the Asfarviridae family (Chapman et al. 2011). It can spread through direct or indirect contact with infected pigs or contaminated materials such as feed, water, clothing, or equipment. It can also be spread by soft ticks belonging to genera *Ornithodoros* (Pietschmann et al. 2016). Signs of ASF are fever, loss of appetite, lethargy swollen lymph nodes, vomiting, bloody diarrhea, redness, and swelling of the skin. Sometimes abortion and sudden death can occur in extreme cases (Olesen et al. 2020). There is no known cure or vaccine against ASF and that is why precautionary measures must be strictly followed (Arias et al. 2002).

### 7.4.6 Kyasanur Forest Disease

Kyasanur Forest disease (KFD) is a tick-borne viral hemorrhagic fever that is caused by the virus belonging to the Flavivirus family. It was first identified in 1957 in the villages of the Kyasanur Forest region of India and is hence named after it. This disease primarily affected monkeys and resulted in a significant number of deaths (Holbrook 2012). Monkeys are often considered reservoir hosts because they harbor the virus without showing severe symptoms; ticks (*Haemaphysalis spinigera*) can acquire the virus from them and are involved in transmitting the virus to other animals and potentially to humans (Gupta et al. 2022). Initial symptoms of KFD include fever, headache, muscle pain, chill, fatigue, weakness, and nausea (Banerjee 2019). Gastrointestinal issues have also been documented in a few cases (Sadanandane et al. 2017). KFD fever is characterized by a biphasic component in certain individuals, and neurological symptoms are typically found in the second phase. Leucopenia, thrombocytopenia, and increased transaminases are the characteristic features of the initial stage of KFD (Gupta et al. 2022). Currently, there is no specific antiviral drug therapy available for KFD. The primary treatment approach involves supportive care, focusing on maintaining proper hydration and circulation. This may include the administration of intravenous fluids, colloids, or blood products based on the patient's clinical signs and symptoms.

### 7.4.7 Omsk Hemorrhagic Fever

Omsk hemorrhagic fever (OHF) is endemic to the Omsk region of Siberia (Karan et al. 2014) and is caused by the Omsk hemorrhagic fever virus (OHFV) that has a close genomic resemblance to the tick-borne encephalitis virus (TBEV) of flaviviruses, which are part of the Flaviviridae family and *Flavivirus* genus (Kovalev and Okulovskaya 2024). Additionally, OHFV capacity to induce hemorrhagic fever is a characteristic that it shares with KFDV (Holbrook 2012). The virus can be transmitted mainly by *Dermacentor reticulates* ticks, but people are mainly infected by having contact with infected muskrats (Kovalev and Mazurina 2022). Humans can contract illnesses either by coming into touch with the blood, excrement, or urine of an infected, sick, or deceased animal. There is no evidence of transmission between humans (Karan et al. 2014).

### 7.4.8 Powassan Encephalitis

Powassan virus (POWV) is a lethal neurotropic virus, classified as a "flavivirus," and is the sole member of the tick-borne encephalitis serogroup found in North America (Hermance and Thangamani 2017). POWV primarily spreads through ticks (*Ixodes scapularis*) and can acquire the virus when they ingest blood from groundhogs, mice, squirrels, or other rodents that carry the virus (Mlera and Bloom 2018). Infected ticks can transmit the POWV to humans and other animals through their bites. Initial symptoms may consist of fever, altered consciousness, seizures, and focal neurological deficits (Choi and Taylor 2012). The reported fatality rate ranges from 10% to 15%, with approximately 50% of survivors experiencing residual neurological deficits (Kemenesi and Bányai 2018).

### 7.4.9 Severe Fever with Thrombocytopenia Syndrome

Severe fever with thrombocytopenia syndrome (SFTS) is among the recently reported pathological condition caused by severe fever with thrombocytopenia syndrome virus (SFTSV) belonging to the genus Phlebovirus in the family Bunyaviridae(Seo et al. 2021). SFTFV is spread by the *Haemaphysalis longicornis* tick and is prevalent in central and eastern China, South Korea, and Japan, causing hundreds of cases each year (Choi et al. 2016). SFTS manifests as an indistinct feverish condition with a low platelet count that has the potential to advance to multiple-organ dysfunction, resulting in a mortality rate that ranges from 12% to 30% (Endy 2020). Patients with SFTS have received a variety of therapies, including steroids, intravenous immunoglobulin (IVIG), antiviral medications, and therapeutic plasma exchange (TPE) (Seo et al. 2021). There is currently no confirmed antiviral treatment available; supportive care is primarily required for recovery.

### 7.4.10 Tick-Borne Encephalitis

Tick-borne encephalitis (TBE) was first identified as a distinct clinical entity in the late 1930s in the far eastern part of Russia (Gritsun et al. 2003). Tick-borne encephalitis virus (TBEV) infected ticks, usually the *Ixodes* spp. (Table 7.3), spread the disease. The initial phase of the illness usually manifests with flu-like symptoms, including fever, headache, fatigue, muscle pain, and sometimes gastrointestinal issues (Bogovič et al. 2022). However, in some cases, the virus then progresses to a second phase that affects the central nervous system. This can result in various neurological symptoms such as meningitis, encephalitis, or meningoencephalitis (Michelitsch et al. 2019). These conditions involve inflammation of the membranes around the brain and spinal cord, or inflammation of the brain itself. While many individuals fully recover from TBE, some cases can lead to severe and long-term neurological complications or even be fatal. It is also important to note that, though rare, TBE can be contracted by consuming unpasteurized dairy products from the infected animals (Klaus et al. 2012). Vaccination against TBE is available in some countries and is recommended for people in or traveling to areas with a high prevalence of the disease (Steffen 2019).

## 7.5 Conclusion

Tick-borne diseases are present worldwide, and their distribution is continuously expanding due to the expansion of tick species, driven by changes in micro-and macroclimate, human behavior, land use, vector population, population growth, and various other factors including human traveling and transportation of wild and domesticated animals from one part of the world to the others. As science is progressing, new parasite-infecting usual and unusual hosts are uncovered and it is crucial to comprehend the transmission of pathogens across hosts, so the control strategies must be designed and implemented against ticks and TBDs.

## References


Abdally MH, Al-Marri TM, Abdally HM, Al-Jabr OA (2020) Incidence and prevalence of hard ticks in ruminants of Al-Ahsa oasis region, Kingdom of Saudi Arabia. World's Vet J 10(3):276–285

Abdulhaq AA, Hershan AA, Karunamoorthi K, Al-Mekhlafi HM (2022) Human Alkhumra hemorrhagic fever: emergence, history and epidemiological and clinical profiles. Saudi J Biol Sci 29(3):1900–1910

Aguiar DM, Cavalcante GT, Pinter A, Gennari SM, Camargo LMA, Labruna MB (2007) Prevalence of *Ehrlichia canis* (Rickettsiales: Anaplasmataceae) in dogs and *Rhipicephalus sanguineus* (Acari: Ixodidae) ticks from Brazil. J Med Entomol 44(1):126–132

Aktas M, Altay K, Dumanli N (2006) PCR-based detection of *Theileria ovis* in *Rhipicephalus bursa* adult ticks. Vet Parasitol 140(3–4):259–263

Aktas M, Altay K, Dumanli N (2011) Molecular detection and identification of *Anaplasma* and *Ehrlichia* species in cattle from Turkey. Ticks tick-borne diseases 2(1):62–65

Aktas M, Vatansever Z, Altay K, Aydin MF, Dumanli N (2010) Molecular evidence for *Anaplasma phagocytophilum* in *Ixodes ricinus* from Turkey. Trans R Soc Trop Med Hyg 104(1):10–15

Allsopp BA (2010) Natural history of *Ehrlichia ruminantium*. Vet Parasitol 167(2–4):123–135

Altay K, Aktas M, Dumanli N (2008) Detection of *Babesia ovis* by PCR in *Rhipicephalus bursa* collected from naturally infested sheep and goats. Res Vet Sci 85(1):116–119

Anderson JF, Armstrong PM (2012) Prevalence and genetic characterization of Powassan virus strains infecting *Ixodes scapularis* in Connecticut. Am J Trop Med Hygiene 87(4):754

Anstead GM (2020) History, rats, fleas, and opossums: the ascendency of flea-borne typhus in the United States, 1910–1944. Trop Med Infect Dis 5(1):37

Aouadi A, Leulmi H, Boucheikhchoukh M, Benakhla A, Raoult D, Parola P (2017) Molecular evidence of tick-borne hemoprotozoan-parasites (*Theileria ovis* and *Babesia ovis*) and bacteria in ticks and blood from small ruminants in Northern Algeria. Comp Immunol Microbiol Infect Dis 50:34–39

Arias M, Sánchez-Vizcaíno JM, Morilla A, Yoon K, Zimmerman J (2002) African swine fever. In: Trends in emerging viral infections of swine. Iowa State Press, Ames, pp 119–124

Atif FA (2015) *Anaplasma marginale* and *Anaplasma phagocytophilum*: Rickettsiales pathogens of veterinary and public health significance. Parasitol Res 114:3941–3957

Ayoob AL, Prittie J, Hackner SG (2010) Feline babesiosis. J Vet Emerg Crit Care 20(1):90–97

Baek BK, Soo KB, Kim JH, Hur J, Lee BO, Jung JM, Onuma M, Oluoch AO, Kim C-H, Kakoma I (2003) Verification by polymerase chain reaction of vertical transmission of *Theileria sergenti* in cows. Can J Vet Res 67(4):278

Bai L, Goel P, Jhambh R, Kumar P, Joshi V (2017) Molecular prevalence and haemato-biochemical profile of canine monocytic ehrlichiosis in dogs in and around Hisar, Haryana, India. J Parasit Dis 41:647–654

Bajer A, Beck A, Beck R, Behnke JM, Dwużnik-Szarek D, Eichenberger RM, Farkas R, Fuehrer H-P, Heddergott M, Jokelainen P (2022) Babesiosis in Southeastern, Central and Northeastern Europe: an emerging and re-emerging tick-borne disease of humans and animals. Microorganisms 10(5):945

Bakken JS, Dumler JS (2015) Human granulocytic anaplasmosis. Infect Dis Clin 29(2):341–355

Banerjee K (2019) Kyasanur forest disease. In: Arboviruses. CRC, Boca Raton, pp 93–116

Barel M, Charbit A (2019) *Francisella tularensis*: causative agent of tularemia and biothreat agent. In: Defense against biological attacks, vol 2. Springer, Cham, pp 239–250

Barmaki A, Rafinejad J, Vatandoost H, Telmadarraiy Z, Mohtarami F, Leghaei S, Oshaghi M (2010) Study on presence of *Borrelia persica* in soft ticks in Western Iran. Ir J Arthropod-borne Dis 4(2):19

Baron MD, Holzer B (2015) Nairobi sheep disease virus/Ganjam virus. Rev Sci TechnOff Int Épizoot 34(2):411–417

Battsetseg B, Xuan X, Ikadai H, Bautista JLR, Byambaa B, Boldbaatar D, Battur B, Battsetseg G, Batsukh Z, Igarashi I, Nagasawa H, Mikami T, Fujisaki K (2001) Detection of *Babesia caballi* and *Babesia equi* in *Dermacentor nuttalli* adult ticks. Int J Parasitol 31(4):384–386. https://doi.org/10.1016/S0020-7519(01)00120-5

Bawm S, Kakisaka K, Thu MJ, Chel HM, Oo YMN, Soe NC, Katakura K (2018) First molecular detection of *Theileria luwenshuni* from goats in Myanmar. Parasitol Res 117:3361–3364

Beall MJ, Mainville CA, Arguello-Marin A, Clark G, Lemieux C, Saucier J, Thatcher B, Breitschwerdt EB, Cohn LA, Qurollo BA (2022) An improved point-of-care ELISA for the diagnosis of anaplasmosis and ehrlichiosis during the acute phase of tick-borne infections in dogs. Top Companion Anim Med 51:100735

Bekloo AJ, Bakhshi H, Soufizadeh A, Sedaghat MM, Bekloo RJ, Ramzgouyan MR, Chegeni AH, Faghihi F, Telmadarraiy Z (2017) Ticks circulate *Anaplasma, Ehrlichia*, Babesia and *Theileria* parasites in North of Iran. Vet Parasitol 248:21–24

Bente DA, Forrester NL, Watts DM, McAuley AJ, Whitehouse CA, Bray M (2013) Crimean-Congo hemorrhagic fever: history, epidemiology, pathogenesis, clinical syndrome and genetic diversity. Antivir Res 100(1):159–189

Bhatia B, Feldmann H, Marzi A (2020) Kyasanur forest disease and Alkhurma hemorrhagic fever virus—two neglected zoonotic pathogens. Microorganisms 8(9):1406

Biesiada G, Czepiel J, Leśniak MR, Garlicki A, Mach T (2012) State of the art paper Lyme disease. Arch Med Sci 8(6):978–982

Biguezoton A, Noel V, Adehan S, Adakal H, Dayo G-K, Zoungrana S, Farougou S, Chevillon C (2016) *Ehrlichia ruminantium* infects *Rhipicephalus microplus* in West Africa. Parasit Vectors 9:1–4

Blanco J, Oteo J (2002) Human granulocytic ehrlichiosis in Europe. Clin Microbiol Infect 8(12):763–772

Bloch EM, Mrango Z, Kasubi M, Weaver J, Mihailovic A, Munoz B, Weimer A, Levin A, Tonnetti L, Linnen JM (2019) The *Babesia* observational antibody (BAOBAB) study: a cross-sectional evaluation of *Babesia* in two communities in Kilosa district, Tanzania. PLoS Neglected Trop Dis 13(8):e0007632

Bogovič P, Kastrin A, Lotrič-Furlan S, Ogrinc K, Županc TA, Korva M, Knap N, Strle F (2022) Clinical and laboratory characteristics and outcome of illness caused by tick-borne encephalitis virus without central nervous system involvement. Emerg Infect Dis 28(2):291

Bonnet S, Boulanger N (2017) Ixodes tick saliva: a potent controller at the skin Interface of early *Borrelia burgdorferi sensu lato* transmission. In: Arthropod vector: controller of disease transmission, vol 2. Elsevier, Oxford, pp 231–248

Boulanger N, Boyer P, Talagrand-Reboul E, Hansmann Y (2019) Ticks and tick-borne diseases. Med Mal Infect 49(2):87–97

Bowen GS (2019) Colorado tick fever. In: The arboviruses. CRC Press, pp 159–176

Boyle WK, Wilder HK, Lawrence AM, Lopez JE (2014) Transmission dynamics of *Borrelia turicatae* from the arthropod vector. PLoS Negl Trop Dis 8(4):e2767

Bratton RL, Corey GR (2005) Tick-borne disease. Am Fam Physician 71(12):2323–2330

Breitschwerdt EB, Hegarty BC, Maggi RG, Lantos PM, Aslett DM, Bradley JM (2011) *Rickettsia rickettsii* transmission by a lone star tick, North Carolina. Emerg Infect Dis 17(5):873

Brites-Neto J, Duarte KMR, Martins TF (2015) Tick-borne infections in human and animal population worldwide. Vet World 8(3):301

Brocklesby DW, Sellwood SA (1973) *Babesia major* in Britain: tick transmitted infections in splenectomised calves. Res Vet Sci 14(1):47–52

Bullard JMP, Ahsanuddin AN, Perry AM, Lindsay LR, Iranpour M, Dibernardo A, Van Caeseele PG (2014) The first case of locally acquired tick-borne *Babesia microti* infection in Canada. Can J Infect Dis Med Microbiol 25:209521

Burri C, Dupasquier C, Bastic V, Gern L (2011) Pathogens of emerging tick-borne diseases, *Anaplasma phagocytophilum, rickettsia* spp., and *Babesia* spp., in *ixodes* ticks collected from rodents at four sites in Switzerland (Canton of Bern). Vector-Borne Zoonotic Diseases 11(7):939–944

Busch A, Thomas P, Zuchantke E, Brendebach H, Neubert K, Gruetzke J, Al Dahouk S, Peters M, Hotzel H, Neubauer H (2018) Revisiting *Francisella tularensis* subsp. *holarctica*, causative agent of tularemia in Germany with bioinformatics: new insights in genome structure, DNA methylation and comparative phylogenetic analysis. Front Microbiol 9:344

Carrade D, Foley J, Borjesson D, Sykes J (2009) Canine granulocytic anaplasmosis: a review. J Vet Intern Med 23(6):1129–1141

Celli J, Zahrt TC (2013) Mechanisms of *Francisella tularensis* intracellular pathogenesis. Cold Spring Harb Perspect Med 3(4):a010314

Chao LL, Lu CW, Lin YF, Shih CM (2017) Molecular and morphological identification of a human biting tick, *Amblyomma testudinarium* (Acari: Ixodidae), in Taiwan. Exp Appl Acarol 71:401–414

Chapman DA, Darby AC, Da Silva M, Upton C, Radford AD, Dixon LK (2011) Genomic analysis of highly virulent Georgia 2007/1 isolate of African swine fever virus. Emerg Infect Dis 17(4):599

Charrel RN, Fagbo S, Moureau G, Alqahtani MH, Temmam S, De Lamballerie X (2007) Alkhurma hemorrhagic fever virus in *Ornithodoros savignyi* ticks. Emerg Infect Dis 13(1):153

Charrel RN, Zaki AM, Attoui H, Fakeeh M, Billoir F, Yousef AI, de Lamballerie X (2001) Complete coding sequence of the Alkhurma virus, a tick-borne flavivirus causing severe hemorrhagic fever in humans in Saudi Arabia. Biochem Biophys Res Commun 287(2):455–461

Chochlakis D, Giadinis N, Petridou E, Filioussis G, Tselentis Y, Psaroulaki A, Ioannidou E, Papanikolopoulou V, Karatzias H (2020) Molecular evidence of *Anaplasma phagocytophilum* in aborted goat fetuses and placenta. Vet Ital 56(4):302–303

Chochlakis D, Ioannou I, Tselentis Y, Psaroulaki A (2010) Human anaplasmosis and *Anaplasma ovis* variant. Emerg Infect Dis 16(6):1031

Choi EEJ, Taylor RA (2012) A case of Powassan viral hemorrhagic encephalitis involving bilateral thalami. Clin Neurol Neurosurg 114(2):172–175

Choi SJ, Park S-W, Bae I-G, Kim S-H, Ryu SY, Kim HA, Jang H-C, Hur J, Jun J-B, Jung Y (2016) Severe fever with thrombocytopenia syndrome in South Korea, 2013-2015. PLoS Neglected Trop Dis 10(12):e0005264

Clark JJ, Gilray J, Orton RJ, Baird M, Wilkie G, Filipe ADS, Johnson N, McInnes CJ, Kohl A, Biek R (2020) Population genomics of louping ill virus provide new insights into the evolution of tick-borne flaviviruses. PLoS Negl Trop Dis 14(9):e0008133

Cohen SB, Yabsley MJ, Freye JD, Dunlap BG, Rowland ME, Huang J, Dunn JR, Jones TF, Moncayo AC (2010) Prevalence of *Ehrlichia chaffeensis* and *Ehrlichia ewingii* in ticks from Tennessee. Vector-Borne Zoonotic Diseases 10(5):435–440

Crippa M, Rais O, Gern L (2002) Investigations on the mode and dynamics of transmission and infectivity of *Borrelia burgdorferi sensu stricto* and *Borrelia afzelii* in *Ixodes ricinus* ticks. Vector Borne Zoonotic Dis 2(1):3–9

Cutler SJ, Rudenko N, Golovchenko M, Cramaro WJ, Kirpach J, Savic S, Christova I, Amaro A (2017) Diagnosing borreliosis. Vector-Borne Zoonotic Diseases 17(1):2–11

Dantas-Torres F, Chomel BB, Otranto D (2012) Ticks and tick-borne diseases: a one health perspective. Trends Parasitol 28(10):437–446

Dawson JE, Warner CK, Standaert S, Olson JG (1996) The interface between research and the diagnosis of an emerging tick-borne disease, human ehrlichiosis due to *Ehrlichia chaffeensis*. Arch Intern Med 156(2):137–142

De Marco MDMF, Hernández-Triana LM, Phipps LP, Hansford K, Mitchell ES, Cull B, Swainsbury CS, Fooks AR, Medlock JM, Johnson N (2017) Emergence of *Babesia canis* in southern England. Parasit Vectors 10:1–9

Demessie Y, Derso S (2015) Tick borne hemoparasitic diseases of ruminants: a review. Adv Biol Res 9(4):210–224

Dipeolu O, Otesile E, Adetunji A, Fagbemi B (1983) Studies on blood parasites of pigs in Nigeria: pathogenicity of *Babesia trautmanni* in experimentally infected pigs. Zentralbl Veterinarmed B 30(1–10):97–102

Dobler G (2010) Zoonotic tick-borne flaviviruses. Vet Microbiol 140(3–4):221–228

Dumler JS, Choi KS, Garcia-Garcia JC, Barat NS, Scorpio DG, Garyu JW, Bakken JS (2005) Human granulocytic anaplasmosis and *Anaplasma phagocytophilum*. Emerg Infect Dis 11(12):1828

Eisen L, Lane RS (2002) Vectors of *Borrelia burgdorferi sensu lato*. In: Lyme borreliosis: biology, epidemiology and control, pp 91–115

Eisen RJ, Eisen L, Ogden NH, Beard CB (2016) Linkages of weather and climate with *Ixodes scapularis* and *Ixodes pacificus* (Acari: Ixodidae), enzootic transmission of *Borrelia burgdorferi*, and Lyme disease in North America. J Med Entomol 53(2):250–261

Endy TP (2020) Viral febrile illnesses and emerging pathogens. In: Hunter's tropical medicine and emerging infectious diseases. Elsevier, pp 325–350

Erdemir A, Aktas M, Dumanli N, Turgut-Balik D (2012) Isolation, cloning and sequence analysis of the lactate dehydrogenase gene from *Theileria annulata* may lead to design of new antitheilerial drugs. Vet Med 57(10):559–567

Fanelli A (2021) A historical review of *Babesia* spp. associated with deer in Europe: *Babesia divergens*/*Babesia divergens*-like, *Babesia capreoli*, *Babesia venatorum*, *Babesia* cf. *odocoilei*. Vet Parasitol 294:109433

Farooq I, Moriarty TJ (2021) The impact of tick-borne diseases on the bone. Microorganisms 9(3):663

Feldman KA (2003) Tularemia. J Am Vet Med Assoc 222(6):725–730

Fonseca JP, Bruhn FRP, Ribeiro MJM, Hirsch C, Rocha CMBM, Guedes E, Guimarães AM (2017) Hematological parameters and seroprevalence of *Ehrlichia canis* and *Babesia vogeli* in dogs. Ciência Anim Bras 18:e36095

Fritz CL, Payne JR, Schwan TG (2013) Serologic evidence for *Borrelia hermsii* infection in rodents on federally owned recreational areas in California. Vector-Borne Zoonotic Diseases 13(6):376–381

Gargili A, Estrada-Peña A, Spengler JR, Lukashev A, Nuttall PA, Bente DA (2017) The role of ticks in the maintenance and transmission of Crimean-Congo hemorrhagic fever virus: a review of published field and laboratory studies. Antivir Res 144:93–119

Geissler AL, Thorp E, Van Houten C, Lanciotti RS, Panella N, Cadwell BL, Staples JE (2014) Infection with Colorado tick fever virus among humans and ticks in a national park and forest, Wyoming, 2010. Vector-Borne Zoonotic Diseases 14(9):675–680

Goud KS, Vijayakumar K, Davis KJ, Tresamol P, Devada K (2020) Efficacy of different treatment regimens against oriental theileriosis in naturally infected cattle. Indian J Vet Med 40(2):14–19

Gritsun T, Lashkevich V, Gould E (2003) Tick-borne encephalitis. Antivir Res 57(1–2):129–146

Gupta N, Wilson W, Neumayr A, Saravu K (2022) Kyasanur forest disease: a state-of-the-art review. An Int J Med 115(6):351–358
Gyuranecz M, Rigó K, Dán Á, Földvári G, Makrai L, Dénes B, Fodor L, Majoros G, Tirják L, Erdélyi K (2011) Investigation of the ecology of *Francisella tularensis* during an inter-epizootic period. Vector-Borne and Zoonotic Diseases 11(8):1031–1035
Hawman DW, Feldmann H (2023) Crimean–Congo haemorrhagic fever virus. Nat Rev Microbiol 21(7):463–477
He L, Liu Q, Yao B, Zhou Y, Hu M, Fang R, Zhao J (2017) A historical overview of research on *Babesia orientalis*, a protozoan parasite infecting water buffalo. Front Microbiol 8:1323
Hermance ME, Thangamani S (2017) Powassan virus: an emerging arbovirus of public health concern in North America. Vector-Borne Zoonotic Diseases 17(7):453–462
Hestvik G, Warns-Petit E, Smith L, Fox N, Uhlhorn H, Artois M, Hannant D, Hutchings M, Mattsson R, Yon L (2015) The status of tularemia in Europe in a one-health context: a review. Epidemiol Infect 143(10):2137–2160
Holbrook MR (2012) Kyasanur forest disease. Antivir Res 96(3):353–362
Hong SH, Kim SY, Song BG, Roh JY, Cho CR, Kim CN, Lee SE (2019) Detection and characterization of an emerging type of *Babesia* sp. similar to *Babesia motasi* for the first case of human babesiosis and ticks in Korea. Emerg Microb Infect 8(1):869–878
Hornok S, Abichu G, Meli ML, Tánczos B, Sulyok KM, Gyuranecz M, Gönczi E, Farkas R, Hofmann-Lehmann R (2014) Influence of the biotope on the tick infestation of cattle and on the tick-borne pathogen repertoire of cattle ticks in Ethiopia. PLoS One 9(9):e106452
Horowitz HW, Hsieh T-C, Aguero-Rosenfeld ME, Kalantarpour F, Chowdhury I, Wormser GP, Wu JM (2001) Antimicrobial susceptibility of *Ehrlichia phagocytophila*. Antimicrob Agents Chemother 45(3):786–788
Horton KC, Fahmy NT, Watany N, Zayed A, Mohamed A, Ahmed AA, Rollin PE, Dueger EL (2016) Crimean Congo hemorrhagic fever virus and Alkhurma (Alkhumra) virus in ticks in Djibouti. Vector-Borne Zoonotic Diseases 16(10):680–682
Inci A, Yildirim A, Duzlu O, Doganay M, Aksoy S (2016) Tick-borne diseases in Turkey: a review based on one health perspective. PLoS Negl Trop Dis 10(12):e0005021
Jääskeläinen AE, Tikkakoski T, Uzcátegui NY, Alekseev AN, Vaheri A, Vapalahti O (2006) Siberian subtype tickborne encephalitis virus, Finland. Emerg Infect Dis 12(10):1568
Jain SH (2018) Rickettsia an overview. Arch Infect Dis Ther 2(3):1–7
Jakab Á, Kahlig P, Kuenzli E, Neumayr A (2022) Tick borne relapsing fever-a systematic review and analysis of the literature. PLoS Negl Trop Dis 16(2):e0010212
Jay R, Armstrong P (2020) Clinical characteristics of Rocky Mountain spotted fever in the United States: a literature review. J Vector Borne Dis 57(2):114–114
John M, Raman M, Ryan K (2017) A tiny tick can cause a big health problem. Indian J Ophthalmol 65(11):1228–1232
Jongejan F, Uilenberg G (2004) The global importance of ticks. Parasitology 129(S1):S3–S14
Jongejan F, Ringenier M, Putting M, Berger L, Burgers S, Kortekaas R, Lenssen J, Van Roessel M, Wijnveld M, Madder M (2015) Novel foci of *Dermacentor reticulatus* ticks infected with *Babesia canis* and *Babesia caballi* in The Netherlands and in Belgium. Parasit Vectors 8:1–10
Kalal MN (2019) Crimean-Congo haemorrhagic fever: a global perspective. Int J Res Med Sci 7(12):4812
Karan LS, Ciccozzi M, Yakimenko VV, Presti AL, Cella E, Zehender G, Rezza G, Platonov AE (2014) The deduced evolution history of Omsk hemorrhagic fever virus. J Med Virol 86(7):1181–1187
Karim S, Budachetri K, Mukherjee N, Williams J, Kausar A, Hassan MJ, Adamson S, Dowd SE, Apanskevich D, Arijo A (2017) A study of ticks and tick-borne livestock pathogens in Pakistan. PLoS Negl Trop Dis 11(6):e0005681
Kelly PJ, Beati L, Mason PR, Matthewman LA, Roux V, Raoult D (1996) *Rickettsia africae* sp. nov., the etiological agent of African tick bite fever. Int J Syst Evol Microbiol 46(2):611–614
Kemenesi G, Bányai K (2018) Tick-borne flaviviruses, with a focus on Powassan virus. Clin Microbiol Rev 32(1):00106-00117. https://doi.org/10.1128/cmr

Klaus C, Beer M, Saier R, Schau U, Moog U, Hoffmann B, Diller R, Süss J (2012) Goats and sheep as sentinels for tick-borne encephalitis (TBE) virus–epidemiological studies in areas endemic and non-endemic for TBE virus in Germany. Ticks Tick-borne Diseases 3(1):27–37

Kocan KM, Blouin EF, Barbet AF (2000) Anaplasmosis control: past, present, and future. Ann N Y Acad Sci 916(1):501–509

Kocan KM, de la Fuente J, Guglielmone AA, Meléndez RD (2003) Antigens and alternatives for control of *Anaplasma marginale* infection in cattle. Clin Microbiol Rev 16(4):698–712

Konnai S, Imamura S, Nakajima C, Witola WH, Yamada S, Simuunza M, Onuma M (2006) Acquisition and transmission of *Theileria parva* by vector tick, *Rhipicephalus appendiculatus*. Acta tropica 99(1):34–41

Kovalev SY, Mazurina EA (2022) Omsk hemorrhagic fever virus is a tick-borne encephalitis virus adapted to muskrat through host-jumping. J Med Virol 94(6):2510–2518

Kovalev SY, Okulovskaya VY (2024) The first record of Omsk hemorrhagic FeverVirus and tick-borne encephalitis virus of Baltic lineage from the Kemerovo region of Russia. Vector-Borne Zoonotic Diseases 24:443

Krasteva S, Jara M, Frias-De-Diego A, Machado G (2020) Nairobi sheep disease virus: a historical and epidemiological perspective. Front Vet Sci 7:419

Kubiak K, Szczotko M, Dmitryjuk M (2021) *Borrelia miyamotoi*—an emerging human tick-borne pathogen in Europe. Microorganisms 9(1):154

Kuhn JH, Wiley MR, Rodriguez SE, Bào Y, Prieto K, Travassos da Rosa AP, Guzman H, Savji N, Ladner JT, Tesh RB (2016) Genomic characterization of the genus Nairovirus (family Bunyaviridae). Viruses 8(6):164

Labruna MB, Terassini F, Camargo LMA (2009) Notes on population dynamics of *Amblyomma* ticks (Acari: Ixodidae) in Brazil. J Parasitol 95(4):1016–1018

Laferl H, Hogrefe W, Köck T, Pichler H (1999) A further case of acute human granulocytic ehrlichiosis in Slovenia. Eur J Clin Microbiol Infect Dis 18(5):385–386

Lakew BT, Eastwood S, Walkden-Brown SW (2023) Epidemiology and transmission of *Theileria orientalis* in Australasia. Pathogens 12(10):1187

Larcombe SD, Kolte SW, Ponnudurai G, Kurkure N, Magar S, Velusamy R, Shiels BR (2019) The impact of tick-borne pathogen infection in Indian bovines is determined by host type but not the genotype of *Theileria annulata*. Infect Genet Evol 75:103972

Lasecka L, Bin-Tarif A, Bridgen A, Juleff N, Waters RA, Baron MD (2015) Antibodies to the core proteins of Nairobi sheep disease virus/Ganjam virus reveal details of the distribution of the proteins in infected cells and tissues. PLoS One 10(4):e0124966

Leal B, Zamora E, Fuentes A, Thomas DB, Dearth RK (2020) Questing by tick larvae (Acari: Ixodidae): a review of the influences that affect off-host survival. Ann Entomol Soc Am 113(6):425–438

Lempereur L, Beck R, Fonseca I, Marques C, Duarte A, Santos M, Zúquete S, Gomes J, Walder G, Domingos A (2017) Guidelines for the detection of *Babesia* and *Theileria* parasites. Vector-Borne Zoonotic Diseases 17(1):51–65

Levin M, Studer E, Killmaster L, Zemtsova G, Mumcuoglu K (2012) Crossbreeding between different geographical populations of the brown dog tick, *Rhipicephalus sanguineus* (Acari: Ixodidae). Exp Appl Acarol 58:51–68

Lewis EA (1946) Nairobi sheep disease: the survival of the virus in the tick *Rhipicephalus appendiculatus*. Parasitology 37(1–2):55–59

Li Y, Luo J, Guan G, Ma M, Liu A, Liu J, Ren Q, Niu Q, Lu B, Gao J (2009) Experimental transmission of *Theileria uilenbergi* infective for small ruminants by *Haemaphysalis longicornis* and *Haemaphysalis qinghaiensis*. Parasitol Res 104:1227–1231

Little SE (2017) Ehrlichiosis. In: Arthropod borne diseases. Springer, Cham, pp 205–213

Liu Q, He B, Huang SY, Wei F, Zhu XQ (2014) Severe fever with thrombocytopenia syndrome, an emerging tick-borne zoonosis. Lancet Infect Dis 14(8):763–772

Liu Q, Zhao JL, Zhou YQ, Liu EY, Yao BA, Fu Y (2005) Study on some molecular characterization of *Babesia orientalis*. Vet Parasitol 130(3):191–198. https://doi.org/10.1016/j.vetpar.2005.03.021

Luskin MS, Meijaard E, Surya S, Sheherazade W, C., & Linkie, M. (2021) African swine fever threatens Southeast Asia's 11 endemic wild pig species. Conserv Lett 14(3):e12784

Madani TA, Abuelzein E-TM (2021) Alkhumra hemorrhagic fever virus infection. Arch Virol 166(9):2357–2367

Madani TA, Kao M, Abuelzein E-TM, Azhar EI, Al-Bar HM, Abu-Araki H, Bokhary RY, Ksiazek TG (2014) Propagation and titration of Alkhumra hemorrhagic fever virus in the brains of newborn Wistar rats. J Virol Methods 199:39–45

Madison-Antenucci S, Kramer LD, Gebhardt LL, Kauffman E (2020) Emerging tick-borne diseases. Clin Microbiol Rev 33(2):00083-00018. https://doi.org/10.1128/cmr

Maeda H, Hatta T, Alim MA, Tsubokawa D, Mikami F, Matsubayashi M, Tanaka T (2016) Establishment of a novel tick-*Babesia* experimental infection model. Sci Rep 6(1):37039

Masters EJ, Olson GS, Weiner SJ, Paddock CD (2003) Rocky Mountain spotted fever: a clinician's dilemma. Arch Intern Med 163(7):769–774

Maurin M (2020) *Francisella tularensis*, tularemia and serological diagnosis. Front Cell Infect Microbiol 10:512090

Michelitsch A, Wernike K, Klaus C, Dobler G, Beer M (2019) Exploring the reservoir hosts of tick-borne encephalitis virus. Viruses 11(7):669

Milutinović M, Masuzawa T, Tomanović S, Radulović Ž, Fukui T, Okamoto Y (2008) *Borrelia burgdorferi sensu lato, Anaplasma phagocytophilum, Francisella tularensis* and their co-infections in host-seeking *Ixodes ricinus* ticks collected in Serbia. Exp Appl Acarol 45:171–183

Mlera L, Bloom ME (2018) The role of mammalian reservoir hosts in tick-borne flavivirus biology. Front Cell Infect Microbiol 8:298

Morters MK, Archer J, Ma D, Matthee O, Goddard A, Leisewitz AL, Schoeman JP (2020) Long-term follow-up of owned, free-roaming dogs in South Africa naturally exposed to *Babesia rossi*. Int J Parasitol 50(2):103–110

Moutailler S, Valiente Moro C, Vaumourin E, Michelet L, Tran FH, Devillers E, Vayssier-Taussat M (2016) Co-infection of ticks: the rule rather than the exception. PLoS Negl Trop Dis 10(3):e0004539

Mustafa BHS (2017) Pathogenicity of Boophilus species hard tick among engorged female in naturally infested cattle with Ixodidae Piroplasmosis in Sulaimani Province-Kurdistan region/Iraq. Tikrit J Agric Sci 17:1

Negredo A, de la Calle-Prieto F, Palencia-Herrejón E, Mora-Rillo M, Astray-Mochales J, Sánchez-Seco MP, Bermejo Lopez E, Menárguez J, Fernández-Cruz A, Sánchez-Artola B (2017) Autochthonous Crimean–Congo Hemorrhagic Fever in Spain. N Engl J Med 377(2):154–161

Niu Q, Liu Z, Yang J, Yu P, Pan Y, Zhai B, Yin H (2016) Genetic diversity and molecular characterization of *Babesia motasi*-like in small ruminants and ixodid ticks from China. Infect Genet Evol 41:8–15

Norval RAI, Fivaz BH, Lawrence JA, Brown AF (1985) Epidemiology of tick-borne diseases of cattle in Zimbabwe. III. *Theileria parva* group. Trop Anim Health Prod 17:19–28

Ogden NH, Artsob H, Margos G, Tsao J, Sonenshine D, Roe M (2011) Non-rickettsial tick-borne bacteria and the diseases they cause. Biol Ticks 2:278–312

Ola-Fadunsin SD, Sharma RSK, Abdullah DA, Gimba FI, Abdullah FFJ, Sani RA (2021) The molecular prevalence, distribution and risk factors associated with *Babesia bigemina* infection in peninsular Malaysia. Ticks Tick-borne Diseases 12(3):101653

Olesen AS, Belsham GJ, Bruun Rasmussen T, Lohse L, Bødker R, Halasa T, Boklund A, Bøtner A (2020) Potential routes for indirect transmission of African swine fever virus into domestic pig herds. Transbound Emerg Dis 67(4):1472–1484

Ouedraogo AS, Zannou OM, Biguezoton AS, Yao KP, Belem AMG, Farougou S, Lempereur L (2021) Cross border transhumance involvement in ticks and tick-borne pathogens dissemination and first evidence of Anaplasma Centrale in Burkina Faso. Ticks Tick-borne Diseases 12(5):101781

Owen S, Gaffney C, Grado L, Woodson ML, King JA, Balaraman RP, Bechelli J (2021) Colorado tick fever virus induces apoptosis in human endothelial cells to facilitate viral replication. Ticks Tick-borne Diseases 12(5):101775

Paddock CD, Folk SM, Shore GM, Machado LJ, Huycke MM, Slater LN, Liddell AM, Buller RS, Storch GA, Monson TP (2001) Infections with *Ehrlichia chaffeensis* and *Ehrlichia ewingii* in persons coinfected with human immunodeficiency virus. Clin Infect Dis 33(9):1586–1594

Padgett KA, Kjemtrup A, Novak M, Velez JO, Panella N (2022) Colorado tick fever virus in the far west: forgotten, but not gone. Vector-Borne Zoonotic Diseases 22(8):443–448

Passos LMF, Geiger SM, Ribeiro MFB, Pfister K, Zahler-Rinder M (2005) First molecular detection of *Babesia vogeli* in dogs from Brazil. Vet Parasitol 127(1):81–85

Penrith ML, Vosloo W (2009) Review of African swine fever: transmission, spread and control. J S Afr Vet Assoc 80(2):58–62

Petersen J, Carlson J, Yockey B, Pillai S, Kuske C, Garbalena G, Pottumarthy S, Chalcraft L (2009) Direct isolation of *Francisella* spp. from environmental samples. Lett Appl Microbiol 48(6):663–667

Phipps LP, Hernández-Triana LM, Goharriz H, Welchman D, Johnson N (2016) Detection of *Theileria luwenshuni* in sheep from Great Britain. Parasit Vectors 9:1–4

Pienaar R, Neitz AW, Mans BJ (2018) Tick paralysis: solving an enigma. Vet Sci 5(2):53

Piesman J, Eisen L (2008) Prevention of tick-borne diseases. Annu Rev Entomol 53:323–343

Pietschmann J, Mur L, Blome S, Beer M, Pérez-Sánchez R, Oleaga A, Sánchez-Vizcaíno JM (2016) African swine fever virus transmission cycles in Central Europe: evaluation of wild boar-soft tick contacts through detection of antibodies against *Ornithodoros erraticus* saliva antigen. BMC Vet Res 12:1–5

Qayyum A, Farooq U, Samad H, Chauhdry H (2010) Prevalence, clinicotherapeutic and prophylactic studies on theileriosis in district Sahiwal (Pakistan). J Anim Sci 20:266

Qin XR, Han HJ, Han FJ, Zhao FM, Zhang ZT, Xue ZF, Ma DQ, Qi R, Zhao M, Wang LJ, Zhao L, Yu H, Liu JW, Yu XJ (2019) *Rickettsia japonica* and novel rickettsia species in ticks, China. Emerg Infect Dis 25(5):992–995. https://doi.org/10.3201/eid2505.171745

Quessada T, Martial-Convert F, Arnaud S, Leudet De La Vallee H, Gilot B, Pichot J (2003) Prevalence of *Borrelia burgdorferi* species and identification of *Borrelia valaisiana* in questing *Ixodes ricinus* in the Lyon region of France as determined by polymerase chain reaction-restriction fragment length polymorphism. Eur J Clin Microbiol Infect Dis 22:165–173

Ragagli C, Bertolotti L, Giacobini M, Mannelli A, Bisanzio D, Amore G, Tomassone L (2011) Transmission dynamics of *Borrelia lusitaniae* and *Borrelia afzelii* among *Ixodes ricinus*, lizards, and mice in Tuscany, Central Italy. Vector-Borne Zoonotic Diseases 11(1):21–28

Rajapakse P, Bakirhan K (2021) Autoimmune hemolytic anemia associated with human babesiosis. J Hematol 10(2):41

Ranjbar R, Behzadi P, Mammina C (2016) Respiratory tularemia: *Francisella tularensis* and microarray probe designing. Open Microbiol J 10:176

Raoult D, Fournier PE, Fenollar F, Jensenius M, Prioe T, de Pina JJ, Caruso G, Jones N, Laferl H, Rosenblatt JE (2001) *Rickettsia africae*, a tick-borne pathogen in travelers to sub-Saharan Africa. N Engl J Med 344(20):1504–1510

René M, Chêne J, Beaufils J, Moro CV, Bourdoiseau G, Mavingui P, Chabanne L (2012) First evidence and molecular characterization of *Babesia vogeli* in naturally infected dogs and *Rhipicephalus sanguineus* ticks in southern France. Vet Parasitol 187(3–4):399–407

Renneker S, Abdo J, Bakheit M, Kullmann B, Beyer D, Ahmed J, Seitzer U (2013) Coinfection of sheep with Anaplasma, Theileria and Babesia species in the Kurdistan region, Iraq. Transbound Emerg Dis 60:113–118

Riaz M, Nazir MM, Tasawar Z, Ahmed AN, Ayaz MM, Akram Q, Lindsay DS (2019) Molecular epidemiology and prevalence of *Theileria lestoquardi* and *Theileria ovis* infection in goats infested with tick vectors from Multan, Pakistan. J Med Entomol 56(3):844–848

Rjeibi MR, Ayadi O, Rekik M, Gharbi M (2018) Molecular survey and genetic characterization of *Anaplasma centrale*, *A. Marginale* and *A. Bovis* in cattle from Algeria. Transbound Emerg Dis 65(2):456–464

Růžek D, Yakimenko VV, Karan LS, Tkachev SE (2010) Omsk haemorrhagic fever. Lancet 376(9758):2104–2113

Sadanandane C, Elango A, Marja N, Sasidharan P, Raju K, Jambulingam P (2017) An outbreak of Kyasanur forest disease in the Wayanad and Malappuram districts of Kerala, India. Ticks Tick-borne Diseases 8(1):25–30

Safdie G, Farrah IY, Yahia R, Marva E, Wilamowski A, Sawalha SS, Wald N, Schmiedel J, Moter A, Göbel UB (2010) Molecular characterization of *Borrelia persica*, the agent of tick borne relapsing fever in Israel and The Palestinian Authority. PLoS One 5(11):e14105

Sainz Á, Roura X, Miró G, Estrada-Peña A, Kohn B, Harrus S, Solano-Gallego L (2015) Guideline for veterinary practitioners on canine ehrlichiosis and anaplasmosis in Europe. Parasit Vectors 8:1–20

Schoeman JP (2009) Canine babesiosis: tick-borne diseases. Onderstepoort J Vet Res 76(1):59–66

Schott M, Grosskinsky S, Brenner C, Kraiczy P, Wallich R (2010) Molecular characterization of the interaction of *Borrelia parkeri* and *Borrelia turicatae* with human complement regulators. Infect Immun 78(5):2199–2208

Schwan TG, Raffel SJ, Schrumpf ME, Policastro PF, Rawlings JA, Lane RS, Breitschwerdt EB, Porcella SF (2005) Phylogenetic analysis of the spirochetes *Borrelia parkeri* and *Borrelia turicatae* and the potential for tick-borne relapsing fever in Florida. J Clin Microbiol 43(8):3851–3859

Schwan TG, Raffel SJ, Schrumpf ME, Webster LS, Marques AR, Spano R, Rood M, Burns J, Hu R (2009) Tick-borne relapsing fever and *Borrelia hermsii*, Los Angeles County, California, USA. Emerg Infect Dis 15(7):1026

Scoles GA, Lohmeyer KH, Ueti MW, Bonilla D, Lahmers KK, Piccione J, Rogovskyy AS (2021) Stray Mexico origin cattle captured crossing into southern Texas carry *Babesia bovis* and other tick-borne pathogens. Ticks Tick-borne Diseases 12(5):101708

Seo J-W, Kim D, Yun N, Kim D-M (2021) Clinical update of severe fever with thrombocytopenia syndrome. Viruses 13(7):1213

Shabangu N, Penzhorn BL, Oosthuizen MC, Vorster I, van Schalkwyk OL, Harrison-White RF, Matjila PT (2021) A shared pathogen: *Babesia rossi* in domestic dogs, black-backed jackals (Canis mesomelas) and African wild dogs (Lycaon pictus) in South Africa. Vet Parasitol 291:109381

Shah SZ, Jabbar B, Ahmed N, Rehman A, Nasir H, Nadeem S, Jabbar I, Rahman ZU, Azam S (2018) Epidemiology, pathogenesis, and control of a tick-borne disease-Kyasanur Forest disease: current status and future directions. Front Cell Infect Microbiol 8:149

Silva-Ramos CR, Hidalgo M, Faccini-Martínez ÁA (2021) Clinical, epidemiological, and laboratory features of *Rickettsia parkeri* rickettsiosis: a systematic review. Ticks Tick-borne Diseases 12(4):101734

Simuunza MC (2009) Differential diagnosis of tick-borne diseases and population genetic analysis of *Babesia bovis* and *Babesia bigemina* (Doctoral dissertation, University of Glasgow

Singh K, Kumar S, Sharma AK, Jacob S, RamVerma M, Singh NK, Shakya M, Sankar M, Ghosh S (2022) Economic impact of predominant ticks and tick-borne diseases on Indian dairy production systems. Exp Parasitol 243:108408

Sivakumar T, Igarashi I, Yokoyama N (2016) *Babesia ovata*: taxonomy, phylogeny and epidemiology. Vet Parasitol 229:99–106

Skotarczak B, Wodecka B (2005) Identification of *Borrelia burgdorferi* genospecies inducing Lyme disease in dogs from western Poland. Acta Vet Hung 53(1):13–21

Socolovschi C, Kernif T, Raoult D, Parola P (2012) Borrelia, rickettsia, and Ehrlichia species in bat ticks, France, 2010. Emerg Infect Dis 18(12):1966

Sojka D, Jalovecká M, Perner J (2022) Babesia, Theileria, plasmodium and hemoglobin. Microorganisms 10(8):1651

Springer A, Höltershinken M, Lienhart F, Ermel S, Rehage J, Hülskötter K, Lehmbecker A, Wohlsein P, Barutzki D, Gietl C (2020) Emergence and epidemiology of bovine babesiosis due to *Babesia divergens* on a northern German beef production farm. Front Vet Sci 7:649

Steere AC, Strle F, Wormser GP, Hu LT, Branda JA, Hovius JW, Li X, Mead PS (2016) Lyme borreliosis. Nat Rev Dis Prim 2(1):1–19

Steffen R (2019) Tick-borne encephalitis (TBE) in children in Europe: epidemiology, clinical outcome and comparison of vaccination recommendations. Ticks Tick-borne Dis 10(1):100–110

Steiner DJ, Furuya Y (2014) Metzger DW (2014) Host–pathogen interactions and immune evasion strategies in *Francisella tularensis* pathogenicity. Infect Drug Resist 7:239–251

Stich B, Möhring J, Piepho HP, Heckenberger M, Buckler ES, Melchinger AE (2008) Comparison of mixed-model approaches for association mapping. Genetics 178(3):1745–1754

Stone BL, Brissette CA (2017) Host immune evasion by Lyme and relapsing fever Borreliae: findings to lead future studies for *Borrelia miyamotoi*. Front Immunol 8:12

Tajeri S, Razmi G, Haghparast A (2016) Establishment of an artificial tick feeding system to study *Theileria lestoquardi* infection. PLoS One 11(12):e0169053

Tarif AB, Lasecka L, Holzer B, Baron MD (2012) Ganjam virus/Nairobi sheep disease virus induces a pro-inflammatory response in infected sheep. Vet Res 43(1):1–12

Teodorowski O, Kalinowski M, Winiarczyk D, Dokuzeylül B, Winiarczyk S, Adaszek Ł (2022) *Babesia gibsoni* infection in dogs-a European perspective. Animals 12(6):730

Thirumalapura NR, Walker DH (2015) Ehrlichia. In: molecular medical microbiology, vol 3 Acad Press, pp 2011–2032

Thomas S, Alexander W, Gilligan J, Rikihisa Y (2016) The importance of Rickettsiales infections. In: Rickettsiales: biology, molecular biology, epidemiology, and vaccine development. Springer Cham, pp 3–21

Tonetti N, Voordouw MJ, Durand J, Monnier S, Gern L (2015) Genetic variation in transmission success of the Lyme borreliosis pathogen *Borrelia afzelii*. Ticks Tick-borne Dis 6(3):334–343

Trapido H, Rajagopalan P, Work T, Varma M (1959) Kyasanur Forest disease Part VIII Isolation of Kyasanur Forest disease virus from naturally infected ticks of the genus Haemaphysalis. Indian J Med Res 47(2):133–138

Trevisan G, Cinco M, Trevisini S, di Meo N, Ruscio M, Forgione P, Bonin S (2021) Borreliae part 2: *Borrelia* relapsing fever group and unclassified *Borrelia*. Biology 10(11):1117

Trevisan G, Cinco M, Ruscio M, Forgione P, Nazario Bonoldi VL, Falkingham E, Trevisini S, Tranchini P, Bonin S, Yoshinari NH (2022) Borrelia Lyme Group. J Dermatol Res Rev Rep 3(3):1–12

Tveten AK (2013) Prevalence of *Borrelia burgdorferi sensu stricto, Borrelia afzelii, Borrelia garinii,* and *Borrelia valaisiana* in *Ixodes ricinus* ticks from the northwest of Norway. Scand J Infect Dis 45(9):681–687

Vaca DJ, Dobler G, Fischer SF, Keller C, Konrad M, von Loewenich FD, Orenga S, Sapre SU, van Belkum A, Kempf VA (2022) Contemporary diagnostics for medically relevant fastidious microorganisms belonging to the genera *Anaplasma, Bartonella, Coxiella, Orientia* and *Rickettsia*. FEMS Microbiol Rev 46(4):fuac013

Vatansever Z, Uzun R, Estrada-Pena A, Ergonul O (2007) Crimean-Congo Hemorrhagic Fever in Turkey In: Crimean-Congo Hemorrhagic Fever, A Global Perspective, Springer Dordrecht, pp 59–74

Vercruysse J, Parent R (1981) An outbreak of porcine babesiosis in Senegal due to *Babesia perroncitoi*. Ann Soc Belg Med Trop 61(1):125–131

Verdiere-de NC, Hamane S, Assous MV, Sertour N, Ferquel E, Cornet M (2011) Tickborne relapsing fever caused by *Borrelia persica*. Uzbekistan and Tajikistan Emerg Infect Dis 17(7):1325

Wagemakers A, Staarink PJ, Sprong H, Hovius JW (2015) *Borrelia miyamotoi*: a widespread tick-borne relapsing fever spirochete. Trends Parasitol 31(6):260–269

Wang G, Van Dam AP, Schwartz I, Dankert J (1999) Molecular typing of *Borrelia burgdorferi sensu lato*: taxonomic, epidemiological, and clinical implications. Clin Microbiol Rev 12(4):633–653

Watts JG, Playford MC, Hickey KL (2016) *Theileria orientalis*: a review. N Z Vet J 64(1):3–9

Williamson BN, Fischer RJ, Lopez JE, Ebihara H, Schwan TG (2019) Prevalence and strains of Colorado tick fever virus in Rocky Mountain wood ticks in the Bitterroot Valley. Montana Vector Borne Zoonotic Dis 19(9):694–702

Yagupsky P, Moses S (1985) Neonatal *Borrelia* species infection (relapsing fever). Am J Dis Child 139(1):74–76

Yeni DK, Büyük F, Ashraf A, Shah MSUD (2021) Tularemia: a re-emerging tick-borne infectious disease. Folia Microbiol 66(1):1–14

Yeom JS, Rhie K, Park JS, Seo JH, Park ES, Lim JY, Park CH, Woo HO, Youn HS (2015) The first pediatric case of tularemia in Korea: manifested with pneumonia and possible infective endocarditis. Korean J Pediatr 58(10):398

Zaeemi M, Haddadzadeh H, Khazraiinia P, Kazemi B, Bandehpour M (2011) Identification of different *Theileria* species (*Theileria lestoquardi, Theileria ovis,* and *Theileria annulata*) in naturally infected sheep using nested PCR–RFLP. Parasitol Res 108:837–843

Zakkyeh T, Ali OM, Nasibeh HV, Reza YEM, Farhang B, Fatemeh M (2012) First molecular detection of *Theileria ovis* in *Rhipicephalus sanguineus* tick in Iran. Asian Pac J Trop Med 5(1):29–32

Ziam H, Kernif T, Saidani K, Kelanemer R, Hammaz Z, Geysen D (2020) Bovine piroplasmosisanaplasmosis and clinical signs of tropical theileriosis in the plains of Djurdjura (north Algeria). Veterinary Medicine and Science, 6(4):720–729.

Zintl, A, Mulcahy G, Skerrett Helen E, Taylor Stuart M, Gray Jeremy S (2003) Babesia divergens, a Bovine Blood Parasite of Veterinary and Zoonotic Importance. Clinical Microbiology Reviews, 16(4):622–636. https://doi.org/10.1128/cmr.16.4.622-636.2003

# Unlocking Tick Resistance with Transcriptome-Based Bioinformatics

8

Raquel Cossío-Bayúgar, Itzel Amaro-Estrada, Estefan Miranda-Miranda, Hugo Aguilar-Diaz, and Sachin Kumar

**Abstract**

The tick *Rhipicephalus microplus* and the diseases it causes, such as anaplasmosis and babesiosis, are critical factors that severely impact cattle production and related industries globally. The prevalence of tick infestations in livestock has increased due to the increasing resistance of ticks to pesticides. Evidence shows that specific genes and their encoded proteins are central to tick resistance to chemical acaricides. Fast molecular tests are necessary to address the limitations of outdated bioassays and to identify the molecular mechanisms underlying acaricide resistance in cattle ticks. This resistance is genetically inherited and involves the expression of one or more genes. The development of effective molecular tests for various acaricide chemical formulations requires understanding these mechanisms. Transcriptomic analysis, a relatively new field, allows the study of the complete set of mRNA molecules in an organism, thereby shedding light on the roles of different proteins. This information is invaluable for developing new pest control methods and molecular procedures to identify acaricide-resistant ticks. Currently, several *Rhipicephalus microplus* transcriptomes are available in public databases, offering a wealth of information that has led to extensive

R. Cossío-Bayúgar (✉) · E. Miranda-Miranda
Instituto Nacional de Investigaciones, Agrícolas y Pecuarias, Mexico City, Mexico
e-mail: cossio.raquel@inifap.gob.mx

I. Amaro-Estrada · H. Aguilar-Diaz
National Center for Disciplinary Research in Animal Health and Safety, INIFAP, Carretera Federal Cuernavaca-Cuautla 8534, Jiutepec, Morelos, Mexico
e-mail: cossio.raquel@inifap.gob.mx

S. Kumar
Entomology Laboratory, Division of Parasitology, ICAR-Indian Veterinary Research Institute, Izzatnagar, Bareilly, Uttar Pradesh, India

Constituent Government College, Meerapur Banger, Bijnor, Uttar Pradesh, India



S. Kumar et al. (eds.), *Acaricides Resistance in Ticks*,
https://doi.org/10.1007/978-981-97-7411-1_8

analyses and publications. This chapter lists the datasets of the *Rhipicephalus microplus* transcriptome available in the databases and presents examples of the importance and scope of this type of analysis. Some essential points in the use of these methodologies are also discussed. Although the results are promising, the present challenge is to analyze the information in depth and, with this knowledge, to achieve a breakthrough in the control of pests and cattle diseases.

**Keywords**

Genome · Transcriptome · Databanks · PDB · Omics techniques

## 8.1 Introduction

Ixodid ticks are medically significant vectors responsible for transmitting serious diseases to both humans and livestock. These blood-sucking ectoparasites cause zoonotic illnesses, such as Lyme disease, which affect wildlife and humans in the Northern Hemisphere (Eisen et al. 2017). Additionally, ticks are vectors of infectious bovine diseases, including theileriosis, babesiosis, anaplasmosis, and cowdriosis, which negatively impact cattle and small ruminant production in regions such as Latin America, Australia, and Africa (Domingos et al. 2013).

The cattle tick *Rhipicephalus microplus* is the subject of numerous scientific research projects due to its significant economic impact on the cattle industry and the urgent need for effective, scientifically based control measures. Molecular biology approaches for studying this important livestock pest include various omics techniques (Guerrero et al. 2021; Garcia et al. 2020; Shi et al. 2021; Zhang et al. 2014). For the purposes of this chapter, we will focus specifically on the transcriptomics of *R. microplus* (Garcia et al. 2020). This discipline provides insights into various aspects of the tick biology, including the tick microbiome (Zhang et al. 2022), host interactions, feeding behavior, life cycle stages (Garcia et al. 2020), and intrinsic resistance to pesticides (Giachetto et al. 2020).

Pesticides, known as acaricides, which are used to prevent tick infestations in cattle, constitute either the sole or a major component of integrated tick control methods worldwide (Domingos et al. 2013). The primary reasons for relying on these chemicals to manage tick and tick-borne diseases (TTBDs) are their relative nontoxicity to mammals and their ability to offer a quick and cost-effective method for suppressing tick populations (Abbas et al. 2014). However, the prolonged use of acaricides presents a significant disadvantage. As large tick populations are repeatedly exposed to various acaricide formulations, Darwinian selection favors acaricide-tolerant and acaricide-resistant ticks, eventually leading to homogenous populations resistant to nearly all major classes of acaricides (Rodriguez-Vivas et al. 2018). Once acaricide resistance is established in a cattle grazing area, tick control becomes severely compromised, adversely affecting cattle production and the capacity to manage this blood-sucking parasite.

The intensive and prolonged use of acaricides for tick control has a significant disadvantage: It exposes large populations of ticks to various acaricide formulations, leading to Darwinian selection of acaricide-tolerant and resistant ticks. Over time, this process results in the emergence of homogenous resistant tick populations across nearly all major classes of acaricides (Rodriguez-Vivas et al. 2018). Once acaricide resistance occurs in a cattle grazing area, it severely compromises tick control efforts, negatively impacting cattle production and the ability to manage these blood-sucking parasites. Consequently, identifying and preventing the spread of acaricide resistance has become a major challenge, especially when tick control relies solely on pesticide treatments for cattle.

To effectively circumvent acaricide resistance, it is essential to monitor the presence or absence of ticks that are resistant to specific acaricides. By making the selection of pesticide formulations for a particular area a scientifically informed decision, we can avoid the possibility of pesticide use. The Insecticide Resistance Action Committee (IRAC) defines resistance as "a heritable change in the sensitivity of a pest population that is reflected in the repeated failure of a product to achieve the expected level of control when used according to the label recommendation for that pest species" (IRAC 2020). The cattle tick is among the top 12 arthropod species to develop resistance to various pesticide products and has shown resistance to more than 44 chemical formulations. By 2014, there were 167 reported cases of resistance to one or more acaricide compounds (Sparks and Nauen 2015).

When reporting results from acaricide resistance bioassays, it is customary to distinguish between two types of resistance: phenotypic and molecular. Phenotypic resistance refers to the toxicological profiles of tick strains or field isolates against specific acaricide formulations. This type of resistance is typically used in field surveillance reports to identify acaricides that fail to effectively control ticks under laboratory conditions. The results are reported as the mortality rate of tick larvae exposed to various acaricide concentrations and are compared against reference-sensitive and resistant tick strains (Martinez Ibañez et al. 2021).

The second type of resistance involves the molecular mechanisms underlying resistance. This encompasses changes in the expression levels or structural alterations of gene products associated with resistance, as determined by molecular detection assays such as gene sequencing, polymerase chain reaction (PCR), or proteomic analysis (Cossio-Bayugar et al. 2021).

This second type of resistance presents a significant scientific challenge, as it necessitates the identification and characterization of the molecular mechanisms underlying the observed phenotypic resistance to various acaricides. The rationale for investigating molecular resistance lies in the potential to pinpoint the specific molecules responsible for each type of acaricide resistance. This could eventually lead to faster and more cost-effective diagnostics using molecular tests. In theory, understanding the precise mechanisms that confer resistance should enable the development of strategies to deploy alternative acaricides or to implement integrated methods for controlling acaricide-resistant ticks. Additionally, this approach provides the ability to monitor the emergence of resistance alleles and predict which acaricides will become ineffective in tick control for a given region, ultimately leading to more efficient use of acaricides.

New-generation sequencing technologies have made it possible to obtain longer reads, which facilitate the assembly of larger genomes. Several reference genomes and transcriptomes of *Rhipicephalus microplus* are now available in public databases, serving as valuable resources for any transcriptomic project. These databases are crucial for comparing and identifying polymorphisms in genes obtained through high-throughput sequencing and are also suitable for phylogenetic analyses. Furthermore, this information can be conveniently utilized as a reference for transcriptome assembly and gene ontology enrichment analysis (Amaro-Estrada et al. 2023). Transcriptome assembly from high-throughput nucleic acid sequencing raw data requires advanced computational skills or access to specialized software, which is typically compatible with Unix file formats. Several specialized vendors offer computational resources and expertise for raw data processing. Additionally, many bioinformatics analyses such as multiple sequence alignment, phylogenetic analysis, single nucleotide polymorphism (SNP) detection, and insertion/deletion identification may be available from various providers (Nowrousian 2014). Several transcriptomic datasets of cattle ticks are available in public databases for reference comparisons and data mining. Table 8.1 lists the transcriptomic data of *Rhipicephalus microplus* available in GenBank.

## 8.2 Molecular Basis of Acaricide Resistance

Acaricides, which are pesticides specifically designed to target ticks and mites, play a crucial role in managing blood-sucking ectoparasites that pose significant threats to both livestock and human health. However, the overuse and misuse of these chemicals have led to the emergence of resistance in tick populations, thereby diminishing the efficacy of acaricides over time (Cossio-Bayugar et al. 2021).

The primary acaricides used for tick control are detailed in Table 8.2 and are categorized based on the Insecticide Resistance Action Committee (IRAC) classification (IRAC 2020; Sparks and Nauen 2015). The initial generation of ixodicides consisted of arsenic salt compounds, which were rapidly discontinued due to their detrimental effects on cattle and the environment (George et al. 2004). The subsequent generation included synthetic organochlorines closely related to DDT, carbamates, and organophosphates. The third generation included synthetic pyrethroids and amidines. The most recent generation comprises phenypyrazoles, insect growth regulators (IGRs), and macrocyclic lactones, with these compounds currently being the predominant class of acaricides used globally for tick control programs (Rodriguez-Vivas et al. 2018; Abbas et al. 2014). These ixodicides primarily target various physiological aspects of tick function, such as the nervous system, affecting sites such as acetylcholinesterase, voltage-gated para-sodium channels (Dong et al. 2014), glutamate-gated chloride channels (Glu-GCCs) (Lumaret et al. 2012; Omura 2008), and g-aminobutyric acid-gated chloride channels (GABA-GCCs) (Bloomquist 2003).

The identification and understanding of the molecular basis of underlying acaricide resistance pose significant scientific challenges. Transcriptome-based bioinformatics approaches are powerful tools for revealing the genetic mechanisms underlying tick resistance but are crucial for developing strategies to address

**Table 8.1** The *Rhipicephalus microplus* transcriptome datasets available at GenBank

| GenBank Bioproject | Description | Data type | Submission | Publications |
|---|---|---|---|---|
| PRJNA82295 | Expressed gene sequences from larval genes overexpressed upon *Babesia bovis* infection of *R. microplus* | Transcriptome or gene expression Scope: monoisolate | Registration date: 30-Jan-2012 USDA-ARS | NA |
| PRJNA884635 | *Rhipicephalus microplus* raw ovary gene expression sequence reads | Transcriptome or gene expression Scope: multiisolate | Registration date: 27-Sep-2022 Instituto de Biotecnologia, UNAM | NA |
| PRJNA103873; GEO: GSE9880 | *Babesia* infected/ control LongSAGE libraries for *Boophilus microplus* ovary tissue | Transcriptome or gene expression Scope: multiisolate | Registration date: 1-Mar-2009 Agriculture Research Service, Agriculture, USDA | NA |
| PRJNA108259; GEO: GSE10109 | SAGE in *Rhipicephalus* (*Boophilus*) *microplus* following OP treatment of larvae from OP resistant/susceptible strains | Transcriptome or gene expression Scope: multiisolate | Registration date: 14-May-2008 Agriculture research service, agriculture, USDA | Guerrero et al. (2007) |
| PRJNA125857; GEO: GSE21690 | Temporal characterization of the organ-specific *Rhipicephalus microplus* transcriptional response to *Anaplasma marginale* infection | Transcriptome or gene expression Scope: multiisolate | Registration date: 13-Apr-2011 College of veterinary medicine, Washington State University | Mercado-Curiel et al. (2011) |
| PRJNA162847 | Synganglia transcriptome of adult Mexican cattle ticks | Transcriptome or gene expression Scope: multiisolate | Registration date: 2-May-2012 USDA-ARS | Guerrero et al. (2016) |

(continued)

**Table 8.1** (continued)

| GenBank Bioproject | Description | Data type | Submission | Publications |
|---|---|---|---|---|
| PRJNA162849 | Transcriptome of synganglia from adult Australian cattle tick monoisolate | Transcriptome or gene expression Scope: multiisolate | Registration date: 2-May-2012 USDA-ARS | NA |
| PRJNA162923; GEO: GSE37728 | Transcriptome analysis of the immature lifestages in feeding *Rhipicephalus microplus* cattle ticks | Transcriptome or gene expression Scope: multiisolate | Registration date: 16-Feb-2012 Molecular parasitology, biochemistry, University of Pretoria | NA |
| PRJNA193287; GEO: GSE35867 | Gene expression profiling of adult female tissues in feeding ticks. Transcriptional profiling of salivary gland, midgut, and ovary tissues isolated from *R. microplus* females on day 20 post infestation | Transcriptome or gene expression Scope: multiisolate | Registration date: 16-Feb-2012 Molecular parasitology, Biochemistry, University of Pretoria | Stutzer et al. (2013) |
| PRJNA232001 | *R. microplus* (Porto Alegre strain). Seven organs/tissues (ovary, synganglion, salivary gland, fat body, gut) of *R. microplus*, obtained at various stages of development (embryo, semiengorged and engorged female) | Transcriptome or gene expression Scope: multiisolate | Registration date: 18-Dec-2013 Instituto Nacional de Ciência e Tecnologia de Entomologia Molecular Instituto Nacional de Ciencia e Tecnologia de Entomologia Molecular | Xavier et al. (2019) and Tirloni et al. (2014) |
| PRJNA288687 | *Rhipicephalus microplus* strain: Deutch. Different developmental stages of the gene's organ | Transcriptome or gene expression Scope: multiisolate | Registration date: 1-Jul-2015 USDA | NA |

(continued)

**Table 8.1** (continued)

| GenBank Bioproject | Description | Data type | Submission | Publications |
|---|---|---|---|---|
| PRJNA313345 | Salivary gland transcriptome Characterize the salivary gland transcriptome of adult female ticks during the feeding process | Raw sequence reads, transcriptome or gene expression Scope: monoisolate | Registration date: 27-Feb-2016 Agricultural Research Council/ Biotechnology Platform, Agricultural Research Council, South Africa | NA |
| PRJNA329522 | Salivary transcriptome. Global tick salivary transcriptome when feeding of susceptible or resistant breeds of bovines when they underwent a primary infestation | Transcriptome or gene expression Scope: monoisolate | Registration date: 18-Jul-2016 National Institute of Allergy and Infectious Diseases | NA |
| PRJNA338961 | RNASeq of larvae Transcriptional responses in bovine skin and tick salivary glands during blood feeding are reciprocal and differ according to the host genotype | Transcriptome or gene expression Scope: monoisolate | Registration date: 15-Aug-2016 National Institute of Allergy and Infectious Diseases | |
| PRJNA431211 | Transcriptome of fed and unfed adult females | Transcriptome or gene expression Scope: monoisolate | Registration date: 23-Jan-2018 USDA-Agricultural Research Service, USA | Bendele et al. (2019) |

(continued)

**Table 8.1** (continued)

| GenBank Bioproject | Description | Data type | Submission | Publications |
|---|---|---|---|---|
| PRJNA438314 | *Rhipicephalus microplus* raw sequence reads RNA/transcriptome sequencing was performed on 11 libraries from three localities in Brazil. All libraries were sequenced on a multiples lanes (paired-end, 125 bp read-length) on an Illumina HiSeq 2500 platform. Revelance virus transcriptomics | Raw sequence reads. Scope: monoisolate | Registration date: 14-Mar-2018 Universidade de Sao Paulo | NA |
| PRJNA596777 | *Rhipicephalus* (*Boophilus*) *microplus* cattle tick salivary gland transcriptome of engorged females fed on susceptible or resistant hosts was performed | Raw sequence reads Scope: multispecies | Registration date: 19-Dec-2019 EMBRAPA Informatica Agropecuaria | NA |
| PRJNA607772 | Transcriptome of BME26 cells treated with dorsal, relish, or stat specific dsRNAs Transcriptome was assessed by RNA-seq | Transcriptome or gene expression Scope: monoisolate | Registration date: 20-Feb-2020 NIH | NA |
| PRJNA660356 | *Rhipicephalus microplus* physiology in absence or presence of the endosymbiotic Coxiella | Transcriptome or gene expression Scope: multispecies | Registration date: 31-Aug-2020 Institutos Nacionais de Ciencia e Tecnologia em Entomologia Molecular | NA |

(continued)

**Table 8.1** (continued)

| GenBank Bioproject | Description | Data type | Submission | Publications |
|---|---|---|---|---|
| PRJNA915116; GEO:GSE221646 | Differential gene expression of ticks that were fed on cattle vaccinated with a multicomponent vaccine (Bm86 and 3 putative Bm86-binding proteins) and adult ticks fed on control nonvaccinated cattle | Transcriptome or gene expression Scope: multispecies | Registration date: 22-Dec-2022 Molecular and Plant Pathogen Interactions, Plant and Soil Science, University of Pretoria | Maritz-Olivier et al. (2023) |
| PRJNA1013468 | RNA-seq of *Rhipicephalus microplus* midgut | Transcriptome or gene expression Scope: multispecies | Registration date: 6-Sep-2023 National Institute of Allergy and Infectious Diseases | NA |

*NA* not available

resistance issues efficiently and potentially predict future trends in resistance development for more judicious acaricide use. Therefore, for the use of these omics techniques, two key mechanisms underlying acaricide resistance must be understood: enhanced metabolic detoxification and target site modification (Fig. 8.1).

### 8.2.1 Enhanced Metabolic Detoxification

Enhanced metabolic detoxification is a common mechanism through which ticks develop resistance to acaricides. Xenobiotic modifying enzymes (XMEs) play a pivotal role in this process by metabolizing acaricides and rendering them less toxic to ticks (Cossio-Bayugar et al. 2008). This increase in detoxification pathways allows ticks to efficiently neutralize and eliminate acaricides before they can exert their toxic effects. Increased enzyme activity can result from gene amplification, upregulation, coding sequence mutations, or a combination of these mechanisms (Karunaratne et al. 2018). Several studies indicate that resistance to pesticides in arthropods is largely mediated by the action of XMEs (Parkinson and Ogilvie 2010). Consequently, most acaricide resistance research has focused extensively on the expression of XMEs, such as cytochrome P450 enzymes, glutathione S-transferases, carboxylesterases, and cholinesterases. For example, significant increases in the expression of AChE2, ranging from 8.52 to almost 80 tenfold, have been reported in field-isolated OP acaricide-resistant Mexican ticks with overexpression levels (Cossío-Bayúgar et al. 2009, 2024).

**Table 8.2** Categorization of major acaricide classes for tick control according to the IRAC

| IRAC main group<br>MOA group description<br>Primary site of action | Chemical group | Commercial acaricides brands |
|---|---|---|
| Acetylcholinesterase (AChE) inhibitors<br>Inhibiting acetylcholinesterase (AChE) leads to muscle hyperexcitation or tetanization. AChE is the enzyme responsible for terminating the action of the excitatory neurotransmitter acetylcholine at nerve synapses<br>Nerve action | Carbamates | Carbaryl, Propoxur |
| | Organophosphates | Chlorpyrifos, Chlorfenvinphos Coumaphos, Diazinon, Ethion |
| GABA gated chloride channel blockers (antagonist)<br>Blocking the GABA-gated chloride channels (GABA-GCC) prevents the action of GABA, the primary inhibitory neurotransmitter in insects. This disruption leads to hyperexcitation and convulsions<br>Nerve action | Cyclodiene organochlorines | Chlordane, Lindane, Dieldrin |
| | Phenylpyrazoles | Fipronil, Pyripol |
| Voltage gated sodium channel modulator<br>By keeping sodium channels open, hyperexcitation occurs and, in some cases, results in nerve block. Sodium channels play a crucial role in the propagation of action potentials along nerve axons<br>Nerve action | Pyrethroids and Pyrethrins | Cypermethrin, Deltamethrin, Cyhalothrin, Flumethrin, Permethrin, Cyfluthrin |
| Glutamate chloride channel activators<br>Allosterically activate glutamate-gated chloride channels (Glu-GCC), glutamate is an important inhibitory neurotransmitter in insect causing paralysis<br>Nerve and muscle targets | Avermectins | Ivermectin Doramectin, Selamectin, Abamectin, and Eprinomectin |
| | Milbemycins | Milbemectin Moxidectin, Milbemycin Oxime |
| Octopamine receptor<br>Allosteric activation of glutamate-gated chloride channels (Glu-GCC) results in paralysis. In insects, glutamate functions as a crucial inhibitory neurotransmitter<br>Nerve action | Formamidines | Amitraz |
| These inhibitors target chitin biosynthesis by specifically affecting chitin synthase 1 (CHS1) | Benzoylureas | Fuazuron |

Adapted from Cossio-Bayugar et al. (2021)

XMEs biochemically transform both endogenous and exogenous xenobiotics. For example, the ixodicide permethrin is metabolized into phenoxyphenyl-methanol and dichloroethenyl-dimethylcyclopropanecarboxylate, which are less toxic and more easily eliminated. This metabolic process, known as biotransformation, is a process in which the first line of XMEs modify pesticides, which are then eliminated and secreted (Fig. 8.1).

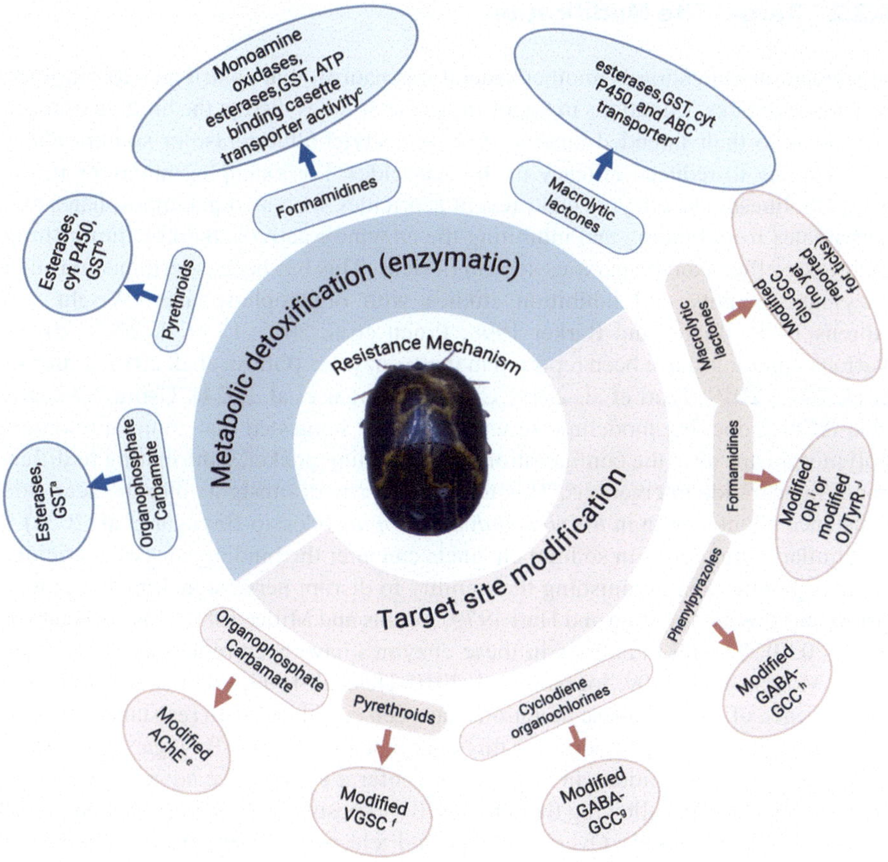


**Fig. 8.1** Mechanisms underlying acaricide resistance in ticks. *AChE* acetylcholinesterase, *VGSC* voltage gated sodium channel modulator, *GABA-GCC* GABA-gated chloride channel, *OR* octopamine receptor, *O/TyrR* octopamine/tyramine receptor, *Glu-GCC* glutamate-gated chloride channel; [a](Fular et al. 2020; Baxter and Barker 2002; Miranda-Miranda et al. 2009; Baffi et al. 2008; Cossio-Bayugar et al. 2024), [b](Cossío-Bayúgar et al. 2018; Cossío-Bayúgar et al. 2009; De Jersey et al. 1985; Baffi et al. 2008), [c](Jonsson et al. 2018; Lara et al. 2015), [d](Le Gall et al. 2018), [e](Temeyer et al. 2007, 2019; Cossio-Bayugar et al. 2024), [f](Stone et al. 2014; Morgan et al. 2009; He et al. 1999; Cossío-Bayúgar et al. 2020), [g](Tian et al. 2019), [h](Tian et al. 2019), [i](Baron et al. 2015), [j](Corley et al. 2013; Jonsson et al. 2018). (Image created by Biorender.com)

The impact of enhanced metabolic detoxification on resistance development is significant. When exposed to acaricides, ticks with upregulated XMEs can effectively breakdown and eliminate the chemicals before they can reach their target sites within the tick's body. This rapid detoxification process reduces the concentration of acaricides to sublethal levels, thereby diminishing their effectiveness in controlling tick populations. Over time, repeated exposure to acaricides leads to the selection of ticks with heightened metabolic detoxification capabilities, ultimately resulting in widespread resistance.

### 8.2.2 Target Site Modification

Target site modification is another crucial mechanism that contributes to acaricide resistance in ticks. Mutations in target sites of acaricides disrupt the binding of these chemicals to their intended targets, such as acetylcholinesterase or sodium channels, leading to reduced efficacy of the acaricides. For example, mutations in the acetylcholinesterase enzyme can prevent acaricides such as organophosphates and carbamates from binding and inhibiting the enzyme's activity, thereby diminishing their toxic effects on the nervous system of ticks. This has been determined through enzymatic activity and inhibition studies with organophosphates (Wright and Ahrens 1988; Baxter and Barker 1998; Pruett et al. 2002; Li et al. 2003, 2005). Various mutations have been reported in these enzymes (Ghosh et al. 2015; Temeyer et al. 2007, 2019; Jyoti et al. 2016; Cossio-Bayugar et al. 2024). Using 3D acaricide-AChE2 docking modeling, researchers have suggested that some amino acid polymorphisms alter the configuration of the binding pocket, contributing to differences in acaricide interactions. This ultimately provides insights into the acaricide resistance phenomenon in *Rhipicephalus microplus* (Cossio-Bayugar et al. 2024).

Similarly, mutations in sodium channels can alter the binding sites of acaricides such as pyrethroids, diminishing their ability to disrupt nerve signaling and induce paralysis in ticks (Osborne and Hart 1979; Adams and Miller 1980; Cossío-Bayúgar et al. 2020). Several mutations in these enzymes have been reported (Stone et al. 2014; Morgan et al. 2009; Jonsson et al. 2010; He et al. 1999; Villar et al. 2020), and the presence of some of these mutations has been correlated with resistance, providing a physiological explanation for this phenomenon (Cossío-Bayúgar et al. 2020) (Fig. 8.1). These alterations in target sites confer a competitive advantage to ticks with resistant alleles, allowing them to survive exposure to acaricides that are lethal to susceptible individuals. Over time, repeated selection pressure from acaricide use increases the prevalence of resistant ticks in populations, posing significant challenges to tick control efforts.

In conclusion, the molecular basis of acaricide resistance involves complex interplay between enhanced metabolic detoxification pathways and target site modifications in ticks. Understanding these mechanisms is crucial for developing effective strategies to manage and prevent acaricide resistance. By revealing the genetic and biochemical pathways involved in resistance development, researchers can work toward the development of new acaricides or integrated pest management approaches to mitigate the impact of tick resistance on livestock and human health.

## 8.3 Obtaining and Preparation of Biological Samples

Efforts in scientific research involving omics technologies must intensify significantly to achieve comprehensive control of cattle ticks in the coming years. It is particularly important to maintain effective and ongoing communication with service providers. The goals of the experiment and the source of the samples before

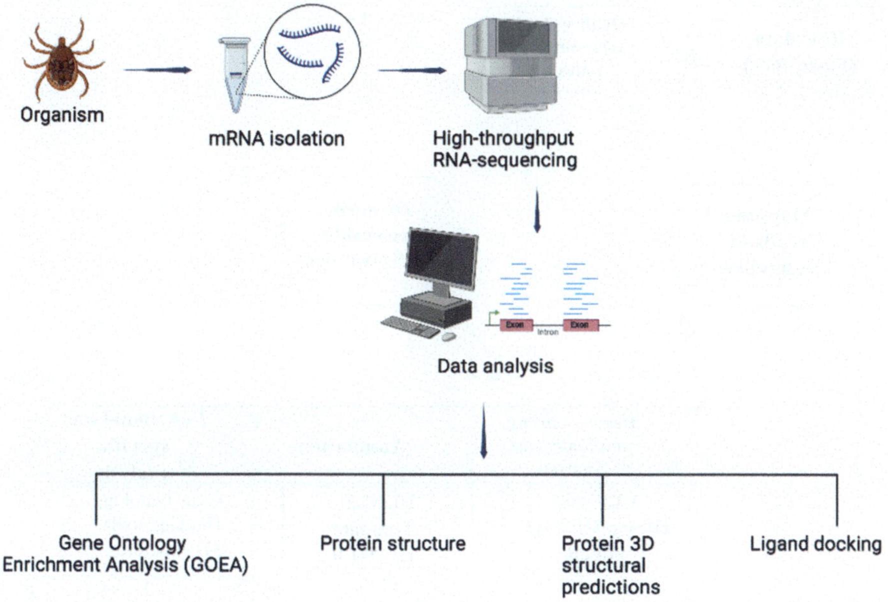


**Fig. 8.2** Schematic diagram of high-throughput sequencing data generation and their analysis. (Created with BioRender.com)

starting the process would be clearly explained. Accordingly, effective routes for data analysis could be defined. The general method is shown in Figs. 8.2 and 8.3.

## 8.4 Workflow for Transcriptomic Studies

The vast amount of data generated from high-throughput sequencing necessitates substantial computational capacity, specialized algorithms, applications (software), and bioinformatics expertise to process raw data and transform it into interpretable information that addresses the initial research objectives. Figure 8.3 illustrates the main steps and some of the commonly used tools for data management.

Gene Ontology Enrichment Analysis (GOEA) has made substantial progress, in part due to increased computational capabilities since it became a mainstream scientific discipline in the early 2000s (Gene Ontology Consortium 2021). Multiple scientific disciplines now converge on the GOEA for insights into protein function, as well as for developing novel therapies and drug treatments Chabrun et al. (2020), leveraging powerful algorithms available as free online services or downloadable shareware (Ashburner et al. 2000). GOEA is now integral to most functional protein research that seeks to describe the basic molecular functions of proteins.

An exponential increase in publications on the subject has been observed over the past decade (Góngora-Castillo et al. 2020). The availability of these tools has significantly expanded the literature on predicted protein functionality, reflecting an

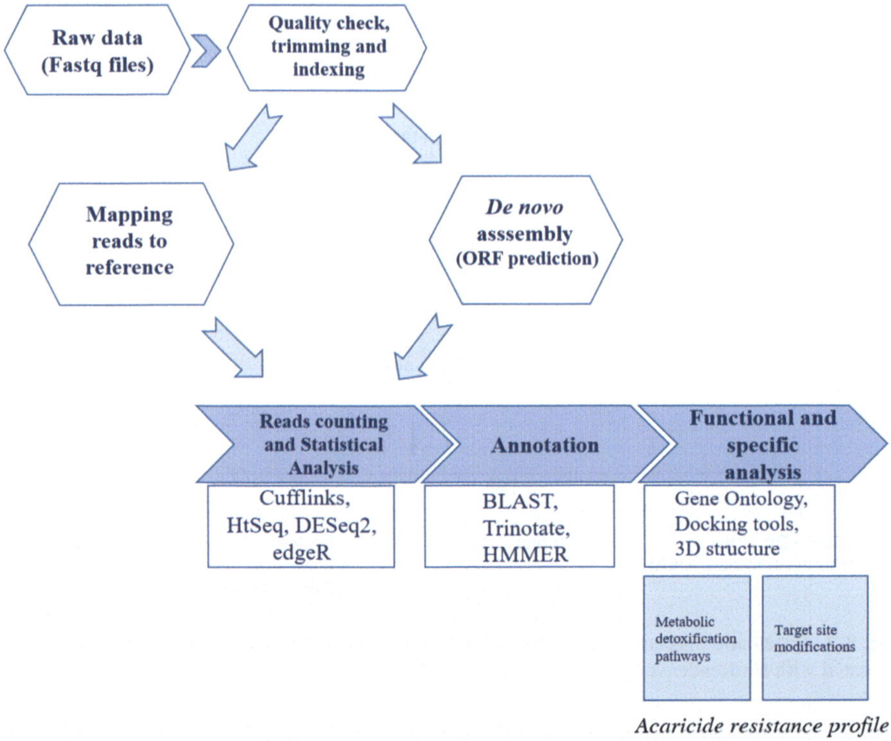


**Fig. 8.3** The workflow for RNAseq data analysis, which can be applied for *R. microplus* transcriptome analysis and identification of related resistance elements

increasing appreciation among protein researchers and spurring further development of protein modeling techniques (Gene Ontology Consortium 2021). Currently, such analysis is considered an essential assessment for most scientific research involving the characterization of proteins, receptors, and enzymes, particularly when these entities are reported for the first time in *R. microplus* or other medically important arthropods. Most of these algorithms are employed in protein discovery projects (Zeng and Extavour 2012). Since computational simulations can predict interactions between the binding sites of proteins and small molecules that may trigger biochemical responses, this type of analysis has become a mandatory step before conducting any in vivo experimentation (Lopez et al. 2007).

Gene Ontology enrichment analysis (GOEA) is valuable because of its ability to assess related protein orthologs, which can predict how pesticide resistance genes may evolve under pesticide pressure in cattle grazing areas (Fang et al. 2010). This is particularly valuable when designing tick control strategies and eradication campaigns for *Rhipicephalus microplus* (Cossio-Bayugar et al. 2021). The comprehensive nature of *R. microplus* transcriptome data encompassing transcripts expressed under various conditions makes data mining a standard preexperimental step for chemical compound screening and formulation selection. Fortunately for protein researchers, most algorithms assist scientists in elucidating the functions of compounds and their interactions with proteins at the molecular level (Góngora-Castillo et al. 2020). The availability of free online algorithms has enabled scientists without specialized bioinformatics or computational analysis expertise to obtain reliable results in enzyme docking simulations (EDS). Unless the three-dimensional (3D) protein structure has been precisely determined through X-ray diffraction or NMR spectroscopy, most algorithms generate a 3D approximation model. This is accomplished by starting with the amino acid sequence and identifying a preexisting 3D model that best matches the structure and function of the protein in question. Consequently, it is important to recognize that protein-ligand docking analyses are based on virtual approximations, which may differ from actual effects observed in real-world scenarios. Table 8.3 lists the PDB databases worldwide where most Protein Data Bank (PDB) (PDBe-KB consortium et al. 2022) models are stored and explains how programmable logic device (PLD) algorithms search for the closest match to any protein query (Berman et al. 2003).

## 8.5 Enzyme Docking Simulation Algorithms

Most algorithms predict protein structure based on molecular flexibility, irrespective of their underlying premises. All of these algorithms require a PDB model as well as parameters such as electric charges, torsional movements, and bond angles between atoms (Lopez et al. 2007). These physical properties are collectively referred to as modeling criteria. The simulation process is generally similar across

**Table 8.3** The PDB 3D protein model databanks

| PDB database | Description | Reference | Online accession |
|---|---|---|---|
| The worldwide PDB (wwPDB) | Publicly available Protein Data Bank Archive (PDB Archive) of macromolecular structures solved either by X-ray crystallography or nuclear magnetic resonance (NMR) spectroscopy | Berman et al. (2003) | http://www.pdb.org |
| Biological Magnetic Resonance Data Bank BMRB | Data derived from NMR spectroscopic investigations of biologically relevant molecules | Ulrich et al. (2007) | https://bmrb.io |
| The protein data bank RCSB PDB | Protein data Bank archive-information about the 3D shapes of proteins, nucleic acids, and complex assemblies | Berman (2000) | https://www.rcsb.org |
| Protein Data Bank Europe PDNe | Macromolecular structures and related data make it available to the biomedical community | PDBe-KB consortium et al. (2022) | https://www.ebi.ac.uk/pdbe/ |
| Structure NCBI | Protein Data Bank archive-information about the 3D shapes of proteins, nucleic acids, and complex assemblies | Wang et al. (2020) | https://www.ncbi.nlm.nih.gov/structure |

different algorithms, representing surface electrostatic fields to identify probable ligand binding sites and cavities (Halperin et al. 2002).

A routine procedure for any protein researcher involves an exhaustive search for proteins of interest—in this case, within the *Rhipicephalus microplus* transcriptomes. Once an amino acid sequence meeting the study criteria is identified from the protein databank, a matching PDB file can be obtained by submitting these sequences to a preferred 3D viewer algorithm. Several algorithms can convert a FASTA amino acid sequence into a corresponding PDB file based on models preloaded in protein data bank repositories. Finding a matching PDB file from an amino acid sequence is only one part of the analysis. Most algorithms also provide a detailed description of the protein folding patterns and structural arrangements within the polypeptide chain. These structural patterns often include binding pockets that exhibit affinity for known drugs, offering insights into the potential function of specific proteins (Ehrt et al. 2016). Modern 3D modeling algorithms can accurately predict multiple binding pockets and describe the amino acid residues that interact with specific ligands.

## References

Abbas RZ, Zaman MA, Colwell DD, Gilleard J, Iqbal Z (2014) Acaricide resistance in cattle ticks and approaches to its management: the state of play. Vet Parasitol 203(1-2):6–20. https://doi.org/10.1016/j.vetpar.2014.03.006

Adams ME, Miller TA (1980) Neural and behavioral correlates of pyrethroid and DDT-type poisoning in the house fly, *Musca domestica* L. Pestic Biochem Physiol 13:137–147. https://doi.org/10.1016/0048-3575(80)90065-6

Amaro-Estrada I, Miranda Miranda E, Cossío-Bayúgar R, Sachman-Ruiz B (2023) Chapter 11: Comparative genomics and transcriptomics in the cattle tick *Rhipicephalus microplus*. In: Cossio-Bayugar R, Miranda-Miranda E, Kumar S (eds) A laboratory Manual on *Rhipicephalus microplus*. Cambridge Scholars Publishing. Lady Stephenson Library, Newcastle upon Tyne, pp 170–189. ISBN (10): 1-5275-0418-2 ISBN (13): 978-1-5275-0418-9

Ashburner M, Ball CA, Blake JA, Botstein D, Butler H, Cherry JM, Davis AP, Dolinski K, Dwight SS, Eppig JT, Harris MA, Hill DP, Issel-Tarver L, Kasarskis A, Lewis S, Matese JC, Richardson JE, Ringwald M, Rubin GM, Sherlock G (2000) Gene ontology: tool for the unification of biology. Nat Genet 25:25–29. https://doi.org/10.1038/75556

Baffi MA, de Souza GR, de Sousa CS, Ceron CR, Bonetti AM (2008) Esterase enzymes involved in pyrethroid and organophosphate resistance in a Brazilian population of *Riphicephallus (Boophilus) microplus* (Acari, Ixodidae). Mol Biochem Parasitol 160(1):70–73. https://doi.org/10.1016/j.molbiopara.2008.03.009

Baron S, van der Merwe NA, Madder M, Maritz-Olivier C (2015) SNP Analysis Infers that Recombination Is Involved in the Evolution of Amitraz Resistance in *Rhipicephalus microplus*. PLoS One 10(7):e0131341. https://doi.org/10.1371/journal.pone.0131341

Baxter GD, Barker SC (1998) Acetylcholinesterase cDNA of the cattle tick, *Boophilus microplus*: characterisation and role in organophosphate resistance. Insect Biochem Mol Biol 28(8):581–589. https://doi.org/10.1016/s0965-1748(98)00034-4

Bendele KG, Guerrero FD, Cameron C, Bodine DM, Miller RJ (2019) Gene expression during the early stages of host perception and attachment in adult female *Rhipicephalus microplus* ticks. Exp Appl Acarol 79:107–124. https://doi.org/10.1007/s10493-019-00420-1

Berman HM (2000) The Protein Data Bank. Nucleic Acids Res 28:235–242. https://doi.org/10.1093/nar/28.1.235

Berman H, Henrick K, Nakamura H (2003) Announcing the worldwide protein data Bank. Nat Struct Mol Biol 10:980–980. https://doi.org/10.1038/nsb1203-980

Bloomquist JR (2003) Chloride channels as tools for developing selective insecticides. Arch Insect Biochem Physiol 54:145–156. https://doi.org/10.1002/arch.10112

Chabrun F, Huetz N, Dieu X, Rousseau G, Bouzillé G, Chao de la Barca JM, Procaccio V, Lenaers G, Blanchet O, Legendre G, Mirebeau-Prunier D, Cuggia M, Guardiola P, Reynier P, Gascoin G (2020) Data-mining approach on transcriptomics and methylomics placental analysis highlights genes in fetal growth restriction. Front Genet 10:1292. https://doi.org/10.3389/fgene.2019.01292

Corley SW, Jonsson NN, Piper EK, Cutullé C, Stear MJ (2013) Seddon JM. Mutation in the RmβAOR gene is associated with amitraz resistance in the cattle tick *Rhipicephalus microplus*. Proc Natl Acad Sci USA 110(42):16772–16777. https://doi.org/10.1073/pnas.1309072110

Cossio-Bayúgar R, Miranda-Miranda E, Ortiz-Nájera A, Neri-Orantes S, Olvera F (2008) Cytochrome P-450 monoxygenase gene expression supports multifactorial origin for acaricide resistance in *Rhipicephalus microplus*. J Parasitol Res 3:59–66. https://scialert.net/abstract/?doi=jp.2008.59.66

Cossío-Bayúgar R, Miranda-Miranda E, Portilla-Salgado D, Osorio-Miranda J (2009) Quantitative PCR detection of cholinesterase and carboxylesterase expression levels in acaricide resistant *Rhipicephalus (Boophilus) microplus*. J Entomol 6(2):117–123. https://doi.org/10.3923/je.2009.117.123

Cossío-Bayúgar R, Martínez-Ibañez F, Aguilar-Díaz H, Miranda-Miranda E (2018) Pyrethroid Acaricide resistance is proportional to P-450 cytochrome oxidase expression in the cattle tick *Rhipicephalus microplus*. Biomed Res Int 2018:1–6. https://doi.org/10.1155/2018/8292465

Cossío-Bayúgar R, Miranda-Miranda E, Martínez-Ibañez F, Narváez-Padilla V, Reynaud E (2020) Physiological evidence that three known mutations in the para-sodium channel gene confer cypermethrin knockdown resistance in *Rhipicephalus microplus*. Parasit Vectors 13(1):370. https://doi.org/10.1186/s13071-020-04227-7

Cossio-Bayugar R, Miranda-Miranda E, Aguilar Díaz H, Reynaud E (2021) Type of resistance. In: The entomological guide to *Rhipicephalus*, insects and other terrestrial arthropods: biology, chemistry and behavior. Nova Scientific, New York, NY, pp 147–176

Cossio-Bayugar R, Martinez-Ibañez F, Aguilar-Diaz H, Miranda-Miranda E (2024) Relationship between acaricide resistance and acetylcholinesterase gene polymorphisms in the cattle tick *Rhipicephalus microplus*. Parasite 31:3. https://doi.org/10.1051/parasite/2024003

De Jersey J, Nolan J, Davey PA, Riddles PW (1985) Separation and characterization of the pyrethroid-hydrolyzing esterases of the cattle tick, *Boophilus microplus*. Pestic Biochem Physiol 23:349–357. https://doi.org/10.1016/0048-3575(85)90096-3

Domingos A, Antunes S, Borges L, Rosário VE (2013) Approaches towards tick and tick-borne diseases control. Rev Soc Bras Med Trop 46(3):265–269. https://doi.org/10.1590/0037-8682-0014-2012

Dong K, Du Y, Rinkevich F, Nomura Y, Xu P, Wang L, Silver K, Zhorov BS (2014) Molecular biology of insect sodium channels and pyrethroid resistance. Insect Biochem Mol Biol 50:1–17. https://doi.org/10.1016/j.ibmb.2014.03.012

Ehrt C, Brinkjost T, Koch O (2016) Impact of binding site comparisons on medicinal chemistry and rational molecular design. J Med Chem 59:4121–4151. https://doi.org/10.1021/acs.jmedchem.6b00078

Eisen RJ, Kugeler KJ, Eisen L, Beard CB, Paddock CD (2017) Tick-Borne Zoonoses in the United States: Persistent and Emerging Threats to Human Health. ILAR J 58(3):319–335. https://doi.org/10.1093/ilar/ilx005

Fang G, Bhardwaj N, Robilotto R, Gerstein MB (2010) Getting started in gene orthology and functional analysis. PLoS Comput Biol 6:e1000703. https://doi.org/10.1371/journal.pcbi.1000703

Fular A, Gupta S, Sharma AK, Kumar S, Upadhaya D, Shakya M, Nagar G, Ghosh S (2020) Standardization of tick specific biochemical tools for estimation of esterases, monooxygenases and glutathione S-transferase for characterization of acaricide resistance. Pestic Biochem Physiol 164:130–139. https://doi.org/10.1016/j.pestbp.2020.01.008

Garcia GR, Marcos J, Ribeiro C, Maruyama SR, Gardinassi LG, Nelson K, Ferreira BR, Andrade TG, Ferreira IK, Santos DM (2020) OPEN a transcriptome and proteome of the tick *Rhipicephalus microplus* shaped by the genetic composition of its hosts and developmental stage. Sci Rep 1:1–23. https://doi.org/10.1038/s41598-020-69793-3

Gene Ontology Consortium (2021) The gene ontology resource: enriching a gold mine. Nucleic Acids Res 49:D325–D334. https://doi.org/10.1093/nar/gkaa1113

George JE, Pound JM, Davey RB (2004) Chemical control of ticks on cattle and the resistance of these parasites to acaricides. Parasitology 129(Suppl):S353–S366. https://doi.org/10.1017/s0031182003004682

Ghosh S, Kumar R, Nagar G, Kumar S, Sharma AK, Srivastava A, Kumar S, Ajith Kumar KG, Saravanan BC (2015) Survey of acaricides resistance status of *Rhipiciphalus* (*Boophilus*) *microplus* collected from selected places of Bihar, an eastern state of India. Ticks Tick Borne Dis 6(5):668–675. https://doi.org/10.1016/j.ttbdis.2015.05.013

Giachetto PF, Cunha RC Jr, Nhani A (2020) Gene expression in the salivary gland of *Rhipicephalus* (*Boophilus*) *microplus* fed on tick-susceptible and tick-resistant hosts. Front Cell Infect Microbiol 9:1–15. https://doi.org/10.3389/fcimb.2019.00477

Góngora-Castillo E, López-Ochoa LA, Apolinar-Hernández MM, Caamal-Pech AM, Contreras-de la Rosa PA, Quiroz-Moreno A, Ramírez-Prado JH, O'Connor-Sánchez A (2020) Data mining of metagenomes to find novel enzymes: a non-computationally intensive method. 3 Biotech 10:78. https://doi.org/10.1007/s13205-019-2044-6

Guerrero FD, Bendele KG, Chen AC, Li AY, Miller RJ, Pleasance E, Varhol R, Rousseau ME, Nene VM (2007) Serial analysis of gene expression in the southern cattle tick following acaricide treatment of larvae from organophosphate resistant and susceptible strains. Insect Mol Biol 16(1):49–60. https://doi.org/10.1111/j.1365-2583.2007.00699.x

Guerrero FD, Kellogg A, Ogrey AN, Heekin AM, Barrero R, Bellgard MI, Dowd SE, Leung MY (2016) Prediction of G protein-coupled receptor encoding sequences from the synganglion transcriptome of the cattle tick, *Rhipicephalus microplus*. Ticks Tick Borne Dis 7(5):670–677. https://doi.org/10.1016/j.ttbdis.2016.02.014

Guerrero FD, Ghaffari N, Bendele KG, Metz RP, Dickens CM, Blood PD, Tidwell J, Miller RJ, Pérez AA, León D, Teel PD, Johnson CD (2021) Raw pacific biosciences and illumina sequencing reads and assembled genome data for the cattle ticks *Rhipicephalus microplus* and *Rhipicephalus annulatus*. Data Brief 35:106852. https://doi.org/10.1016/j.dib.2021.106852

Halperin I, Ma B, Wolfson H, Nussinov R (2002) Principles of docking: an overview of search algorithms and a guide to scoring functions. Proteins Struct Funct Genet 47:409–443. https://doi.org/10.1002/prot.10115

He H, Chen AC, Davey RB, Ivie GW, George JE (1999) Identification of a point mutation in the para-type sodium channel gene from a pyrethroid-resistant cattle tick. Biochem Biophys Res Commun 261(3):558–561. https://doi.org/10.1006/bbrc.1999.1076

IRAC (2020) Insecticide Resistance Action Committee. IRAC Insecticide Resistance Action Committee. www.iraconline.org or enquiries@irac-online.org.

Jonsson NN, Cutullè C, Corley SW, Seddon JM (2010) Identification of a mutation in the para-sodium channel gene of the cattle tick *Rhipicephalus microplus* associated with resistance to flumethrin but not to cypermethrin. Int J Parasitol 40(14):1659–1664. https://doi.org/10.1016/j.ijpara.2010.07.006

Jonsson NN, Klafke G, Corley SW, Tidwell J, Berry CM, Koh-Tan HC (2018) Molecular biology of amitraz resistance in cattle ticks of the genus *Rhipicephalus*. Front Biosci 23(5):796–810. https://doi.org/10.2741/4617

Jyoti, Singh NK, Singh H, Singh NK, Rath SS (2016) Multiple mutations in the acetylcholinesterase 3 gene associated with organophosphate resistance in *Rhipicephalus* (*Boophilus*) *microplus* ticks from Punjab. India Vet Parasitol 216:108–117. https://doi.org/10.1016/j.vetpar.2015.12.004

Karunaratne SHPP, De Silva WAPP, Weeraratne TC, Surendran SN (2018) Insecticide resistance in mosquitoes: development, mechanisms and monitoring. Ceylon J Sci 47:299–309. https://doi.org/10.4038/cjs.v47i4.7547

Lara FA, Pohl PC, Gandara AC, Ferreira Jda S, Nascimento-Silva MC, Bechara GH, Sorgine MH, Almeida IC, Vaz Ida S, Jr OPL (2015) ATP Binding Cassette Transporter Mediates Both Heme and Pesticide Detoxification in Tick Midgut Cells. PLoS One 10(8):e0134779. https://doi.org/10.1371/journal.pone.0134779

Le Gall VL, Klafke GM, Torres TT (2018) Detoxification mechanisms involved in ivermectin resistance in the cattle tick, *Rhipicephalus* (*Boophilus*) *microplus*. Sci Rep 8(1):12401. https://doi.org/10.1038/s41598-018-30907-7

Li AY, Davey RB, Miller RJ, George JE (2003) Resistance to Coumaphos and Diazinon in *Boophilus microplus* (Acari: Ixodidae) and Evidence for the Involvement of an Oxidative Detoxification Mechanism. J Med Entomol 40:482–490. https://doi.org/10.1603/0022-2585-40.4.482

Li AY, Davey LR, George JE (2005) Carbaryl resistance in Mexican strains of the southern cattle tick (Acari: Ixodidae). J Econ Entomol 98(2):552–556. https://doi.org/10.1603/0022-0493-98.2.552

Lopez G, Valencia A, Tress ML (2007) Firestar—prediction of functionally important residues using structural templates and alignment reliability. Nucleic Acids Res 35:W573–W577. https://doi.org/10.1093/nar/gkm297

Lumaret JP, Errouissi F, Floate K, Römbke J, Wardhaugh K (2012) A review on the toxicity and non-target effects of macrocyclic lactones in terrestrial and aquatic environments. Curr Pharm Biotechnol 13(6):1004–1060. https://doi.org/10.2174/138920112800399257

Maritz-Olivier C, Ferreira M, Olivier NA, Crafford J, Stutzer C (2023) Mining gene expression data for rational identification of novel drug targets and vaccine candidates against the cattle tick, *Rhipicephalus microplus*. Exp Appl Acarol 91(2):291–317. https://doi.org/10.1007/s10493-023-00838-8

Martinez Ibañez F, Cossio-Bayugar R, Miranda-Miranda E, Jasso-Villazul CE (2021) Reference tick strains as an important biological material for resistance characterization. In: The entomological guide to *Rhipicephalus*. Nova Scientific, New York, NY, pp 177–200

Mercado-Curiel RF, Palmer GH, Guerrero FD, Brayton KA (2011) Temporal characterisation of the organ-specific *Rhipicephalus microplus* transcriptional response to *Anaplasma marginale* infection. Int J Parasitol Jul 41(8):851–860. https://doi.org/10.1016/j.ijpara.2011.03.003

Miranda-Miranda E, Cossio-Bay R, Quezada-De MDR, Olvera-Valencia F, Neri-Orant S (2009) Age-induced carboxylesterase expression in Acaricide-resistant *Rhipicephalus microplus*. Res J Parasitol 4:70. https://doi.org/10.3923/jp.2009.70.78

Morgan JA, Corley SW, Jackson LA, Lew-Tabor AE, Moolhuijzen PM, Jonsson NN (2009) Identification of a mutation in the para-sodium channel gene of the cattle tick *Rhipicephalus* (*Boophilus*) *microplus* associated with resistance to synthetic pyrethroid acaricides. Int J Parasitol 39(7):775–779. https://doi.org/10.1016/j.ijpara.2008.12.006

Nowrousian M (2014) Next-generation sequencing techniques for eukaryotic microorganisms: sequencing-based solutions to biological problems MINIREVIEW next-generation sequencing techniques for eukaryotic microorganisms: sequencing-based solutions to biological problems. Eukaryot Cell 9:1300–1310. https://doi.org/10.1128/EC.00123-10

Omura S (2008) Ivermectin: 25 years and still going strong. Int J Sci Environ Technol 31:91–98. https://doi.org/10.1016/j.ijantimicag.2007.08.023

Osborne MP, Hart RJ (1979) Neurophysiological studies of the effects of permethrin upon pyrethroid resistant (kdr) and susceptible strains of dipteran larvae. Pestic Sci 10:407–413. https://doi.org/10.1002/ps.2780100507

Parkinson A, Ogilvie BW (2010) Chapter 6. biotransformation of xenobiotics. In: Klaassen CD, Watkins JB, III (eds) Casarett & Doull's Essentials of Toxicology, 2e. The McGraw-Hill Companies

PDBe-KB Consortium, Varadi M, Anyango S, Armstrong D, Berrisford J, Choudhary P, Deshpande M, Nadzirin N, Nair SS, Pravda L, Tanweer A, Al-Lazikani B, Andreini C, Barton GJ, Bednar

D, Berka K, Blundell T, Brock KP, Carazo JM, Damborsky J, David A, Dey S, Dunbrack R, Recio JF, Fraternali F, Gibson T, Helmer-Citterich M, Hoksza D, Hopf T, Jakubec D, Kannan N, Krivak R, Kumar M, Levy ED, London N, Macias JR, Srivatsan MM, Marks DS, Martens L, McGowan SA, McGreig JE, Modi V, Parra RG, Pepe G, Piovesan D, Prilusky J, Putignano V, Radusky LG, Ramasamy P, Rausch AO, Reuter N, Rodriguez LA, Rollins NJ, Rosato A, Rubach P, Serrano L, Singh G, Skoda P, Sorzano COS, Stourac J, Sulkowska JI, Svobodova R, Tichshenko N, Tosatto SCE, Vranken W, Wass MN, Xue D, Zaidman D, Thornton J, Sternberg M, Orengo C, Velankar S (2022) PDBe-KB: collaboratively defining the biological context of structural data. Nucleic Acids Res 50:D534–D542. https://doi.org/10.1093/nar/gkab988

Pruett JH, Guerrero FD, Hernandez R (2002) Isolation and identification of an esterase from a Mexican strain of *Boophilus microplus* (Acari: Ixodidae). J Econ Entomol 95(5):1001–1007. https://doi.org/10.1603/0022-0493-95.5.1001

Rodriguez-Vivas RI, Jonsson NN, Bhushan C (2018) Strategies for the control of *Rhipicephalus microplus* ticks in a world of conventional acaricide and macrocyclic lactone resistance. Parasitol Res 117(1):3–29. https://doi.org/10.1007/s00436-017-5677-6

Shi J, Shen S, Wu H, Zhang Y (2021) Metagenomic profiling of viruses associated with *Rhipicephalus microplus* ticks in Yunnan Province, China. Virol Sin 36:623–635. https://doi.org/10.1007/s12250-020-00319-x

Sparks TC, Nauen R (2015) IRAC: mode of action classification and insecticide resistance management. Pestic Biochem Physiol 121:122–128. https://doi.org/10.1016/j.pestbp.2014.11.014

Stone NE, Olafson PU, Davey RB, Buckmeier G, Bodine D, Sidak-Loftis LC, Giles JR, Duhaime R, Miller RJ, Mosqueda J, Scoles GA, Wagner DM, Busch JD (2014) Multiple mutations in the para-sodium channel gene are associated with pyrethroid resistance in *Rhipicephalus microplus* from the United States and Mexico. Parasit Vectors 1(7):456. https://doi.org/10.1186/s13071-014-0456-z

Stutzer C, van Zyl WA, Olivier NA, Richards S, Maritz-Olivier C (2013) Gene expression profiling of adult female tissues in feeding *Rhipicephalus microplus* cattle ticks. Int J Parasitol 43:541–554. https://doi.org/10.1016/j.ijpara.2013.01.009

Temeyer KB, Pruett JH, Olafson PU, Chen AC (2007) R86Q, a mutation in BmAChE3 yielding a *Rhipicephalus microplus* organophosphate-insensitive acetylcholinesterase. J Med Entomol 44(6):1013–1018. https://doi.org/10.1603/00222585(2007)44[1013:ramiby]2.0.co;2

Temeyer KB, Schlechte KG, McDonough WP (2019) Baculoviral Expression of Presumptive OP Resistance Mutations in BmAChE1 of *Rhipicephalus* (*Boophilus*) *microplus* (Ixodida: Ixodidae) and Biochemical Resistance to OP Inhibition. J Med Entomol 3;56(5):1318–1323. https://doi.org/10.1093/jme/tjz062

Tian Y, Gao Y, Chen Y, Liu G, Ju X (2019) Identification of The Fipronil Resistance Associated Mutations in Nilaparvata lugens GABA Receptors by Molecular Modeling. Molecules 24(22):4116. https://doi.org/10.3390/molecules24224116

Tirloni L, Reck J, Terra RMS, Martins JR, Mulenga A, Sherman NE, Fox JW, Yates JR, Termignoni C, Pinto AFM, da Silva Vaz I (2014) Proteomic analysis of cattle tick *Rhipicephalus* (*Boophilus*) *microplus* saliva: a comparison between partially and fully engorged females. PLoS One 9:e94831. https://doi.org/10.1371/journal.pone.0094831

Ulrich EL, Akutsu H, Doreleijers JF, Harano Y, Ioannidis YE, Lin J, Livny M, Mading S, Maziuk D, Miller Z, Nakatani E, Schulte CF, Tolmie DE, Kent Wenger R, Yao H, Markley JL (2007) BioMagResBank. Nucleic Acids Res 36:D402–D408. https://doi.org/10.1093/nar/gkm957

Villar D, Klafke GM, Rodríguez-Durán A, Bossio F, Miller R, Pérez de León AA, Cortés-Vecino JA, Chaparro-Gutiérrez JJ (2020) Resistance profile and molecular characterization of pyrethroid resistance in a *Rhipicephalus microplus* strain from Colombia. Med Vet Entomol 34(1):105–115. https://doi.org/10.1111/mve.12418

Wang J, Youkharibache P, Zhang D, Lanczycki CJ, Geer RC, Madej T, Phan L, Ward M, Lu S, Marchler GH, Wang Y, Bryant SH, Geer LY, Marchler-Bauer A (2020) iCn3D, a web-based 3D viewer for sharing 1D/2D/3D representations of biomolecular structures. Bioinformatics 36:131–135. https://doi.org/10.1093/bioinformatics/btz502

Wright FC, Ahrens EH (1988) Cholinesterase insensitivity: a mechanism of resistance in Mexican strains of *Boophilus microplus* (Acari: Ixodidae) against coumaphos. J Med Entomol 25(4):234–239. https://doi.org/10.1093/jmedent/25.4.234

Xavier MA, Tirloni L, Pinto AFM, Diedrich JK, Yates JR 3rd, Gonzales S, Farber M, da Silva Vaz I Junior, Termignoni C (2019) Tick Gené's organ engagement in lipid metabolism revealed by a combined transcriptomic and proteomic approach. Ticks Tick Borne Dis 10(4):787–797. https://doi.org/10.1016/j.ttbdis.2019.03.013

Zeng V, Extavour CG (2012) ASGARD: an open-access database of annotated transcriptomes for emerging model arthropod species. In: Database 2012, p bas048. https://doi.org/10.1093/database/bas048

Zhang X, Liu Z, Yang J, Chen Z, Guan G, Ren Q, Liu A, Luo J, Yin H, Li Y (2014) Multiplex PCR for diagnosis of *Theileria uilenbergi*, *Theileria luwenshuni*, and *Theileria ovis* in small ruminants. Parasitol Res 113(2):527–531. https://doi.org/10.1007/s00436-013-3684-9

Zhang XL, Deng YP, Yang T, Li LY, Cheng TY, Liu GH, Duan DY (2022) Metagenomics of the midgut microbiome of *Rhipicephalus microplus* from China. Parasit Vectors 15:1–15. https://doi.org/10.1186/s13071-022-05161-6

# Vaccines Against Ticks

# 9

Juan Mosqueda, Consuelo Almazán,
Daniel Gustavo López-Díaz, Iván Corona-Guerrero,
Aldo Josué Pavón-Rocha, María Martina Esperanza Perez-Soria, Diego Josimar Hernández-Silva,
and Rodrigo Morales-García

**Abstract**

Ticks are the ectoparasites that cause the most damage to the veterinary industry. Because of their hematophagous habits, ticks consume significant amounts of blood, causing debilitating and immunosuppressive effects. In addition, ticks are the major transmitters of pathogens, including viruses, bacteria, and protozoa. Tick infestations are controlled with acaricides; However, the disadvantages of using them, including the increasing resistance of ticks to ixodicides, the negative impact on human and animal health and the ecological damage to the environment, force the use of sustainable alternatives such as immune control through vaccination. Although commercial vaccines against the most important cattle tick, *Rhipicephalus microplus* have been developed, vaccines against other tick species do not exist. In addition, vaccines based on other antigens besides Bm86, an antigen from the surface of tick midgut, have not been developed. This chapter will delve into the vital aspects of the immune response essential for tick antigens, presenting significant findings on vaccine targets, strategies, and innovations. Moreover, this chapter will examine cutting-edge approaches for vaccine development, including the emerging concept of "multi-epitopic" vaccines and vaccines derived from tick microbiota.

**Keywords**

Vaccines · Ticks · Epitopes · Antibodies · Immune response

J. Mosqueda (✉) · C. Almazán · D. G. López-Díaz · I. Corona-Guerrero · A. J. Pavón-Rocha · M. M. E. Perez-Soria · D. J. Hernández-Silva · R. Morales-García
Immunology and Vaccines Laboratory, Faculty of Natural Sciences, Autonomous University of Queretaro, Queretaro, Mexico
e-mail: joel.mosqueda@uaq.mx





S. Kumar et al. (eds.), *Acaricides Resistance in Ticks*,
https://doi.org/10.1007/978-981-97-7411-1_9

## 9.1 Introduction

Ticks pose significant challenges as pervasive pests, creating not only health concerns but also substantial economic burdens. Their role as vectors for various pathogens, amplifies their impact on public health systems globally. Additionally, they inflict severe losses in the livestock industry through direct harm, such as blood loss and hide damage, as well as indirect effects, acting as vectors of tick-borne diseases. Globally, the costs incurred due to tick infestations, including expenses for disease treatment and prevention, productivity loss, and livestock mortality, run into billions of dollars annually (Calvano et al. 2019; Strydom et al. 2023). As such, the economic and health-related implications of ticks underline the urgent need for effective and sustainable control strategies, including the development of comprehensive and integrative tick vaccines (Lew-Tabor and Rodríguez-Valle 2016).

Currently, the control of ticks relies on the use of several chemical acaricides applied by different ways. This kind of control has drawbacks such as the negative impact on human and animal health, the ecological damage on the environment, and the genetic selection of ticks resistant to ixodicides, forcing to the use of new sustainable alternatives such as immune control through vaccination (George et al. 2004; Showler and Saelao 2022). Herein a review on significant findings on vaccine targets, strategies, and innovations including the emerging concept of "multi-epitopic" vaccines and microbiota vaccines is presented.

## 9.2 Mode of Action of Tick Vaccines

Since the beginning of the last century, it is known that exposure to ticks elicits an immune response that protects against subsequent infestations (Johnston and Bancroft 1918). Observations in laboratory animals allowed to conclude that tick infestation produces an immune response that decreases tick numbers after successive infestations (Trager 1939). The initial proof of concept for tick vaccines was demonstrated through the immunization of animals with tick crude extracts. This approach generated a humoral response, which damaged the ticks fed on the treated animals (Allen and Humphreys 1979). The rationale behind tick vaccines is that antibodies targeting proteins responsible of any specific and vital function in ticks are taken within blood meals and block the protein's function (Fig. 9.1). Consequently, ticks that feed on immunized hosts show changes in phenotype, noticed as smaller size, reddish coloration, decrement in reproductive parameters, and in some cases, their death (Agbede and Kemp 1986; Kemp et al. 1986).

Several reports demonstrated that a partial or strong immunity to tick infestations can be induced by inoculation with a variety of antigenic materials, including whole tick homogenates, extracts of salivary glands, internal organs of ticks, tick intestinal material, and cement material, among others (Willadsen 1987; Kemp et al. 1989). Tick vaccine antigens are classified into two groups. The first group includes antigens involved in naturally acquired resistance to tick infestation, those immunogenic materials exposed to a host through normal tick attachment and feeding

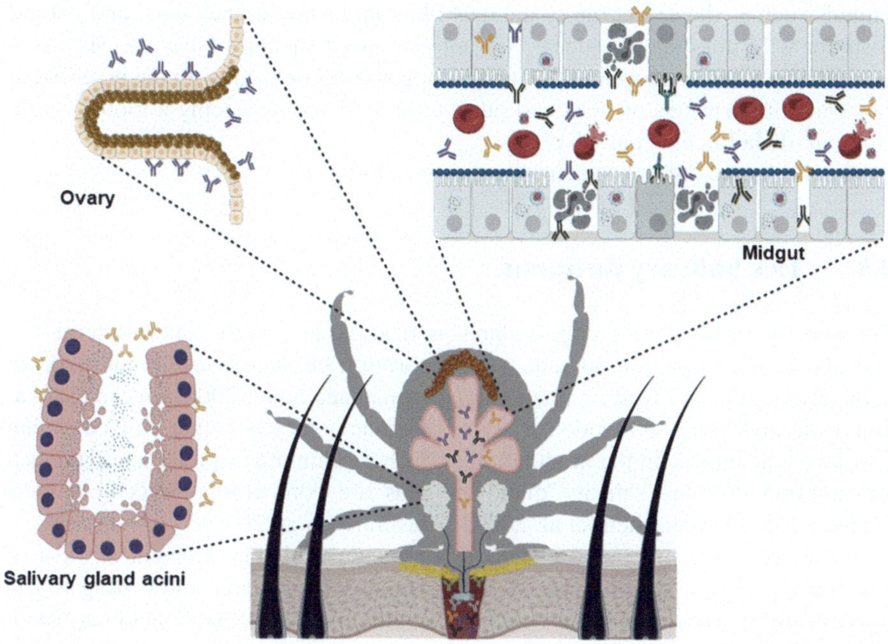


**Fig. 9.1** Mechanism of action of tick vaccines. Ticks acquire host blood through the hypostome. The blood components then pass to the midgut lumen, where intracellular digestion occurs. Antibodies can bind to membrane antigens on digestive cells, inhibiting their functions and trigger complement activation to destroy them, facilitating the passage of antibodies and host cells to the hemolymph. Some immunoglobulins employ other mechanisms and are able to cross the gut without losing their functional structure, hence maintaining their biological activity. The binding to carrier proteins allows the internalization of the antibody into the cells, and even a paracellular movement has been proposed based on reports of a leaky gut. Antibodies reaching the hemolymph recognize their epitopes, interfering with the physiological processes of the proteins. Additionally, it has been revealed that antibodies remain throughout the molting stages. (Created with BioRender.com)

processes. Most of these molecules are anti-hemostatic and modulate the host immune response. The second group of antigens includes those that are "hidden" antigens; that is, those antigens that are not part of the normal host-parasite interaction and, under normal circumstances, do not stimulate an immune response. However, they are necessary for some specific biological function in ticks. They are also called "concealed" antigens, of which Bm86 is the best example. However, several other hidden antigens with various functions have been identified. In general, antibodies that target both exposed and hidden antigens act against specific molecules in the cells of the salivary glands, intestine, ovaries, and other organs (Willadsen and Kemp 1988; Willadsen 2004).

Most of the available data on the efficacy of vaccines against tick infestations under controlled and field conditions have been obtained in cattle. However, results are also available for other farm animals such as sheep and camels, companion animals such as dogs, laboratory animals like rabbits and guinea pigs, and natural hosts for wild ticks such as deer. Tick antigen-based vaccines have also shown to have an effect in reducing infection and pathogen transmission, with the potential to target multiple species of ticks and other arthropod-vectors facing a global health problem (de la Fuente et al. 2017).

The mechanism of tick vaccines is shown in Fig. 9.1.

## 9.3 Tick Salivary Antigens

The salivary glands are the largest glands in ticks situated in the antero-lateral side of the body. Their functions include water absorption and secretion of fluids involved in the attachment and feeding processes (Bowman and Sauer 2004). In each salivation cycle, ticks secrete a wide variety of pharmacologically active molecules that play a significant role in the modulation of the host immune response and pathogen transmission. So, the salivary gland antigens are compelling antigenic targets (Ribeiro 1987; Francischetti et al. 2009; Narasimhan et al. 2020).

There are many functional classes of immunomodulatory molecules, most of which are peptides and proteins. However, lipid derivates and non-coding RNAs have also been discovered in the tick sialome (Ribeiro et al. 1992; Sauer et al. 1995; Wikel 1999).

The serpin superfamily, one of the most abundant protein groups of the tick sialome is comprised of inhibitors of serin proteases from where they obtain their name (Serpin = serine protease inhibitor). These proteases aid in the blood meal acquisition process by disrupting serine-protease-mediated mechanisms, like the coagulation cascade (Law et al. 2006). However, tick serpins are involved in various other biological processes such as oviposition and host immune response modulation (Xu et al. 2020). To date, almost 30 serpins have been described in different tick species, most of them being abundant in salivary glands (Abbas et al. 2022). Vaccination with a serpin derived from *Ixodes ricinus*, IRIS, showed an effect on the nymphs with an increase in mortality of 33%, also significantly decreasing their weight (Prevot et al. 2007). In *R. microplus*, a serpin was isolated and employed as a vaccine, decreasing the engorgement rate and oviposition mass (Jittapalapong et al. 2010). Another *R. microplus* serpin, RmS-17, was immunized into rabbits that were later challenged with *R. microplus* larvae, exhibiting a vaccine efficacy of 79% (Lagunes-Quintanilla et al. 2022). In *R. sanguineus,* three more serpins were expressed and inoculated into mice, and the challenged larvae and nymphs had a higher mortality rate (Zhao et al. 2024).

Another group of serine protease inhibitors, the superfamily of Kunitz-type inhibitors, is highly abundant in salivary gland extracts. These proteins fulfill anti-hemostatic and anti-inflammatory functions in the tick-host interface (Ranasinghe and McManus 2013). Although 22 of these proteins have been reported in ixodid and argasid ticks, only a few have been employed in vaccination trials (Jmel et al. 2023). Examples of Kunitz-type inhibitors used as vaccine antigens are the HA11, which decreased the tick weight, and AsKunitz, which affected the survival and fertility of ticks (Zhang et al. 2017; Costa et al. 2021).

A superfamily of cysteine protease inhibitors, known as cystatins, plays a crucial role in tick physiology. Salivary gland-related cystatins are secreted at the feeding site to facilitate immune evasion. Cystatins expressed in the midgut are related to hemoglobin digestion (Schwarz et al. 2012). To date, 19 tick cystatins have been studied, being part of the type-1 and type-2 cystatins (Chmelař et al. 2017). Sialostatin L2 is a cystatin secreted by saliva and, when evaluated as a vaccine candidate, affected feeding and attachment of *I. scapularis* (Kotsyfakis et al. 2008). Two other cystatins, derived from *Haemaphysalis* and *Hyalomma* ticks, have been analyzed (Song et al. 2022; Zhang et al. 2024). Regarding argasid ticks, an *Ornithodoros moubata* cystatin was characterized, expressed as recombinant protein in a baculovirus system, and evaluated as vaccine antigen in mice. The mortality rate 24% in nymphs fed on vaccinated mice compared with nymphs fed on control mice (Salát et al. 2010).

Metalloproteases (MP) have been identified in several tick species and are essential in many biological processes of blood-sucking organisms, including inhibiting coagulation, degrading extracellular matrix proteins, and blocking host tissue repair due to their antiangiogenic activity (Francischetti et al. 2003; Ali et al. 2015a). A recombinant MP, BrRm-MP4, was tested in cattle against *R. microplus*, obtaining a vaccine efficacy of 60% (Ali et al. 2015b).

Lipocalins are low molecular weight, extracellular proteins that modulate the immune response by interacting with receptors on the cell membrane, capturing small molecules and forming macromolecular complexes through binding to soluble proteins (Flower 1996). Lipocalins have been characterized in the tick *I. persulcatus*, then expressed as a recombinant antigen, and used in a vaccine challenge in mice. The results showed that the effect of antibodies anti-lipocalins 1, 2, and 3 significantly decreased the weight of fully engorged females and delayed the engorgement period by 1 day (Konnai et al. 2011). Recent studies have evaluated a lipocalin from *H. longicornis* in rabbit vaccination challenges, obtaining a vaccine efficacy of 60% (Wang et al. 2021). In a subsequent trial, a DNA plasmid vaccine with the *H. longicornis* lipocalin showed a lower vaccine efficacy (Fan et al. 2022).

Immune cell suppressors have also been pointed as vaccine antigens. Da-p36 and Salp15 are a family of salivary gland-specific proteins acting as immunosuppressants of T-cells. Da-p36 were first discovered in *Dermacentor andersoni* salivary glands and can reduce up to 95% of activated T-cells (Bergman et al. 1998; Alarcon-Chaidez et al. 2003). In *R. haemaphysaloides* ticks, a vaccine trial with the RH-36 recombinant protein significantly reduced engorgement weight and egg-hatching rates (Wang et al. 2017). The Salp15 members are CD4+ T cells immunosuppressants and inhibitors of cytokines derived from dendritic cells (Anguita et al. 2002; Hovius et al. 2008). These proteins have been identified in many *Ixodes* species and are related to *Borrelia burgdorferi* infection (Ramamoorthi et al. 2005; Wang et al. 2014). As vaccine antigens, immunization with Salp15 impaired the transmission of the Lyme disease agent, but no additional tick effects were reported (Dai et al. 2009).

Tick cement is secreted into the injury site within the first minutes after attachment. Cement proteins have also been studied as vaccine antigens (Sauer et al. 1995; de la Fuente et al. 2016). A 29 kDa extracellular matrix-like protein, called p29, was isolated from *H. longicornis* salivary glands. It showed significant structural homology to collagen proteins of vertebrates and invertebrates. Increase mortality of both, nymphs and larvae, as well as reduction in their weight were observed when *H. longicornis* ticks were fed on rabbits immunized with a recombinant p29 (Mulenga et al. 1999). HL34, identified in *H. longicornis* salivary glands, was suggested to be a component of the cement cone. Vaccination of rabbits with recombinant HL34 affected nymphs and reduced female oviposition due to poor blood digestion (Tsuda et al. 2001). Another cement cone protein, 64TRP, has been targeted as a dual action vaccine, decreasing the transmission of tick-borne encephalitis virus (TBEV) and increasing tick mortality (Trimnell et al. 2002; Labuda et al. 2006). Finally, the Rhipicephalus Immuno-dominant Molecule 36, RIM36, induces a high antibody response but its effect on tick fitness has not been described (Bishop et al. 2002).

A flagelliform silk protein called SILK, which was transcriptionally upregulated in male *R. microplus* ticks infected with *Anaplasma marginale*, was expressed as a recombinant protein, purified, and evaluated as a vaccine antigen in cattle. It was found to affect tick survival and bacterial transmission, showing 62% efficacy against *R. microplus* (Merino et al. 2013a, b).

Finally, aquaporins are transmembrane channel proteins specialized in the water transport through osmotic gradients, making them important in tick physiology. Although not specific to the salivary glands, aquaporins have been widely described in these organs. As vaccine antigens, they have been tested in *R. microplus*, where a recombinant aquaporin RmAQP1, expressed in *Pichia pastoris*, induced 68–75% efficacy in a pen trial in cattle. Two *I. ricinus* aquaporins expressed as recombinant antigens showed efficacies from 28 to 80% when nymphs were fed on immunized rabbits (Guerrero et al. 2014; Contreras and de la Fuente 2017).

There are many proteins in the saliva of the tick. The studies on vaccine efficacy with salivary proteins are shown in Table 9.1.

## 9.4 Antigens Derived from the Reproductive System

Sexual maturity of female ixodid ticks occurs through an oogenesis event, which begins in the nymphal stage and ends after engorgement of the adult female, leading to oviposition during the free adult stage (Ogihara and Taylor 2014; Xavier et al. 2018). Oocytes are the female's reproductive cells, and they develop and mature in the ovaries. This process is characterized by morphological changes of oocytes from stage I to stage VI, however, these changes depend on several relevant physiological events such as feeding and mating (de Oliveira et al. 2006; Sreelekha et al. 2015). Some studies in *R. microplus* ticks have shown that during ovary maturation, approximately 3756 proteins are expressed, and out of those, around 80% have a

**Table 9.1** Vaccine efficacy of salivary tick antigens

| Protein | Tick | Vaccine effect | Reference |
|---|---|---|---|
| *Serpins* | | | |
| IRIS | *I. ricinus* | Mortality up to 33% in nymphs | Prevot et al. (2007) |
| rSerpin | *R. microplus* | 83% reduction in adult engorgement and 34% reduction in oviposition mass | Jittapalapong et al. (2010) |
| RMS-3, L7LRK7, L7LTU1 | *R. sanguineus* | 40% and 87% reduction in larvae and nymph engorgement | Zhao et al. (2024) |
| AAS19 | *A. americanum* | Up to 66% ticks failed to lay eggs | Kim et al. (2016) |
| *Kunitz-type inhibitors* | | | |
| HA11 | *H. asiaticum* | Weight and hatching reduction in nymphs | Zhang et al. (2017) |
| AsKunitz | *A. sculptum* | 85–92% vaccine efficacy. Decreased survival and fertility rates | Costa et al. (2021) |
| IrSPI IrLip1 | *I. ricinus* | Significant decrease in tick engorgement | Almazán et al. (2020) |
| *Non-canonical serine protease inhibitors* | | | |
| Longistatin | *H. longicornis* | 73% of vaccine efficacy in nymphs, mainly by decreasing molting and engorgement | Anisuzzaman et al. (2011) |
| *Cystatins* | | | |
| Sialostatin L2 | *I. scapularis* | Significantly reduction of tick weight and attachment rate | Kotsyfakis et al. (2008) |
| OmC2 | *O. moubata* | 30% reduction of nymphal survival | Salát et al. (2010) |
| Bmcys2c | *R. microplus* | Cross-immunity trial on R. *appendiculatus*. 11.5% reduction of engorged females | Parizi et al. (2020) |
| HDcyst-2 | *H. doenitzi* | 51.8% protection to adults | Zhang et al. (2024) |
| HasCPL | *H. asiaticum* | 55% protection against larvae | Song et al. (2022) |
| *Metalloproteases* | | | |
| rBrRm-MP4 | *R. microplus* | 60% overall protection. 43% reduction in tick survival, 15% reduction in egg hatching, and 17.5% oviposition decrease | Ali et al. (2015a, b) |
| Metis 1 | *I. ricinus* | Decreased weight gain and egg laying | Decrem et al. (2008) |
| HLMP1 | *H. longicornis* | 15.6% nymphal mortality and 14.6% adult mortality | Imamura et al. (2009) |
| *Lipocalins* | | | |

(continued)

**Table 9.1** (continued)

| Protein | Tick | Vaccine effect | Reference |
|---|---|---|---|
| LIPERS 1–4 | *I. persulcatus* | Significantly decrease in weight gain and delay of engorging time | Konnai et al. (2011) |
| HlLIP | *H. longicornis* | 60% vaccine efficacy. 12% of increase of feeding period. 12%, 38%, and 27% reduction of weight, oviposition, and egg hatching rates | Wang et al. (2021) |
| pCDNA3.1-HlLIP | *H. longicornis* | 30% vaccine efficacy. 7%, 14%, and 1% reduction of weight, oviposition, and egg hatching rates | Fan et al. (2022) |
| *T-cells immunosuppressants* | | | |
| RH-36 | *R. haemaphysaloides* | Prolonged feeding period. 55% attachment rate, 29.5% engorgement rate, and 57% egg-hatching rate | Wang et al. (2017) |
| Salp15 | *I. scapularis* | Reduced *B. burgdorferi* burden in tissues | Dai et al. (2009) |
| *Cement proteins* | | | |
| p29 | *H. longicornis* | 40% mortality on larvae and 56% mortality on nymphs | Mulenga et al. (1999) |
| HL34 | *H. longicornis* | 14% and 29% mortality of nymphs and adults respectively. 8% of females did not lay eggs | Tsuda et al. (2001) |
| 64TRP | *R. appendiculatus* | 48% mortality of nymphs. Impaired transmission of TBEV | Trimnell et al. (2002) and Labuda et al. (2006) |
| RIM-36 | *R. appendiculatus* | Elicits high antibody titers in cattle | Bishop et al. (2002) |
| *SILK* | | | |
| SILK | *R. microplus* | 62% of overall vaccine efficacy; 58% reduction in tick survival and 9% decrease on oviposition | Merino et al. (Merino et al. 2013a, b) |
| *Aquaporins* | | | |
| RmAQP1 | *R. microplus* | 75% vaccine efficacy | Guerrero et al. (2014) |
| IrAQP | *I. ricinus* | 32% vaccine efficacy | Contreras and de la Fuente (2017) |

function related to basal metabolism (Xavier et al. 2018). In the case of *H. longicornis* ticks, a total of 3031 proteins have been associated to oogenesis (Wang et al. 2020). A wide diversity of proteins is expressed in the ovary; however, only a few have been evaluated as vaccines against ticks. We will show the proteins that have been identified in tick reproductive organs and whose evidence demonstrates that they are immunogenic or that should be evaluated in a vaccine challenge.

Vitellogenins are large proteins, ranging from 200 to 700 kDa, and serve as precursors to the major egg storage protein, vitellin. Vitellogenin is a glycolipophosphoprotein and is synthesized in organs such as the fat body, midgut, and ovaries, and then transported to oocytes by endocytosis, where it accumulates within yolk granules (Rosell and Coons 1992). To fulfill its biological functions, vitellogenin requires a cell receptor. The gene encoding the vitellogenin receptor protein has been sequenced and reported in four tick species, however, evaluations of vaccine efficacy have not been performed (Smith and Reuben Kaufman 2013; Umemiya-Shirafuji et al. 2019).

Vitellin provides a source of nutrients for larval embryogenesis (Sappington and Raikhel 1998). In one study, recombinant *R. microplus* vitellin protein was expressed and evaluated as a vaccine candidate against this tick species. It prompted a strong immune response and demonstrated an overall vaccine efficacy of 68% in a sheep host model (Tellam et al. 2002). Another study revealed the expression of vitellogenin, vitellogenin-2, and yolk cathepsin in *R. microplus* ovarian tissue. Antibodies against these proteins were recognized by larvae proteins in a western blot assay, suggesting these three ovarian proteins as potential vaccine candidates that could impact tick biological parameters from the larval stage onwards (Ramírez Rodríguez et al. 2016). It is critical to highlight that more than one vitellogenin protein is expressed in the tick ovary, suggesting potential biological redundancy among these proteins (Boldbaatar et al. 2010).

Cysteine endopeptidase and yolk protein cathepsin are two antigens that play vital roles in the degradation of yolk protein during tick embryogenesis. They are also implicated in proteolytic activities such as the degradation of hemoglobin and fibrinogen, ensuring the fluidity of ingested blood during the feeding process (Seixas et al. 2003; Xavier et al. 2019). In a vaccine trial targeting *R. microplus* ticks, vitellin-degrading cysteine endopeptidase demonstrated a protective effect of 21%, characterized by a 17.6% decrease in the weight of the fertile egg mass in the vaccinated group (Seixas et al. 2008).

Another protein whose biological function is directly related to reproduction is the male repletion factor or voraxin. This protein was first characterized as a dimer formed by two peptides in *A. hebraeum*. Interestingly, each individual peptide lacked the functional activity. Voraxin stimulates the repletion of female ticks after mating, allowing them to achieve their optimal engorgement weight. When the recombinant voraxin was evaluated, it reduced the female's weight in 72%, also delaying the feeding period (Weiss and Kaufman 2004). Moreover, voraxin has been tested as a vaccine antigen against *R. appendiculatus* ticks, showing a weight reduction effect of 42% in ticks fed on immunized animals. Likewise, it was observed that the vaccinated group ticks failed to lay eggs (Yamada et al. 2009).

There are many proteins in the reproductive system of ticks that have not yet been characterized, especially as vaccine targets. The studies on vaccine efficacy reported in proteins from these organs, are shown in Table 9.2.

**Table 9.2** Vaccine effects of reproductive-associated antigens

| Protein | Tick | Vaccine effect | Reference |
|---|---|---|---|
| *Ovary antigens* | | | |
| Vitellin | *R. microplus* | 68% of efficacy | Tellam et al. (2002) |
| Vitellin-degrading cysteine endopeptidase | *R. microplus* | 21% of efficacy | Seixas et al. (2008) |
| *Male gonad antigens* | | | |
| Voraxin | *A. hebraeum* | Tick weight reduction of 72% and a delay of 3 days in the feeding period | Weiss and Kaufman (2004) |
| | *R. appendiculatus* | Tick weight reduction of 42.7%<br>38.6% ticks did not lay eggs<br>Reduction of 44% in egg mass weight | Yamada et al. (2009) |

## 9.5 Midgut Antigens

Tick midgut contains several proteins with important roles for tick nutrition and that are utilized for pathogens to infect the tick that can be utilized as recombinant antigens in anti-tick vaccines (de la Fuente et al. 2017).

The first protein employed as a recombinant antigen in commercial anti-tick vaccines was the glycoprotein Bm86 from *R. microplus* (de la Fuente et al. 1999; Odongo et al. 2007). Bm86 is a glycoprotein located on the outer surface of the midgut cells in *R. microplus* (Kemp et al. 1986). Immunization with Bm86 stimulates the immune system of the vertebrate host and induces the production of antibodies against the target protein (de la Fuente et al. 1999). Ticks fed on immunized cattle acquire specific antibodies in their blood. These antibodies, when ingested by ticks during feeding, cause lysis of midgut epithelial cells, which in turn reduces tick weight upon repletion and oviposition (Rand et al. 1989). Additionally, vaccination of cattle with Bm86 over time has shown a correlation with the reduction of *R. microplus* abundance in the environment (Hüe et al. 2017).

Following the release of the first commercial recombinant Bm86 vaccines, their success was limited mainly due to the high variability of the antigen between geographically distant isolates (Merino et al. 2013a, b). For this reason, the need of new vaccine candidates arose, and new immune targets were proposed. One of the first strategies to enhance Bm86 vaccine efficacy was the immunization with multi antigenic vaccines containing Bm86 and Bm91. Bm91 is a carboxydipeptidase homologue present in *R. microplus* midgut and salivary glands (Willadsen et al. 1996). It was previously used as a vaccine antigen on its own and confer protection against tick infestations (Jarmey et al. 1995). The results indicated that immunization with a multiantigenic vaccine containing Bm86 and Bm91 produced more antibodies than Bm86 alone, but there is no synergistic effect (Willadsen et al. 1996).

In Argentina, *R. microplus* strain A showed low susceptibility to immunization with Gavac, a commercial vaccine against *R. microplus* produced in Cuba. In response to this, Bm95, a homologue of Bm86, was cloned from *R. microplus* strain A and expressed in a yeast system (García-García et al. 2000). Immunization with Bm95 showed protective effects against *R. microplus* by delaying the infestation. Additionally, animals immunized were treated with acaricidal baths every 60 days in comparison to 27 days for non-immunized animals (García-García et al. 2000). Another homolog of Bm86 studied as a vaccine candidate is the *Rhipicephalus appendiculatus* protein Ra86. Two allelic variants that share 79% amino acid identity have been identified: Ra85A (73% identity with Bm86) and Ra92A (74% identity with Bm86) (Mbulaiteye-Saimo et al. 2011). Ra86 was used as antigen in a vaccine trial in rabbits, showing a 69.7% efficacy in comparison to non-infected, control rabbits, including a 31.5% weight loss on female fed on immunized animals (Mbulaiteye-Saimo et al. 2011).

The voltage dependent anion channel protein (VDAC) is a barrel-shaped channel protein anchored within cell membranes, involved in physiological roles such as regulation of ion and metabolite flow between mitochondria and the cytosol. It is part of the cells' apoptotic mechanism (Colombini 2004). Upregulation of *R. microplus* VDAC (BmVDAC) in midgut cells during *B. bigemina* infection has been reported, suggesting a role of BmVDAC in the invasion process of the parasite (Rodríguez-Hernández et al. 2015). Immunization with recombinant BmVDAC was evaluated and showed efficacy of 80%. However when the ticks we fed on BmVDAC-immunized cattle infected with *B. bigemina*, the efficacy was reduced to 34% (Ortega-Sánchez et al. 2020).

Ferritins (FER) are iron storage proteins that play a vital role in iron metabolism. Since ticks feed on blood, they metabolize large amounts of iron during feeding (Gao et al. 2022). FER2 is necessary during iron replacement to distribute and transport iron from intestinal cells to the hemolymph. It serves as the primary non-heme iron transporter between the tick's intestine, ovaries, and peripheral tissues (Gao et al. 2022; Hajdusek et al. 2010). The reported efficacy in cattle vaccinated with FER2 was 64% and 72% against *R. microplus* and *R. annulatus* respectively (Hajdusek et al. 2010). However, when tested against *I. ricinus* in cattle, significant results were not obtained (Knorr et al. 2018).

The midgut antigens that have been evaluated as vaccines against ticks are shown in Table 9.3.

## 9.6 Ubiquitous Tick Antigens (Other Antigens)

Subolesin, an orthologue of akirin in insects, is an intracellular protein associated with gene expression and involved in several cellular pathways, playing a vital role in regulating genes involved in immune responses, blood digestion, reproduction, and development (de la Fuente et al. 2006a, b; Galindo et al. 2009; Sultana et al. 2015). This protein is necessary for the gene expression of the nuclear factor NF-kB and the regulation of the immune response (Goto et al. 2008). Subolesin was first characterized in *Ixodes scapularis* ticks, later it was demonstrated to be a highly conserved protein expressed in several tick species (Almazán et al. 2003; Almazán

**Table 9.3** Vaccine effects of midgut antigens

| Protein | Tick | Vaccine effect | Reference |
|---|---|---|---|
| Bm86 | *R. microplus* | Lysis on midgut epithelial cells. Reduced ticks engorged weight and oviposition rate. Reduced tick presence in the environment | de la Fuente et al. (1999) and Odongo et al. (2007) |
| Bm91 | *R. microplus* | Enhances the effect of Bm86 vaccines when used in conjunction as a multi-antigenic vaccine | Willadsen et al. (1996) |
| Bm95 | *R. microplus* | Infestation delay | García-García et al. (2000) |
| Ra86 | *R. appendiculatus* | Protection against infestation. Weight and oviposition rate reduction on females fed on immunized animals | Mbulaiteye-Saimo et al. (2011) |
| BmVDAC | *R. microplus* | Protection against infestation. Weight loss and oviposition rate decrease was higher in uninfected ticks compared to ticks infected with Babesia bigemina | Ortega-Sánchez et al. (2020) |
| HDcyst-1 | *H. doenitzi* | 64.1% protection against adult ticks infestation. Reduced egg hatching rates and prolonged engorgement time | Zhang et al. (2024) |

et al. 2005a). Subolesin functions are directly related to the modulation of blood ingestion and reproduction (de la Fuente et al. 2006a, b). This protein has been widely evaluated as a vaccine antigen in several tick species, in some cases demonstrating a high vaccine efficacy (Almazán et al. 2005b). Relevant subolesin vaccination studies are showed in Table 9.4.

Glutathione S-transferase (GST) is a ubiquitous enzyme group that catalyzes the conjugation between glutathione and the first step in the formation of mercapturic acids (Nebert and Vasiliou 2004). GST also forms part of the cellular detoxification pathway of endogenous and xenobiotic compounds, including those from pesticides and acaricides (da Silva Vaz et al. 2004). Given that GST are conserved across different tick species, these proteins have been proposed as multi-species tick vaccines (Ndawula et al. 2020). A recombinant GST from *H. longicornis* was evaluated against *R. appendiculatus* and *R. sanguineus* ticks, achieving a 67% of efficacy against the former and no significant effects against the later (Sabadin et al. 2017). Similar effects were observed with the same antigen used as a vaccine against *R. microplus*, affecting both, engorgement and oviposition rates, and an overall efficacy of 57% (Parizi et al. 2011). Another GST was described in *D. marginatus*. In a vaccine efficacy trial, this antigen decreased the engorgement rate, oviposition and egg hatching, obtaining a vaccine efficacy over 40% (Huercha et al. 2020).

Chitinases are a large family of enzymes that are primarily required during inter-state metamorphosis by hydrolyzing chitin polymers present in the cuticle, breaking the internal N-acetyl glucosamine bonds that make up chitin. Also, these enzymes act as important growth regulators (Arakane and Muthukrishnan 2010). As a vaccine candidate, a chitinase from *H. longicornis* was characterized, which caused a significant decrease in molting, approximately 20%, and increased the feeding

**Table 9.4** Vaccine studies with subolesin

| Vaccine | Tick | Vaccine effect | Reference |
|---|---|---|---|
| Recombinant | *I. scapularis* | 71% efficacy | Almazán et al. (2005a) |
| Recombinant | *R. microplus* | 51% efficacy | Almazán et al. (2010) |
| Recombinant | *R. microplus* | 83% efficacy | Carreón et al. (2012) |
| Recombinant | *R. microplus* | Subolesin (recombinant): 60% efficacy | Merino et al. (2013a, b) |
| Recombinant | *R. microplus* | 44% efficacy in first challenge<br>37.2% efficacy in a second study | Shakya et al. (2014) |
| Recombinant peptide | *R. microplus* | Reduction of engorging females and egg-hatching rates | Lagunes-Quintanilla et al. (2016) |
| Recombinant peptide | *R. microplus* | 45% of tick weight reduction<br>71% of oviposition reduction | Lagunes-Quintanilla et al. (2018) |
| Oral recombinant vaccine + heat-inactivated *Mycobacterium bovis* | *R. microplus* | 65% efficacy | Contreras et al. (2019) |
| Recombinant | *R. appendiculatus* | 47% efficacy in Bos indicus<br>90% efficacy in cross-breed cattle | Kasaija et al. (2020) |
| | *A. variegatum* | 47% efficacy in Bos indicus<br>76% efficacy in cross-breed cattle | |
| | *R. decoloratus* | 71% efficacy in cross-breed cattle | |
| Recombinant peptide | *R. microplus* | 67% efficacy | Mendoza-Martínez et al. (2021) |
| Recombinant | *R. australis* | No significant effect | Trentelman et al. (2019) |
| Recombinant | *H. longicornis* | 37% efficacy | Lee et al. (2020) |
| First dose DNA vaccine and recombinant boost | *H. longicornis* | 79% efficacy | Hassan et al. (2020) |
| Recombinant | *R. sanguineus* s.l. (adults) | 86.3% efficacy | Zeb et al. (2024) |
| Synthetic peptides | *O. erraticus* | 70% efficacy | Manzano-Román et al. (2015) |
| | *O. moubata* | 83% efficacy | |

period by 1.5 days. Furthermore, this antigen reduced oviposition by 13% (You et al. 2003; You and Fujisaki 2009). Recently, a chitinase peptide from *R. microplus* with predicted B-cell epitopes was designed and synthesized and found to be immunogenic. Subsequently, in a challenge trial, where cattle were vaccinated and infested with larvae, the peptide showed an efficacy of 71%, mainly reducing tick survival, oviposition mass, and egg hatching rate (Perez-Soria et al. 2024).

Over 80 proteins are estimated to be expressed in ribosomes. One of these, the P0 ribosomal protein, has been evaluated through gene silencing and as a vaccine antigen against ticks. Remarkable vaccine efficacies have been observed when trials were conducted using a P0 peptide conjugated with the Keyhole Limpet Hemocyanin (KLH) molecule. Efficacies reported were as high as 90% against *R. sanguineus* (Rodríguez-Mallon et al. 2012), 96% against *R. microplus* (Rodríguez-Mallon et al. 2015), and 54% against *A. mixtum* (Rodríguez-Mallon et al. 2020). This makes the P0 ribosomal protein a highly promising anti-tick vaccine antigen. Importantly, histological damage was observed in the ovaries of ticks that fed on blood from cattle immunized with the P0 peptide. This suggests that the anti-P0 antibodies may have a specific cellular target within this tissue (Rodríguez-Mallon et al. 2015).

The enzyme enolase is a glycolytic protein that catalyzes the conversion of D-2-phosphoglycerate (2PGA) and phosphoenol pyruvate (PEP) during glycolysis (ninth step) and gluconeogenesis (first step) respectively, by 2-step dehydration in the presence of Mg2+ ions, which is a vital function for cells. Due to the multiple functions this enzyme has, it is considered a "moonlight" protein. As a vaccine antigen, recombinant enolase isolated from *H. longicornis* was able to increase the mortality of nymphs and larvae by 60% and 83% respectively with an overall efficacy of 90% at preventing tick infestation (Haque et al. 2023).

Triosephosphate isomerase (TIM) is a homodimeric glycolytic enzyme that catalyzes the interconversion of d-glyceraldehyde 3-phosphate and dihydroxyacetone phosphate. TIM has been isolated from several parasites including protozoa and arthropods. This enzyme is expressed in all stages and in all tissues of the *H. longicornis* tick. A recombinant TIM from *H. longicornis* (rHLTIM) was immunized in rabbits and evaluated as a vaccine, showing a 50% overall efficacy (Liang et al. 2022).

## 9.7 Multi-Epitopic and Multi-Antigenic Tick Vaccines

Limited and manageable antigenic differences open up the potential for creating a universal vaccine that could combat multiple tick species. While some tick antigens have demonstrated the ability to invoke cross-protective immunity against various tick species, another approach to enhance the efficacy of anti-tick vaccines is combining two or more antigens (Parizi et al. 2011). A vaccine comprising three tick recombinant proteins from two tick species has been shown to offer partial protection to confined cattle against *R. microplus* infestations in previous single-vaccination studies. The vaccine components included vitellin-degrading cysteine endopeptidase (VTDCE) and *Boophilus* yolk pro-cathepsin (BYC) from *R. microplus*, as well as glutathione S-transferase from *H. longicornis* (GST-Hl). A significant reduction in the number of semi-engorged ticks was observed in vaccinated cattle after two inoculations. This effect persisted for 3 months, ranging from 35.3% to 61.6%. Additionally, the vaccinated animals demonstrated a significantly higher body weight gain compared to the control group. The triple-antigen vaccine, composed of VTDCE, BYC, and GST-Hl, provided higher protection levels against *R. microplus* infestations compared to the single-antigen vaccines (Parizi et al. 2012).

The chimeric protein vaccine BM95-MSP1a, which was constructed using the BM95 antigen of *R. microplus* and Major Surface Protein 1a (MSP1a) of *Anaplasma marginale*, successfully induced significant antibody titers in rabbits. In a cattle trial, this vaccine was observed to reduce *R. microplus* infestations by 54% and showed an overall efficacy of 64% (Almazán et al. 2012).

The Q38 Subolesin-Akirin construct, which is comprised of a fused protective epitope chimera, was found to reduce tick infestations and oviposition, showing vaccine efficacy of 75% in cattle (Merino et al. 2013a, b). The efficacy of Q38 vaccination against larvae of *I. ricinus* was 99.9% and 46.4% against *D. reticulatus* in rabbits. The impact of the Q38 vaccine on larval feeding and molting was found to be essential in reducing tick infestations (Contreras and de la Fuente 2016).

The proteins *R. appendiculatus* serpin-3 (RAS-3), *R. appendiculatus* serpin-4 (RAS-4), and a 36-kDa immuno-dominant protein of *R. appendiculatus* (RIM36), when used as a cocktail vaccine preparation, demonstrated protective immunity against female ticks in a tick infestation challenge, leading to mortality rates of 39.5% (Imamura et al. 2008). Two serine protease inhibitors from *R. appendiculatus*, RAS-1 and RAS-2, conferred significant protective immunity against ticks when used to vaccinate cattle. The combination of rRAS-1 and -2 resulted in a 61.4% reduction in nymph engorgement rate, and increased mortality rates in adult female and male ticks by 28 and 43% respectively (Imamura et al. 2006).

A multi-species GST-cocktail vaccine was studied, comprising five tick species of economic importance to the livestock industry: *R. appendiculatus*, *R. decoloratus*, *R. microplus*, *A. variegatum*, and *H. longicornis*. This vaccine induced an immune response that reduced the number of adult female ticks during infestation by 35.3%, but did not significantly impact adult female weight, reproductive parameters, or hatched larvae. However, the vaccine was successful in reducing the size of the parasite population, likely due to the induction of multiple biological effects (Ndawula Jr et al. 2019).

## 9.8 Tick's Microbiota as Vaccine Antigens

The midgut serves as a crucial site of interaction between ticks and their hosts, where ingested blood meals are stored and processed (Lee et al. 2017). This interaction is partly mediated by the tick microbiota, a community of obligate or facultative mutualistic symbiotic microorganisms inhabiting the host midgut (Lee et al. 2017; Stewart and Bloom 2020). This community exhibits slight variation between individuals and comprises archaea, fungi, protozoans, and viruses (Mateos-Hernández et al. 2021).

Microbiota species perform diverse roles based on their relationship with their hosts. Obligate bacterial symbionts, transmitted transstadially, supplement their host's metabolism by producing vital compounds such as vitamins, amino acids, fatty acids, and enzymes. In contrast, facultative symbionts acquired through host-environment interaction modulate their host's behavior and environmental response (Bonnet and Pollet 2021; Narasimhan et al. 2017). Tick-borne pathogens are also considered part of the tick microbiota (Bonnet and Pollet 2021; Narasimhan et al. 2017).

Pathogenic bacteria can influence their host's microbiota population, causing effects from minor diversity alterations to pathogen-induced dysbiosis. For instance, during its intracellular phase, *A. phagocytophilum* can manipulate their host's metabolic pathways to increase the availability of compounds like heme group, fatty acids, or cholesterol (Cabezas-Cruz et al. 2019). Another example is *B. burgdorferi*, which can modulate the expression of immune response genes in *I. scapularis* to create a less competitive environment by inhibiting the formation of other bacteria's biofilm (Narasimhan et al. 2017).

Apicomplexan parasite infections can also induce dysbiosis in their vectors (Adegoke et al. 2020). Such alteration of microbial communities has been observed in *Theileria*-infected *R. microplus*, where microbial diversity was reduced, and les abundant species became more prevalent. Similar results were observed for *Trypanosoma cruzi*-infected *Triatoma* spp., where the vector also demonstrated reduced microbial diversity (Adegoke et al. 2020; Mann et al. 2020). Technologies like high-throughput sequencing are useful to conduct metagenomic analyses of the microbial population of the tick midgut and their functional composition (Wu-Chuang et al. 2021). Microorganisms with high prevalence and co-occurrence with other symbionts, the keystone species, play the largest role in metabolic regulation for other species in the tick microbiome (Mateos-Hernández et al. 2021). The regulation of gut microbiome diversity by keystone species is based on the metabolic resources they produce, generating microbial co-occurrence networks. Studying these networks is helpful to differentiate true symbionts from environmental contaminants (Stewart and Bloom 2020).

Altering microbiota composition represents a novel strategy proposed for controlling tick populations and the transmission of tick-borne pathogens (Fig. 9.2). Anti-microbiota vaccination, a tool capable of disrupting the overall microbial diversity of ticks by reducing the prevalence of keystone taxa, could consequently harm the vector (Mateos-Hernández et al. 2021).

Anti-microbiota vaccines have been evaluated when live bacteria have been used as vaccine. Using this strategy, the vertebrate host is immunized with pure cultures of a keystone species, eliciting antibodies against bacterial proteins (Aželytė et al. 2022; Mateos-Hernández et al. 2020, 2021). The capacity to produce antibodies depends on its intrinsic genetic background and the composition of its own gut microbiota. If the host naturally harbors a high population of the vaccine's key species, it will not produce antibody titers high enough to impact the tick microbiota (Mateos-Hernández et al. 2020). Ingested in the tick's blood meal, these produced antibodies are stored in the midgut for digestion, where they retain their ability to

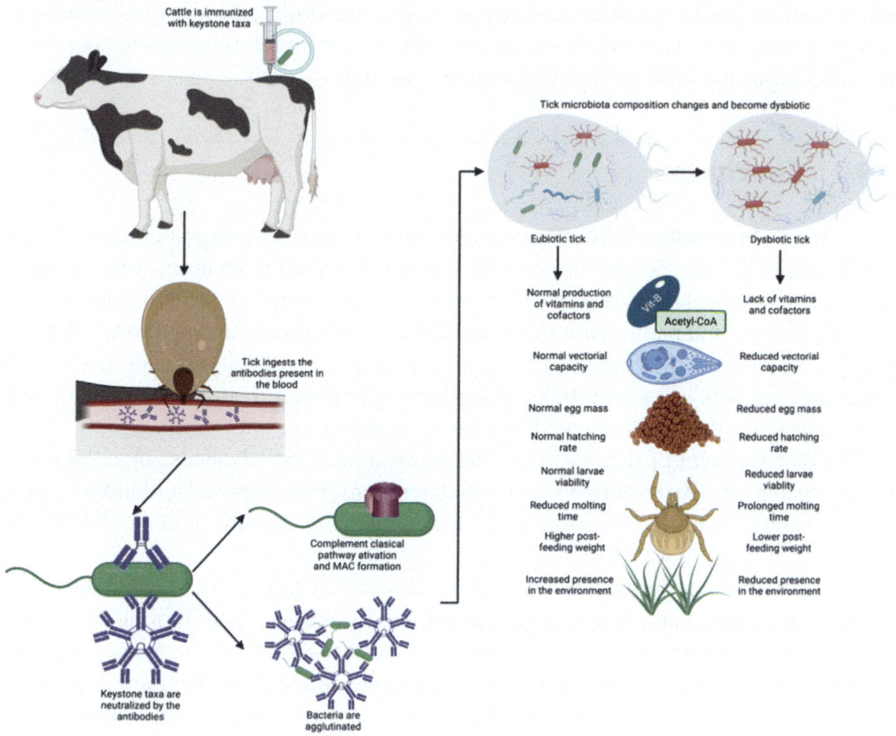


**Fig. 9.2** Mechanism of action of vaccines against tick microbiota. (Created with BioRender.com)

block their respective epitopes (Ackerman et al. 1981). By blocking the activity of keystone bacterial proteins, these antibodies can reduce their abundance and disrupt the microbiota metabolism (Mateos-Hernández et al. 2020).

Anti-microbiota vaccines have proven highly specific and effective in decreasing keystone species prevalence in ticks, causing an immune-induced dysbiosis (Bonnet and Pollet 2021; Mateos-Hernández et al. 2020, 2021). Several factors need consideration when designing anti-microbiota vaccines. For instance, it's essential to select keystone species for immunization, as antibodies against non-keystone taxa will have no significant effect on microbial communities or ticks' health (Mateos-Hernández et al. 2021). Additionally, considerations on community metabolism at a metagenomic level, encompassing both the microbiome and the host genome needs to be considered (Mateos-Hernández et al. 2020). Targeting bacterial species that produce essential nutrients can have the most significant impact on the tick's health (Mateos-Hernández et al. 2021).

While anti-microbiota vaccines offer a safe and effective solution for vector and pathogen control, much remains to be done to fully understand the microbe-microbe and microbe-host relationships in ticks. Future vaccine development efforts must consider the microbiota differences between infected and non-infected vectors to ensure their efficacy under non-controlled conditions. Additionally, the focus should also be on targeting specific enzymes or entire metabolic pathways to impair the complete metabolic network of the vector's midgut, or targeting keystone taxa present across multiple tick species in a region (Fig. 9.2).

## 9.9 Conclusion

There is an obvious need to better vaccines against ticks. The ongoing research and development in tick vaccine antigens highlight the potential for innovative and sustainable tick control measures. By identifying and targeting key proteins involved in tick physiology and pathogen transmission, scientists aim to develop more effective vaccines. These advancements are crucial for addressing the significant health and economic impacts caused by ticks globally, implementing better management and control of tick infestations as well as tick-borne diseases.

The development of tick vaccines has made significant advances since the early twentieth century. By targeting specific tick antigens, both exposed and hidden, vaccines can effectively reduce tick populations and the transmission of tick-borne diseases.

Salivary gland proteins in ticks offer a rich array of targets for vaccine development. From serpins and Kunitz-type inhibitors to cystatins, metalloproteases, lipocalins, immune suppressors, cement proteins, and aquaporins, these molecules play vital roles in tick physiology and host interaction and many of them are expressed not only in salivary glands but in other organs and tissues as well, which might increase the effect when they are used as vaccines.

The exploration of various tick midgut proteins as potential antigens for recombinant anti-tick vaccines has shown promising results in the quest to control tick populations and the diseases they transmit. Among these, the glycoprotein Bm86 from *R. microplus* has been a pioneering antigen in commercial vaccines. Despite the initial success, the geographical variability of Bm86 necessitated the development of alternative strategies, such as multi-antigenic vaccines. Collectively, these efforts highlight the complexity of developing universal anti-tick vaccines and underscore the importance of ongoing research to identify and optimize antigens that can provide broad-spectrum protection against diverse tick species.

Subolesin, an orthologue of akirin in insects, has been shown to be highly conserved across multiple tick species. The conservation and multifunctionality of this antigen highlight its potential as a universal target. This been said, the high homology with the host subolesin, might play against it when it comes to induction of a strong immune response.

Targeting key enzymes and proteins conserved across tick species offers a promising strategy for developing effective multi-species tick vaccines. Glutathione S-transferase (GST), the P0 ribosomal protein, enolase, and triosephosphate isomerase (TIM), have also shown potential as vaccine antigens. These findings underscore the potential of these proteins as targets for innovative anti-tick vaccines.

The development of a universal vaccine targeting multiple tick species could be a reality in the near future. Combining multiple antigens can enhance the efficacy of anti-tick vaccines. Published results on multi-antigenic vaccines underscore their potential in providing broad-spectrum protection against various tick species.

The tick midgut is a pivotal site for tick-host interactions, where the tick microbiota plays a crucial role in modulating these interactions and influencing tick physiology and pathogen transmission. The diverse microbiota, consisting of obligate and facultative symbionts, not only aids in metabolism but also affects the host's immune responses and environmental adaptability. Advances in metagenomic technologies have provided deeper insights into these microbial communities, revealing the significance of keystone species in maintaining microbial balance. Anti-microbiota vaccines, targeting these keystone species, have shown promise in disrupting microbial communities to control tick populations and reduce disease transmission. However, further research is needed to fully understand the complexities of the tick microbiome and optimize vaccine strategies. This knowledge will be essential in developing effective, targeted interventions to combat tick-borne diseases, offering a novel and promising approach to vector control.

## References


Abbas MN, Chlastáková A, Jmel MA, Iliaki-Giannakoudaki E, Chmelar J, Kotsyfakis M (2022) Serpins in tick physiology and tick-host interaction. Front Cell Infect Microbiol 12:892770

Ackerman S, Clare FB, McGill TW, Sonenshine DE (1981) Passage of host serum components, including antibody, across the digestive tract of *Dermacentor variabilis* (Say). J Parasitol 67(5):737. https://doi.org/10.2307/3280459

Adegoke A, Kumar D, Bobo C, Rashid MI, Durrani AZ, Sajid MS, Karim S (2020) Tick-borne pathogens shape the native microbiome within tick vectors. Microorganisms 8(9):1299. https://doi.org/10.3390/microorganisms8091299

Agbede RI, Kemp DH (1986) Immunization of cattle against *Boophilus microplus* using extracts derived from adult female ticks: histopathology of ticks feeding on vaccinated cattle. Int J Parasitol 16(1):35–41. https://doi.org/10.1016/0020-7519(86)90062-7

Alarcon-Chaidez FJ, Muller-Doblies UU, Wikel S (2003) Characterization of a recombinant immunomodulatory protein from the salivary glands of *Dermacentor andersoni*. Parasite Immunol 25(2):69–77. https://doi.org/10.1046/j.1365-3024.2003.00609.x

Ali A, Khan S, Ali I, Karim S, Vaz ID, Termignoni C (2015a) Probing the functional role of tick metalloproteases. Physiol Entomol 40(3):177–188. https://aquila.usm.edu/fac_pubs/15588

Ali A, Parizi LF, Guizzo MG, Tirloni L, Seixas A, Vaz ID, Termignoni C (2015b) Immunoprotective potential of a *Rhipicephalus* (*Boophilus*) microplus metalloprotease. Vet Parasitol 207(1–2):107–114. https://doi.org/10.1016/j.vetpar.2014.11.007

Allen JR, Humphreys SJ (1979) Immunisation of guinea pigs and cattle against ticks. Nature 280(5722):491–493. https://doi.org/10.1038/280491a0

Almazán C, Kocan KM, Bergman DK, Garcia-Garcia JC, Blouin EF, de la Fuente J (2003) Identification of protective antigens for the control of *Ixodes scapularis* infestations using cDNA expression library immunization. Vaccine 21(13–14):1492–1501. https://doi.org/10.1016/s0264-410x(02)00683-7

Almazán C, Blas-Machado U, Kocan KM, Yoshioka JH, Blouin EF, Mangold AJ, de la Fuente J (2005a) Characterization of three *Ixodes scapularis* cDNAs protective against tick infestations. Vaccine 23(35):4403–4416. https://doi.org/10.1016/j.vaccine.2005.04.012

Almazán C, Kocan KM, Blouin EF, de la Fuente J (2005b) Vaccination with recombinant tick antigens for the control of *Ixodes scapularis* adult infestations. Vaccine 23(46–47):5294–5298. https://doi.org/10.1016/j.vaccine.2005.08.004

Almazán C, Lagunes R, Villar M, Canales M, Rosario-Cruz R, Jongejan F, de la Fuente J (2010) Identification and characterization of *Rhipicephalus (Boophilus) microplus* candidate protective antigens for the control of cattle tick infestations. Parasitol Res 106(2):471–479. https://doi.org/10.1007/s00436-009-1689-1

Almazán C, Moreno-Cantú O, Moreno-Cid JA, Galindo RC, Canales M, Villar M, de la Fuente J (2012) Control of tick infestations in cattle vaccinated with bacterial membranes containing surface-exposed tick protective antigens. Vaccine 30(2):265–272. https://doi.org/10.1016/j.vaccine.2011.10.102

Almazán C, Fourniol L, Rakotobe S, Šimo L, Bornères J, Cote M, Peltier S, Maye J, Versillé N, Richardson J, Bonnet SI (2020) Failed disruption of tick feeding, viability, and molting after immunization of mice and sheep with recombinant *Ixodes ricinus* salivary proteins IrSPI and IrLip1. Vaccine 8(3):475. https://doi.org/10.3390/vaccines8030475

Anguita J, Ramamoorthi N, Hovius JWR, Das S, Thomas V, Persinski R, Conze D, Askenase PW, Rincón M, Kantor FS, Fikrig E (2002) Salp15, an *Ixodes scapularis* salivary protein, inhibits CD4+ T cell activation. Immunity 16(6):849–859. https://doi.org/10.1016/S1074-7613(02)00325-4

Anisuzzaman, Islam MK, Alim MA, Miyoshi T, Hatta T, Yamaji K, Matsumoto Y, Fujisaki K, Tsuji N (2011) Longistatin, a plasminogen activator, is key to the availability of blood-meals for ixodid ticks. PLoS Pathog 7(3):e1001312. https://doi.org/10.1371/journal.ppat.1001312

Arakane Y, Muthukrishnan S (2010) Insect chitinase and chitinase-like proteins. Cell Mol Life Sci 67(2):201–216. https://doi.org/10.1007/s00018-009-0161-9

Aželytė J, Wu-Chuang A, Žiegytė R, Platonova E, Mateos-Hernandez L, Maye J, Obregon D, Palinauskas V, Cabezas-Cruz A (2022) Anti-microbiota vaccine reduces avian malaria infection within mosquito vectors. Front Immunol 13:841835. https://doi.org/10.3389/fimmu.2022.841835

Bergman DK, Ramachandra RN, Wikel SK (1998) Characterization of an immunosuppressant protein from *Dermacentor andersoni* (Acari: Ixodidae) salivary glands. J Med Entomol 35(4):505–509. https://doi.org/10.1093/jmedent/35.4.505

Bishop R, Lambson B, Wells C, Pandit P, Osaso J, Nkonge C, Morzaria S, Musoke A, Nene V (2002) A cement protein of the tick Rhipicephalus appendiculatus, located in the secretory e cell granules of the type III salivary gland acini, induces strong antibody responses in cattle. Int J Parasitol 32(7):833–842. https://doi.org/10.1016/s0020-7519(02)00027-9

Boldbaatar D, Umemiya-Shirafuji R, Liao M, Tanaka T, Xuan X, Fujisaki K (2010) Multiple vitellogenins from the *Haemaphysalis longicornis* tick are crucial for ovarian development. J Insect Physiol 56(11):1587–1598. https://doi.org/10.1016/j.jinsphys.2010.05.019

Bonnet SI, Pollet T (2021) Update on the intricate tango between tick microbiomes and tick-borne pathogens. Parasite Immunol 43(5):e12813. https://doi.org/10.1111/pim.12813

Bowman AS, Sauer JR (2004) Tick salivary glands: function, physiology and future. Parasitology 129(Suppl):S67–S81. https://doi.org/10.1017/s0031182004006468

Cabezas-Cruz A, Espinosa P, Alberdi P, de la Fuente J (2019) Tick–pathogen interactions: the metabolic perspective. Trends Parasitol 35(4):316–328. https://doi.org/10.1016/j.pt.2019.01.006

Calvano MPCA, Brumatti RC, Garcia MV, Barros JC, Andreotti R (2019) Economic efficiency of *Rhipicephalus microplus* control and effect on beef cattle performance in the Brazilian Cerrado. Exp Appl Acarol 79(3–4):459–471. https://doi.org/10.1007/s10493-019-00446-5

Carreón D, de la Lastra JM, Almazán C, Canales M, Ruiz-Fons F, Boadella M, Moreno-Cid JA, Villar M, Gortázar C, Reglero M, Villarreal R, de la Fuente J (2012) Vaccination with BM86, subolesin and akirin protective antigens for the control of tick infestations in white tailed deer and red deer. Vaccine 30(2):273–279. https://doi.org/10.1016/j.vaccine.2011.10.099

Chmelař J, Kotál J, Langhansová H, Kotsyfakis M (2017) Protease inhibitors in tick saliva: the role of serpins and cystatins in tick-host-pathogen interaction. Front Cell Infect Microbiol 7:216. https://doi.org/10.3389/fcimb.2017.00216

Colombini M. (2004). VDAC: the channel at the interface between mitochondria and the cytosol. Molecular and cellular biochemistry, 256-257(1-2), 107–115. https://doi.org/10.1023/b:mcbi.0000009862.17396.8d

Contreras M, de la Fuente J (2016) Control of *Ixodes ricinus* and *Dermacentor reticulatus* tick infestations in rabbits vaccinated with the Q38 Subolesin/Akirin chimera. Vaccine 34(27):3010–3013. https://doi.org/10.1016/j.vaccine.2016.04.092

Contreras M, de la Fuente J (2017) Control of infestations by *Ixodes ricinus* tick larvae in rabbits vaccinated with aquaporin recombinant antigens. Vaccine 35(9):1323–1328. https://doi.org/10.1016/j.vaccine.2017.01.052

Contreras M, Kasaija PD, Merino O, de la Cruz-Hernandez NI, Gortazar C, de la Fuente J (2019) Oral vaccination with a formulation combining *Rhipicephalus microplus* subolesin with heat inactivated *Mycobacterium bovis* reduces tick infestations in cattle. Front Cell Infect Microbiol 9:45. https://doi.org/10.3389/fcimb.2019.00045

Costa GCA, Ribeiro ICT, Melo-Junior O, Gontijo NF, Sant'Anna MRV, Pereira MH, Pessoa GCD, Koerich LB, Oliveira F, Valenzuela JG, Giunchetti RC, Fujiwara RT, Bartholomeu DC, Araujo RN (2021) *Amblyomma sculptum* salivary protease inhibitors as potential anti-tick vaccines. Front Immunol 11:611104. https://doi.org/10.3389/fimmu.2020.611104

da Silva Vaz I Jr, Torino Lermen T, Michelon A, Sanchez Ferreira CA, Joaquim de Freitas DR, Termignoni C, Masuda A (2004) Effect of acaricides on the activity of a *Boophilus microplus* glutathione S-transferase. Vet Parasitol 119(2–3):237–245. https://doi.org/10.1016/j.vetpar.2003.11.004

Dai J, Wang P, Adusumilli S, Booth CJ, Narasimhan S, Anguita J, Fikrig E (2009) Antibodies against a tick protein, Salp15, protect mice from the lyme disease agent. Cell Host Microbe 6(5):482–492. https://doi.org/10.1016/j.chom.2009.10.006

de la Fuente J, Rodríguez M, Montero C, Redondo M, García-García JC, Méndez L, Serrano E, Valdés M, Enríquez A, Canales M, Ramos E, Boué O, Machado H, Lleonart R (1999) Vaccination against ticks (*Boophilus* spp.): the experience with the Bm86-based vaccine Gavac™. Genet Anal Biomol Eng 15(3–5):143–148. https://doi.org/10.1016/S1050-3862(99)00018-2

de la Fuente J, Almazán C, Blas-Machado U, Naranjo V, Mangold AJ, Blouin EF, Gortazar C, Kocan KM (2006a) The tick protective antigen, 4D8, is a conserved protein involved in modulation of tick blood ingestion and reproduction. Vaccine 24(19):4082–4095. https://doi.org/10.1016/j.vaccine.2006.02.046

de la Fuente J, Almazán C, Blouin EF, Naranjo V, Kocan KM (2006b) Reduction of tick infections with *Anaplasma marginale* and *A. phagocytophilum* by targeting the tick protective antigen subolesin. Parasitol Res 100(1):85–91. https://doi.org/10.1007/s00436-006-0244-6

de la Fuente J, Kopáček P, Lew-Tabor A, Maritz-Olivier C (2016) Strategies for new and improved vaccines against ticks and tick-borne diseases. Parasite Immunol 38(12):754–769. https://doi.org/10.1111/pim.12339

de la Fuente J, Antunes S, Bonnet S, Cabezas-Cruz A, Domingos AG, Estrada-Peña A, Johnson N, Kocan KM, Mansfield KL, Nijhof AM, Papa A, Rudenko N, Villar M, Alberdi P, Torina A, Ayllón N, Vancova M, Golovchenko M, Grubhoffer L, Caracappa S, Fooks AR, Gortazar C, Rego ROM (2017) Tick-pathogen interactions and vector competence: identification of molecular drivers for tick-borne diseases. Front Cell Infect Microbiol 7:114. https://doi.org/10.3389/fcimb.2017.00114

de Oliveira PR, Camargo Mathias MI, Bechara GH (2006) *Amblyomma triste* (Koch, 1844) (Acari: Ixodidae): morphological description of the ovary and of vitellogenesis. Exp Parasitol 113(3):179–185. https://doi.org/10.1016/j.exppara.2006.01.012

Decrem Y, Mariller M, Lahaye K, Blasioli V, Beaufays J, Zouaoui Boudjeltia K, Vanhaeverbeek M, Cérutti M, Brossard M, Vanhamme L, Godfroid E (2008) The impact of gene knock-down and vaccination against salivary metalloproteases on blood feeding and egg laying by *Ixodes ricinus*. Int J Parasitol 38(5):549–560. https://doi.org/10.1016/j.ijpara.2007.09.003

Fan XY, Xu XC, Wu YX, Liu XY, Yang F, Hu YH (2022) Evaluation of anti-tick efficiency in rabbits induced by DNA vaccines encoding *Haemaphysalis longicornis* lipocalin homologue. Med Vet Entomol 36(4):511–515. https://doi.org/10.1111/mve.12594

Flower DR (1996) The lipocalin protein family: structure and function. Biochem J 318:1–14

Francischetti IM, Mather TN, Ribeiro JM (2003) Cloning of a salivary gland metalloprotease and characterization of gelatinase and fibrin(ogen)lytic activities in the saliva of the Lyme disease tick vector *Ixodes scapularis*. Biochem Biophys Res Commun 305(4):869–875. https://doi.org/10.1016/s0006-291x(03)00857-x

Francischetti IM, Sa-Nunes A, Mans BJ, Santos IM, Ribeiro JM (2009) The role of saliva in tick feeding. Front Biosci 14(6):2051–2088. https://doi.org/10.2741/3363

Galindo RC, Doncel-Pérez E, Zivkovic Z, Naranjo V, Gortazar C, Mangold AJ, Martín-Hernando MP, Kocan KM, de la Fuente J (2009) Tick subolesin is an ortholog of the akirins described in insects and vertebrates. Dev Comp Immunol 33(4):612–617. https://doi.org/10.1016/j.dci.2008.11.002

Gao Z, Zheng P, Wang K, Ji X, Shi Y, Song X, Liu J, Yu Z, Yang X (2022) The molecular and functional characterization of ferritins in the hard tick *Hyalomma rufipes*. Parasit Vectors 15(1):368. https://doi.org/10.1186/s13071-022-05515-0

García-García JC, Montero C, Redondo M, Vargas M, Canales M, Boue O, Rodríguez M, Joglar M, Machado H, González IL, Valdés M, Méndez L, de la Fuente J (2000) Control of ticks resistant to immunization with Bm86 in cattle vaccinated with the recombinant antigen Bm95 isolated from the cattle tick, *Boophilus microplus*. Vaccine 18(21):2275–2287. https://doi.org/10.1016/S0264-410X(99)00548-4

George JE, Pound JM, Davey RB (2004) Chemical control of ticks on cattle and the resistance of these parasites to acaricides. Parasitology 129(Suppl):S353–S366. https://doi.org/10.1017/s0031182003004682

Goto A, Matsushita K, Gesellchen V, El Chamy L, Kuttenkeuler D, Takeuchi O, Hoffmann JA, Akira S, Boutros M, Reichhart JM (2008) Akirins are highly conserved nuclear proteins required for NF-kappaB-dependent gene expression in drosophila and mice. Nat Immunol 9(1):97–104. https://doi.org/10.1038/ni1543

Guerrero FD, Andreotti R, Bendele KG, Cunha RC, Miller RJ, Yeater K, Pérez de León AA (2014) *Rhipicephalus* (*Boophilus*) *microplus* aquaporin as an effective vaccine antigen to protect against cattle tick infestations. Parasit Vectors 7:475. https://doi.org/10.1186/s13071-014-0475-9

Hajdusek O, Almazán C, Loosova G, Villar M, Canales M, Grubhoffer L, Kopacek P, De La Fuente J (2010) Characterization of ferritin 2 for the control of tick infestations. Vaccine 28(17):2993–2998. https://doi.org/10.1016/j.vaccine.2010.02.008

Haque MS, Islam MS, You MJ (2023) Efficacy of recombinant enolase as a candidate vaccine against Haemaphysalis longicornis tick infestation in mice. Parasit Hosts Dis 61(4):439–448. https://doi.org/10.3347/PHD.23075

Hassan IA, Wang Y, Zhou Y, Cao J, Zhang H, Zhou J (2020) Cross protection induced by combined Subolesin-based DNA and protein immunizations against adult *Haemaphysalis longicornis*. Vaccine 38(4):907–915. https://doi.org/10.1016/j.vaccine.2019.10.076

Hovius JWR, De Jong MAWP, Den Dunnen J, Litjens M, Fikrig E, Van Der Poll T, Gringhuis SI, Geijtenbeek TBH (2008) Salp15 Binding to DC-SIGN inhibits cytokine expression by impairing both nucleosome remodeling and mRNA stabilization. PLoS Pathog 4(2):e31. https://doi.org/10.1371/journal.ppat.0040031

Hüe T, Petermann J, Bonnefond R, Mermoud I, Rantoen D, Vuocolo T (2017) Experimental efficacy of a vaccine against *Rhipicephalus australis*. Exp Appl Acarol 73(2):245–256. https://doi.org/10.1007/s10493-017-0184-0

Huercha SR, Li M, Fan X, Hu Z, Wu L, Li Y, Zhang W, Zhang Y, Ma Y, Bayin C (2020) Characterization of glutathione S-transferase of *Dermacantor marginatus* and effect of the recombinant antigen as a potential anti-tick vaccine. Vet Parasitol 279:109043. https://doi.org/10.1016/j.vetpar.2020.109043

Imamura S, Namangala B, Tajima T, Tembo ME, Yasuda J, Ohashi K, Onuma M (2006) Two serine protease inhibitors (serpins) that induce a bovine protective immune response against *Rhipicephalus appendiculatus* ticks. Vaccine 24(13):2230–2237. https://doi.org/10.1016/j.vaccine.2005.10.055

Imamura S, Konnai S, Vaz IDS, Yamada S, Nakajima C, Ito Y, Tajima T, Yasuda J, Simuunza M, Onuma M, Ohashi K (2008) Effects of anti-tick cocktail vaccine against *Rhipicephalus appendiculatus*. Jpn J Vet Res 56(2):85–98

Imamura S, da Silva Vaz I Jr, Konnai S, Yamada S, Nakajima C, Onuma M, Ohashi K (2009) Effect of vaccination with a recombinant metalloprotease from *Haemaphysalis longicornis*. Exp Appl Acarol 48(4):345–358. https://doi.org/10.1007/s10493-009-9245-3

Jarmey JM, Riding GA, Pearson RD, McKenna RV, Willadsen P (1995) Carboxydipeptidase from *Boophilus microplus*: a "concealed" antigen with similarity to angiotensin-converting enzyme. Insect Biochem Mol Biol 25(9):969–974. https://doi.org/10.1016/0965-1748(95)00038-W

Jittapalapong S, Kaewhom P, Pumhom P, Canales M, de la Fuente J, Stich RW (2010) Immunization of rabbits with recombinant serine protease inhibitor reduces the performance of adult female *Rhipicephalus microplus*. Transbound Emerg Dis 57(1–2):103–106. https://doi.org/10.1111/j.1865-1682.2010.01108.x

Jmel MA, Voet H, Araújo RN, Tirloni L, Sá-Nunes A, Kotsyfakis M (2023) Tick salivary Kunitz-type inhibitors: targeting host hemostasis and immunity to mediate successful blood feeding. Int Mol Sci 24(2):1556. https://doi.org/10.3390/ijms24021556

Johnston TH, Bancroft MJ (1918) A tick resistant condition in cattle. Proc R Soc Queensland 30:219–317

Kasaija PD, Contreras M, Kabi F, Mugerwa S, de la Fuente J (2020) Vaccination with recombinant subolesin antigens provides cross-tick species protection in *Bos indicus* and crossbred cattle in Uganda. Vaccine 8(2):319. https://doi.org/10.3390/vaccines8020319

Kemp DH, Agbede RI, Johnston LA, Gough JM (1986) Immunization of cattle against *Boophilus microplus* using extracts derived from adult female ticks: feeding and survival of the parasite on vaccinated cattle. Int J Parasitol 16(2):115–120. https://doi.org/10.1016/0020-7519(86)90096-2

Kemp DH, Pearson RD, Gough JM, Willadsen P (1989) Vaccination against *Boophilus microplus*: localization of antigens on tick gut cells and their interaction with the host immune system. Exp Appl Acarol 7(1):43–58. https://doi.org/10.1007/BF01200452

Kim TK, Radulovic Z, Mulenga A (2016) Target validation of highly conserved *Amblyomma americanum* tick saliva serine protease inhibitor 19. Ticks Tick Borne Dis 7(3):405–414. https://doi.org/10.1016/j.ttbdis.2015.12.017

Knorr S, Anguita J, Cortazar JT, Hajdusek O, Kopáček P, Trentelman JJ, Kershaw O, Hovius JW, Nijhof AM (2018) Preliminary evaluation of tick protein extracts and recombinant Ferritin 2 as anti-tick vaccines targeting *Ixodes ricinus* in cattle. Front Physiol 9:1696. https://doi.org/10.3389/fphys.2018.01696

Konnai S, Nishikado H, Yamada S, Imamura S, Ito T, Onuma M, Murata S, Ohashi K (2011) Molecular identification and expression analysis of lipocalins from blood feeding taiga tick, *Ixodes persulcatus* Schulze. Exp Parasitol 127(2):467–474. https://doi.org/10.1016/j.exppara.2010.10.002

Kotsyfakis M, Anderson JM, Andersen JF, Calvo E, Francischetti IM, Mather TN, Valenzuela JG, Ribeiro JM (2008) Cutting edge: Immunity against a "silent" salivary antigen of the Lyme vector *Ixodes scapular*is impairs its ability to feed. J Immunol 181(8):5209–5212. https://doi.org/10.4049/jimmunol.181.8.5209

Labuda M, Trimnell AR, Licková M, Kazimírová M, Davies GM, Lissina O, Hails RS, Nuttall PA (2006) An antivector vaccine protects against a lethal vector-borne pathogen. PLoS Pathog 2(4):e27. https://doi.org/10.1371/journal.ppat.0020027

Lagunes-Quintanilla R, Domínguez-García D, Quiroz H, Martínez-Velázquez M, Rosario-Cruz R (2016) Potential effects on *Rhipicephalus* microplus tick larvae fed on calves immunized with a Subolesin peptide predicted by epitope analysis. Trop Biomed 33(4):726–738

Lagunes-Quintanilla R, de la Cruz-Hernández NI, Ramírez-Guillen PN, Merino-Charrez JO (2018) Decrease in the cattle tick *Rhipicephalus microplus* biological parameters using anti-subolesin peptide antibodies by artificial capillary feeding. Trop Biomed 35(2):492–500

Lagunes-Quintanilla R, Valdez-Espinoza UM, Hernández-Ortiz R, Castro-Saines E, Merino O, Mendoza-Martínez N (2022) Experimental vaccination in rabbits using the peptide RmS-17 antigen reduces the performance of a Mexican *Rhipicephalus microplus* tick strain. Ticks Tick Borne Dis 13(6):102044. https://doi.org/10.1016/j.ttbdis.2022.102044

Law RH, Zhang Q, McGowan S, Buckle AM, Silverman GA, Wong W, Rosado CJ, Langendorf CG, Pike RN, Bird PI, Whisstock JC (2006) An overview of the serpin superfamily. Genome Biol 7(5):216. https://doi.org/10.1186/gb-2006-7-5-216

Lee J-H, Lee K-A, Lee W-J (2017) Microbiota, gut physiology, and insect immunity. In: Advances in insect physiology, vol 52. Elsevier, Amsterdam, pp 111–138. https://doi.org/10.1016/bs.aiip.2016.11.001

Lee SH, Li J, Moumouni PFA, Okado K, Zheng W, Liu M, Ji S, Kim S, Umemiya-Shirafuji R, Xuan X (2020) Subolesin vaccination inhibits blood feeding and reproduction of *Haemaphysalis longicornis* in rabbits. Parasit Vectors 13(1):478. https://doi.org/10.1186/s13071-020-04359-w

Lew-Tabor GA, Rodríguez-Valle F (2016) A review of reverse vaccinology approaches for the development of vaccines against ticks and tick borne diseases. Ticks Tick Borne Dis 7(6):1236–1237. https://doi.org/10.1016/j.ttbdis.2015.12.012

Liang N, Dong HM, Fan XY, Wu YX, Yang F, Liu XY, Hu YH (2022) Characterization and evaluation of a new triosephosphate isomerase homologue from *Haemaphysalis longicornis* as a candidate vaccine against tick infection. Ticks Tick Borne Dis 13(4):101968. https://doi.org/10.1016/j.ttbdis.2022.101968

Mann AE, Mitchell EA, Zhang Y, Curtis-Robles R, Thapa S, Hamer SA, Allen MS (2020) Comparison of the bacterial gut microbiome of north American *Triatoma* spp. with and without *Trypanosoma cruzi*. Front Microbiol 11:364. https://doi.org/10.3389/fmicb.2020.00364

Manzano-Román R, Díaz-Martín V, Oleaga A, Pérez-Sánchez R (2015) Identification of protective linear B-cell epitopes on the subolesin/akirin orthologues of *Ornithodoros* spp. soft ticks. Vaccine 33(8):1046–1055. https://doi.org/10.1016/j.vaccine.2015.01.015

Mateos-Hernández L, Obregón D, Maye J, Borneres J, Versille N, de la Fuente J, Estrada-Peña A, Hodžić A, Šimo L, Cabezas-Cruz A (2020) Anti-tick microbiota vaccine impacts *ixodes ricinus* performance during feeding. Vaccine 8(4):702. https://doi.org/10.3390/vaccines8040702

Mateos-Hernández L, Obregón D, Wu-Chuang A, Maye J, Bornères J, Versillé N, de la Fuente J, Díaz-Sánchez S, Bermúdez-Humarán LG, Torres-Maravilla E, Estrada-Peña A, Hodžić A, Šimo L, Cabezas-Cruz A (2021) Anti-microbiota vaccines modulate the tick microbiome in a taxon-specific manner. Front Immunol 12:704621. https://doi.org/10.3389/fimmu.2021.704621

Mbulaiteye-Saimo M, Odongo M, Bishop V, Musoke L, Oers V, Lubega GW (2011) Recombinant *Rhipicephalus appendiculatus* gut (Ra86) and salivary gland cement (Trp64) proteins as candidate antigens for inclusion in tick vaccines: Protective effects of Ra86 on infestation with adult *R. appendiculatus*. Vaccine 1:1–23. https://doi.org/10.2147/VDT.S20827

Mendoza-Martínez N, Alonso-Díaz MA, Merino O, Fernández-Salas A, Lagunes-Quintanilla R (2021) Protective efficacy of the peptide Subolesin antigen against the cattle tick *Rhipicephalus microplus* under natural infestation. Vet Parasitol 299:109577. https://doi.org/10.1016/j.vetpar.2021.109577

Merino O, Alberdi P, Pérez De La Lastra JM, De La Fuente J (2013a) Tick vaccines and the control of tick-borne pathogens. Front Cell Infect Microbiol 3:30. https://doi.org/10.3389/fcimb.2013.00030

Merino O, Antunes S, Mosqueda J, Moreno-Cid JA, Pérez de la Lastra JM, Rosario-Cruz R, Rodríguez S, Domingos A, de la Fuente J (2013b) Vaccination with proteins involved in tick-pathogen interactions reduces vector infestations and pathogen infection. Vaccine 31(49):5889–5896. https://doi.org/10.1016/j.vaccine.2013.09.037

Mulenga A, Sugimoto C, Sako Y, Ohashi K, Musoke A, Shubash M, Onuma M (1999) Molecular characterization of a *Haemaphysalis longicornis* tick salivary gland-associated 29-kilodalton protein and its effect as a vaccine against tick infestation in rabbits. Infect Immun 67(4):1652–1658. https://doi.org/10.1128/IAI.67.4.1652-1658.1999

Narasimhan S, Schuijt TJ, Abraham NM, Rajeevan N, Coumou J, Graham M, Robson A, Wu M-J, Daffre S, Hovius JW, Fikrig E (2017) Modulation of the tick gut milieu by a secreted tick protein favors *Borrelia burgdorferi* colonization. Nat Commun 8(1):184. https://doi.org/10.1038/s41467-017-00208-0

Narasimhan S, Kurokawa C, Diktas H, Strank NO, Černý J, Murfin K, Cao Y, Lynn G, Trentleman J, Wu MJ, DePonte K, Kantor F, Anguita J, Hovius J, Fikrig E (2020) *Ixodes scapularis* saliva components that elicit responses associated with acquired tick-resistance. Ticks Tick Borne Dis 11(3):101369. https://doi.org/10.1016/j.ttbdis.2019.101369

Ndawula C Jr, Sabadin GA, Parizi LF, da Silva Vaz I Jr (2019) Constituting a glutathione S-transferase-cocktail vaccine against tick infestation. Vaccine 37(14):1918–1927. https://doi.org/10.1016/j.vaccine.2019.02.039

Ndawula C Jr, Amaral Xavier M, Villavicencio B, Cortez Lopes F, Juliano MA, Parizi LF, Verli H, da Silva Vaz I Jr, Ligabue-Braun R (2020) Prediction, mapping and validation of tick glutathione S-transferase B-cell epitopes. Ticks Tick Borne Dis 11(4):101445. https://doi.org/10.1016/j.ttbdis.2020.101445

Nebert DW, Vasiliou V (2004) Analysis of the glutathione S-transferase (GST) gene family. Hum Genomics 1(6):460–464. https://doi.org/10.1186/1479-7364-1-6-460

Odongo D, Kamau L, Skilton R, Mwaura S, Nitsch C, Musoke A, Taracha E, Daubenberger C, Bishop R (2007) Vaccination of cattle with TickGARD induces cross-reactive antibodies binding to conserved linear peptides of Bm86 homologues in *Boophilus decoloratus*. Vaccine 25(7):1287–1296. https://doi.org/10.1016/j.vaccine.2006.09.085

Ogihara MH, Taylor D (2014) Female reproductive system: anatomy, physiology, and molecular biology. In: Sonenshine DE, Roe RM (eds) Biology of ticks, vol 1. Oxford University Press, New York, NY

Ortega-Sánchez R, Camacho-Nuez M, Castañeda-Ortiz EJ, Martínez-Benítez MB, Hernández-Silva DJ, Aguilar-Tipacamú G, Mosqueda J (2020) Vaccine efficacy of recombinant BmVDAC on *Rhipicephalus microplus* fed on *Babesia bigemina*-infected and uninfected cattle. Vaccine 38(19):3618–3625. https://doi.org/10.1016/j.vaccine.2019.12.040

Parizi LF, Utiumi KU, Imamura S et al (2011) Cross immunity with *Haemaphysalis longicornis* glutathione S-transferase reduces an experimental *Rhipicephalus* (Boophilus) microplus infestation. Exp Parasitol 127(1):113–118. https://doi.org/10.1016/j.exppara.2010.07.001

Parizi LF, Reck J Jr, Oldiges DP, Guizzo MG, Seixas A, Logullo C, de Oliveira PL, Termignoni C, Martins JR, da Vaz IS Jr (2012) Multi-antigenic vaccine against the cattle tick *Rhipicephalus (Boophilus) microplus*: a field evaluation. Vaccine 30(48):6912–6917. https://doi.org/10.1016/j.vaccine.2012.08.078

Parizi LF, Rangel CK, Sabadin GA, Saggin BF, Kiio I, Xavier MA, da Silva Matos R, Camargo-Mathias MI, Seixas A, Konnai S, Ohashi K, Githaka NW, da Silva Vaz I Jr (2020) *Rhipicephalus microplus* cystatin as a potential cross-protective tick vaccine against *Rhipicephalus appendiculatus*. Ticks Tick Borne Dis 11(3):101378. https://doi.org/10.1016/j.ttbdis.2020.101378

Perez-Soria MME, López-Díaz DG, Jiménez-Ocampo R, Aguilar-Tipacamú G, Ueti MW, Mosqueda J (2024) Immunization of cattle with a *Rhipicephalus microplus* chitinase peptide containing predicted B-cell epitopes reduces tick biological fitness. Parasitology 5:1–10. https://doi.org/10.1017/S0031182024000143

Prevot PP, Couvreur B, Denis V, Brossard M, Vanhamme L, Godfroid E (2007) Protective immunity against *Ixodes ricinus* induced by a salivary serpin. Vaccine 25(17):3284–3292. https://doi.org/10.1016/j.vaccine.2007.01.008

Ramamoorthi N, Narasimhan S, Pal U, Bao F, Yang XF, Fish D, Anguita J, Norgard MV, Kantor FS, Anderson JF, Koski RA, Fikrig E (2005) The Lyme disease agent exploits a tick protein to infect the mammalian host. Nature 436(7050):573–577. https://doi.org/10.1038/nature03812

Ramírez Rodríguez PB, Rosario Cruz R, Domínguez García DI, Hernández Gutiérrez R, Lagunes Quintanilla RE, Ortuño Sahagún D, González Castillo C, Gutiérrez Ortega A, Herrera Rodríguez SE, Vallejo Cardona A, Martínez Velázquez M (2016) Identification of immunogenic proteins from ovarian tissue and recognized in larval extracts of *Rhipicephalus (Boophilus) microplus*, through an immunoproteomic approach. Exp Parasitol 170:227–235. https://doi.org/10.1016/j.exppara.2016.10.005

Ranasinghe S, McManus DP (2013) Structure and function of invertebrate Kunitz serine protease inhibitors. Dev Comp Immunol 39(3):219–227. https://doi.org/10.1016/j.dci.2012.10.005

Rand KN, Moore T, Sriskantha A, Spring K, Tellam R, Willadsen P, Cobon GS (1989) Cloning and expression of a protective antigen from the cattle tick *Boophilus microplus*. Proc Natl Acad Sci 86(24):9657–9661. https://doi.org/10.1073/pnas.86.24.9657

Ribeiro JM (1987) *Ixodes dammini*: salivary anti-complement activity. Exp Parasitol 64(3):347–353. https://doi.org/10.1016/0014-4894(87)90046-4

Ribeiro JM, Evans PM, MacSwain JL, Sauer J (1992) Amblyomma americanum: characterization of salivary prostaglandins E2 and F2 alpha by RP-HPLC/bioassay and gas chromatography-mass spectrometry. Exp Parasitol 74(1):112–116. https://doi.org/10.1016/0014-4894(92)90145-z. PMID: 1730268

Rodríguez-Hernández E, Mosqueda J, León-Ávila G, Castañeda-Ortiz EJ, Álvarez-Sánchez ME, Camacho AD, Ramos A, Camacho-Nuez M (2015) BmVDAC upregulation in the midgut of *Rhipicephalus microplus*, during infection with *Babesia bigemina*. Vet Parasitol 212(3–4):368–374. https://doi.org/10.1016/j.vetpar.2015.06.016

Rodríguez-Mallon A, Fernández E, Encinosa PE, Bello Y, Méndez-Pérez L, Ruiz LC, Pérez D, González M, Garay H, Reyes O, Méndez L, Estrada MP (2012) A novel tick antigen shows high vaccine efficacy against the dog tick, *Rhipicephalus sanguineus*. Vaccine 30(10):1782–1789. https://doi.org/10.1016/j.vaccine.2012.01.011

Rodríguez-Mallon A, Encinosa PE, Méndez-Pérez L, Bello Y, Rodríguez Fernández R, Garay H, Cabrales A, Méndez L, Borroto C, Estrada MP (2015) High efficacy of a 20 amino acid peptide of the acidic ribosomal protein P0 against the cattle tick, *Rhipicephalus microplus*. Ticks Tick Borne Dis 6(4):530–537. https://doi.org/10.1016/j.ttbdis.2015.04.007

Rodríguez-Mallon A, Encinosa Guzmán PE, Bello Soto Y, Rosales Perdomo K, Montero Espinosa C, Vargas M, Estrada García MP (2020) A chemical conjugate of the tick P0 peptide is efficacious against *Amblyomma mixtum*. Transbound Emerg Dis 67(Suppl 2):175–177. https://doi.org/10.1111/tbed.13455

Rosell R, Coons LB (1992) The role of the fat body, midgut and ovary in vitellogenin production and vitellogenesis in the female tick, *Dermacentor variabilis*. Int J Parasitol 22(3):341–349. https://doi.org/10.1016/s0020-7519(05)80012-8

Sabadin GA, Parizi LF, Kiio I, Xavier MA, da Silva Matos R, Camargo-Mathias MI, Githaka NW, Nene V, da Silva Vaz I Jr (2017) Effect of recombinant glutathione S-transferase as vaccine antigen against *Rhipicephalus appendiculatus* and *Rhipicephalus sanguineus* infestation. Vaccine 35(48 Pt B):6649–6656. https://doi.org/10.1016/j.vaccine.2017.10.026

Salát J, Paesen GC, Rezácová P, Kotsyfakis M, Kovárová Z, Sanda M, Majtán J, Grunclová L, Horká H, Andersen JF, Brynda J, Horn M, Nunn MA, Kopácek P, Kopecký J, Mares M (2010) Crystal structure and functional characterization of an immunomodulatory salivary cystatin from the soft tick *Ornithodoros moubata*. Biochem J 429(1):103–112. https://doi.org/10.1042/BJ20100280

Sappington TW, Raikhel AS (1998) Molecular characteristics of insect vitellogenins and vitellogenin receptors. Insect Biochem Mol Biol *28*(5–6):277–300. https://doi.org/10.1016/s0965-1748(97)00110-0

Sauer JR, McSwain JL, Bowman AS, Essenberg RC (1995) Tick salivary gland physiology. Annu Rev Entomol 40:245–267. https://doi.org/10.1146/annurev.en.40.010195.001333

Schwarz A, Valdés JJ, Kotsyfakis M (2012) The role of cystatins in tick physiology and blood feeding. Ticks Tick Borne Dis 3(3):117–127. https://doi.org/10.1016/j.ttbdis.2012.03.004

Seixas A, Dos Santos PC, Velloso FF, Da Silva Vaz I Jr, Masuda A, Horn F, Termignoni C (2003) A *Boophilus microplus* vitellin-degrading cysteine endopeptidase. Parasitology 126(Pt 2):155–163. https://doi.org/10.1017/s0031182002002731

Seixas A, Leal AT, Nascimento-Silva MC, Masuda A, Termignoni C, da Silva Vaz I Jr (2008) Vaccine potential of a tick vitellin-degrading enzyme (VTDCE). Vet Immunol Immunopathol 124(3–4):332–340. https://doi.org/10.1016/j.vetimm.2008.04.001

Shakya M, Kumar B, Nagar G, de la Fuente J, Ghosh S (2014) Subolesin: a candidate vaccine antigen for the control of cattle tick infestations in Indian situation. Vaccine 32(28):3488–3494. https://doi.org/10.1016/j.vaccine.2014.04.053

Showler AT, Saelao P (2022) Integrative alternative tactics for ixodid control. Insects 13(3):302. https://doi.org/10.3390/insects13030302

Smith AD, Reuben Kaufman W (2013) Molecular characterization of the vitellogenin receptor from the tick, *Amblyomma hebraeum* (Acari: Ixodidae). Insect Biochem Mol Biol 43(12):1133–1141. https://doi.org/10.1016/j.ibmb.2013.10.002

Song R, Ge T, Hu E, Fan X, Zhang Y, Zhai X, Li M, Zhang W, Wu L, Cheung AKL, Chahan B (2022) Recombinant cysteine proteinase as anti-tick targeting Hyalomma asiaticum infestation. Exp Parasitol 235:108234. https://doi.org/10.1016/j.exppara.2022.108234

Sreelekha KP, Chandrasekhar L, Jyothimol G, Lenka DR, Aswathi V, Adarshkrishna TP, Ajithkumar KG, Nair SN, Ravindran R, Juliet S, Ghosh S (2015) Histoarchitecture of ovary of *Haemaphysalis bispinosa* during engorgement period. Trop Biomed 32(3):497–503

Stewart PE, Bloom ME (2020) Sharing the ride: *Ixodes scapularis* symbionts and their interactions. Front Cell Infect Microbiol 10:142. https://doi.org/10.3389/fcimb.2020.00142

Strydom T, Lavan RP, Torres S, Heaney K (2023) The economic impact of parasitism from nematodes, trematodes and ticks on beef cattle production. Animals 13(10):1599. https://doi.org/10.3390/ani13101599

Sultana H, Patel U, Sonenshine DE, Neelakanta G (2015) Identification and comparative analysis of subolesin/akirin ortholog from *Ornithodoros turicata* ticks. Parasit Vectors 8:132. https://doi.org/10.1186/s13071-015-0749-x

Tellam RL, Kemp D, Riding G, Briscoe S, Smith D, Sharp P, Irving D, Willadsen P (2002) Reduced oviposition of *Boophilus microplus* feeding on sheep vaccinated with vitellin. Vet Parasitol 103(1–2):141–156. https://doi.org/10.1016/s0304-4017(01)00573-8

Trager W (1939) Acquired immunity to ticks. J Parasitol 25(1):57–81. https://doi.org/10.2307/3272160

Trentelman JJA, Teunissen H, Kleuskens JAGM, van de Crommert J, de la Fuente J, Hovius JWR, Schetters TPM (2019) A combination of antibodies against Bm86 and Subolesin inhibits engorgement of *Rhipicephalus australis* (formerly *Rhipicephalus microplus*) larvae in vitro. Parasit Vectors 12(1):362. https://doi.org/10.1186/s13071-019-3616-3

Trimnell AR, Hails RS, Nuttall PA (2002) Dual action ectoparasite vaccine targeting 'exposed' and 'concealed' antigens. Vaccine 20(29–30):3560–3568. https://doi.org/10.1016/s0264-410x(02)00334-1

Tsuda A, Mulenga A, Sugimoto C, Nakajima M, Ohashi K, Onuma M (2001) cDNA cloning, characterization and vaccine effect analysis of *Haemaphysalis longicornis* tick saliva proteins. Vaccine 19(30):4287–4296. https://doi.org/10.1016/s0264-410x(01)00148-7

Umemiya-Shirafuji R, Mihara R, Fujisaki K, Suzuki H (2019) Intracellular localization of vitellogenin receptor mRNA and protein during oogenesis of a parthenogenetic tick, *Haemaphysalis longicornis*. Parasit Vectors 12(1):205. https://doi.org/10.1186/s13071-019-3469-9

Wang X, Huang Y, Niu SB, Jiang BG, Jia N, van der Geest L, Ni XB, Sun Y, Cao WC (2014) Genetic diversity of Salp15 in the *Ixodes ricinus* complex (Acari: *Ixodidae*). PLoS One 9(4):e94131. https://doi.org/10.1371/journal.pone.0094131

Wang F, Lu X, Guo F, Gong H, Zhang H, Zhou Y, Cao J, Zhou J (2017) The immunomodulatory protein RH36 is relating to blood-feeding success and oviposition in hard ticks. Vet Parasitol 240:49–59. https://doi.org/10.1016/j.vetpar.2017.03.017

Wang M, Hu Y, Li M, Xu Q, Zhang X, Wang X, Xue X, Xiao Q, Liu J, Wang H (2020) A proteomics analysis of the ovarian development in females of *Haemaphysalis longicornis*. Exp Appl Acarol 80(2):289–309. https://doi.org/10.1007/s10493-020-00469-3

Wang D, Xu X, Lv L, Wu P, Dong H, Xiao S, Liu J, Hu Y (2021) Gene cloning, analysis and effect of a new lipocalin homologue from *Haemaphysalis longicornis* as a protective antigen for an anti-tick vaccine. Vet Parasitol 290:109358. https://doi.org/10.1016/j.vetpar.2021.109358

Weiss BL, Kaufman WR (2004) Two feeding-induced proteins from the male gonad trigger engorgement of the female tick *Amblyomma hebraeum*. Proc Natl Acad Sci U S A 101(16):5874–5879. https://doi.org/10.1073/pnas.0307529101

Wikel SK (1999) Tick modulation of host immunity: an important factor in pathogen transmission. Int J Parasitol 29(6):851–859. https://doi.org/10.1016/S0020-7519(99)00042-9

Willadsen P (1987) Immunological approaches to the control of ticks. Int J Parasitol 17(2):671–677. https://doi.org/10.1016/0020-7519(87)90145-7

Willadsen P (2004) Anti-tick vaccines. Parasitology 129(Suppl):S367–S387. https://doi.org/10.1017/s0031182003004657

Willadsen P, Kemp DH (1988) Vaccination with 'concealed' antigens for tick control. Parasitol Today 4(7):196–198. https://doi.org/10.1016/0169-4758(88)90084-1

Willadsen P, Smith D, Cobon G, McKenna RV (1996) Comparative vaccination of cattle against *Boophilus microplus* with recombinant antigen Bm86 alone or in combination with recombinant Bm91. Parasite Immunol 18(5):241–246. https://doi.org/10.1046/j.1365-3024.1996.d01-90.x

Wu-Chuang A, Hodžić A, Mateos-Hernández L, Estrada-Peña A, Obregon D, Cabezas-Cruz A (2021) Current debates and advances in tick microbiome research. Curr Res Parasitol Vector Borne Dis 1:100036. https://doi.org/10.1016/j.crpvbd.2021.100036

Xavier MA, Tirloni L, Pinto AFM, Diedrich JK, Yates JR 3rd, Mulenga A, Logullo C, da Silva Vaz I Jr, Seixas A, Termignoni C (2018) A proteomic insight into vitellogenesis during tick ovary maturation. Sci Rep 8(1):4698. https://doi.org/10.1038/s41598-018-23090-2

Xavier MA, Tirloni L, Torquato R, Tanaka A, Pinto AFM, Diedrich JK, Yates JR 3rd, da Silva Vaz I Jr, Seixas A, Termignoni C (2019) Blood anticlotting activity of a *Rhipicephalus microplus* cathepsin L-like enzyme. Biochimie 163:12–20. https://doi.org/10.1016/j.biochi.2019.04.025

Xu Z, Yan Y, Cao J, Zhou Y, Zhang H, Xu Q, Zhou J (2020) A family of serine protease inhibitors (serpins) and its expression profiles in the ovaries of *Rhipicephalus haemaphysaloides*. Infect Genet Evol 84:104346. https://doi.org/10.1016/j.meegid.2020.104346

Yamada S, Konnai S, Imamura S, Ito T, Onuma M, Ohashi K (2009) Cloning and characterization of *Rhipicephalus appendiculatus voraxinalpha* and its effect as anti-tick vaccine. Vaccine 27(43):5989–5997. https://doi.org/10.1016/j.vaccine.2009.07.072

You M, Fujisaki K (2009) Vaccination effects of recombinant chitinase protein from the hard tick *Haemaphysalis longicornis* (Acari: Ixodidae). J Vet Med Sci 71(6):709–712. https://doi.org/10.1292/jvms.71.709

You M, Xuan X, Tsuji N, Kamio T, Taylor D, Suzuki N, Fujisaki K (2003) Identification and molecular characterization of a chitinase from the hard tick *Haemaphysalis longicornis*. J Biol Chem 278(10):8556–8563. https://doi.org/10.1074/jbc.M206831200

Zeb I, Parizi LF, Israr M, da Silva Vaz I Jr, Ali A (2024) Cross-species immunoprotective antigens (subolesin, ferritin 2 and P0) provide protection against *Rhipicephalus sanguineus* sensu lato. Parasit Vectors 17(1):3. https://doi.org/10.1186/s13071-023-06079-3

Zhang H, Qiao R, Gong H, Cao J, Zhou Y, Zhou J (2017) Identification and anticoagulant activity of a novel Kunitz-type protein HA11 from the salivary gland of the tick Hyalomma asiaticum. Exp Appl Acarol 71(1):71–85. https://doi.org/10.1007/s10493-017-0106-1

Zhang S-B, Gao Z-H, Wang Y-K, Lv W-X, Dong K-X, Guo F-D, Wang R-Y, Yang X-L (2024) The evaluation of cystatin protein vaccines based on the stress response of ticks triggered by low-temperature and toxin stress in *Haemaphysalis doenitzi*. Pest Manag Sci 80:3957. https://doi.org/10.1002/ps.8099

Zhao X, Zhao J, Wang J, Liao C, Guan Q, Han Q (2024) Immune protection of three serine protease inhibitors vaccine in mice against *Rhipicephalus sanguineus*. Sci Rep 14(1):7703. https://doi.org/10.1038/s41598-024-58303-4

# Tick Immunoendrocrinology: A Novel Approach to Develop Strategies to Control and Prevent Tick Infestations

10

Hugo Aguilar-Diaz, Rosa Estela Quiroz-Castañeda, Ixchel Guadalupe Díaz-Esquivel, Angel Salvador Ortega-Catalán, Raquel Cossío-Bayúgar, and Edgar Castro-Saines

**Abstract**

Infections by the *Rhipicephalus microplus* tick represent a serious health problem in the global livestock industry, mainly due to direct damage and the vector's capacity to transmit various pathogens. Currently, tick infections have been increasing due to the emergence of populations resistant to ixodicides. Therefore, the search for new targets that contribute to the control of this ectoparasite is a priority. At the same time, studying biological interactions between host, vector, and pathogen, including the microbiota, is a novel but little-explored field. In relation, we know that the immunoendocrine system plays a primary role in these interactions since it is responsible for regulating the health-disease process. Additionally, this macrosystem is related to various immune mechanisms for controlling pathogens and processes associated with the reproduction and development of ticks. Therefore, the study of the immunoendocrine system provides an excellent field in searching for regulatory molecules with vaccine potential or as targets for developing new drugs.

**Keywords**

Pest control · Hormones · Omics · Vaccines targets

Hugo Aguilar-Diaz and Rosa Estela Quiroz-Castañeda contributed equally to this chapter.

H. Aguilar-Diaz (✉) · R. E. Quiroz-Castañeda · I. G. Díaz-Esquivel · A. S. Ortega-Catalán · R. Cossío-Bayúgar · E. Castro-Saines
National Center for Disciplinary Research in Animal Health and Safety, INIFAP, Carretera Federal Cuernavaca-Cuautla 8534, Jiutepec, Morelos, Mexico
e-mail: aguilar.hugo@inifap.gob.mx

R. Cossío-Bayúgar
Instituto Nacional de Investigaciones, Agrícolas y Pecuarias, Mexico City, Mexico
e-mail: aguilar.hugo@inifap.gob.mx


S. Kumar et al. (eds.), *Acaricides Resistance in Ticks*,
https://doi.org/10.1007/978-981-97-7411-1_10

## 10.1 Introduction

The cattle tick, *Rhipicephalus microplus*, is an obligate hematophagous ectoparasite that causes economic losses in the livestock industry, estimated at 22 to 30 billion dollars annually. About 80% of the world's cattle are estimated to be in contact with ticks (FAO 2004; Lew-Tabor and Valle 2016). The damage caused to livestock includes skin lesions, blood loss, toxic effects, decreased milk production, anemia in calves, as well as the transmission of hemoparasites to cattle such as *Babesia bigemina, Babesia bovis,* and *Anaplasma marginale*. This damage produces additional costs in control and treatment since chemical acaricides are the primary tool for controlling infestations. However, the inappropriate use of these products has resulted in the development of resistant tick populations and their impact on the environment (Rodríguez-Vivas 2018).

Additionally, global warming has enhanced the expansion of ticks to new ecological niches, with the consequent increase in the number of diseases they transmit. Therefore, developing new, more effective, and environmentally friendly control strategies is imperative (Estrada-Peña and de la Fuente 2014). In Mexico, estimated economic losses attributed to *R. microplus* are approximately 57,361 million dollars annually, mainly attributed to pathogens transmitted by the tick to cattle (Rodríguez-Vivas et al. 2017; Brayton 2012). Currently, the spatial distribution and annual oscillations in tick abundance are determined mainly by biological variables, such as host availability, and environmental factors, such as temperature and humidity (Chevillon et al. 2013; Estrada-Peña 1999). However, research indicates that environmental aspects, such as temperature and precipitation regimes, can significantly influence the colonization of the *R. microplus* population (Estrada-Peña 2001; Estrada-Peña et al. 2005). On the other hand, recent studies have shown that the adaptation of ticks to their specific environments is closely linked to the composition of their microbiome, which can vary in response to different abiotic factors (Fig. 10.1) (Minard et al. 2015). This approach allows us to understand better how pathogens interact with the immune and endocrine systems of the host and the tick itself, offering alternatives for the most effective control of these diseases (Aguilar-Díaz and Cossío-Bayúgar 2018).

## 10.2 Arthropod Immune System

Arthropods have a sophisticated network of innate defense mechanisms that effectively confront pathogens in their environment (Marín and Salazar-Lugo 2009). This innate immune response is based mainly on physical barriers, accompanied by cellular and humoral responses that protect the organism (Antón-Marín 2009). The first line of defense in many invertebrates is the exoskeleton or cuticle, a rigid structure that protects against mechanical damage and prevents the penetration of pathogens (Antón-Marín 2009). On the other hand, the cellular response is based on specialized cells called hemocytes, which can present phagocytic activity, engulfing the pathogen, in a similar way to macrophages in vertebrates, or they can release

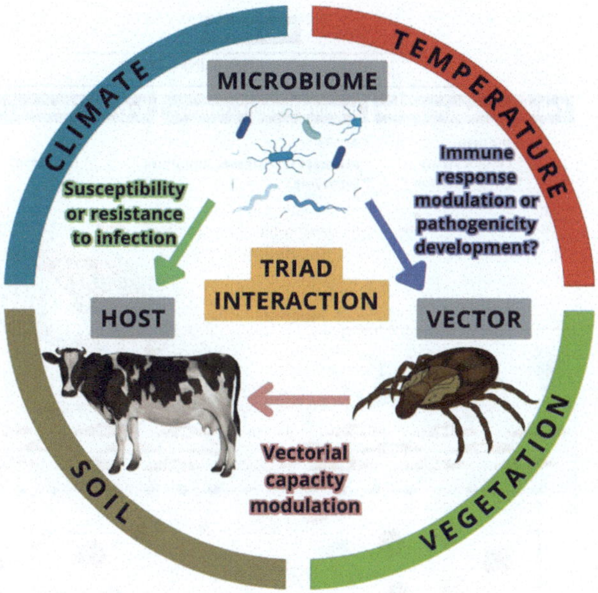


**Fig. 10.1** Host-vector-microbiome triad. Environmental factors influence this interaction, and there is close communication between the triad elements that trigger interaction mechanisms between them. (Fig. created in Canva https://www.canva.com/)

various substances, molecules with microbicidal activity, such as the so-called peptides. Antimicrobials peptides (AMPs) recognize specific patterns that neutralize or eliminate pathogens (Aguilar-Díaz and Cossío-Bayúgar 2018). Finally, another immune protection mechanism is melanization, a process by which a melanized capsule forms around invading pathogens, preventing their spread and, consequently, their death (Ulvedal et al. 2017).

## 10.3 Immune Response in Ticks

The immune response in ticks is a pivotal and intricate process involving cellular and humoral mechanisms. In this context, the hemolymph, intestine, salivary glands, and fat body assume a critical role in immune defense. The fat body, for instance, is the site of synthesis for most of the AMPs produced by ticks. The intestine and salivary glands, on the other hand, produce and release regulatory molecules of the immune response. Finally, the hemolymph acts as a medium to transport the immune cells and effector molecules, thereby facilitating the immune response (Fig. 10.2) (Aguilar-Díaz et al. 2021a; Strand 2008).

Additionally, the immune response varies depending on the type of pathogen, tissue, sex, life cycle phase, and tick species. In this regard, innate immunity activates when membrane receptors recognize bacterial components such as

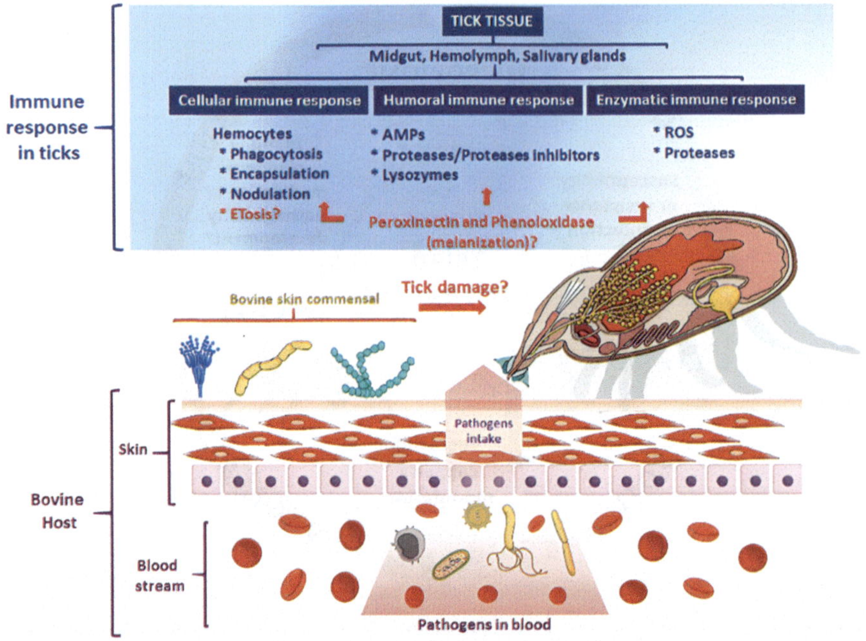


**Fig. 10.2** The general scenario of the immune response in the cattle ticks *R. microplus*. The immune response in a tick involves a cellular, humoral, and enzymatic response. The participation of the host's microbiota also occurs at the level of the skin and the pathogens that circulate in its blood. (Aguilar-Díaz et al., 2021 Pathogens, 10(11), 1511)

peptidoglycans or lipoteichoic acid, triggering the synthesis of AMPs such as defensins, cecropins, attacins, and lysozyme. These AMPs are inserted into the membrane and/or cell wall, causing the pathogen to die. Other components of the bacterial cell wall, known as pathogen-associated molecular patterns (PAMPs), are formed by beta-1-3-glucans and Lipopolysaccharides (LPS), which also activate the immune response through the synthesis of soluble lectins (Aguilar-Díaz et al. 2021a) (Fig. 10.2).

### 10.3.1 Cellular Immune Response

In ticks, hemocytes are the main effectors of the cellular immune response since they control pathogens through encapsulation and nodule formation. Additionally, PAMPs on the microbial surface can activate this primary cellular response by recognizing and destroying pathogens through phagocytosis. Mainly, this process could be regulated by a complement-analogous system, which includes thioester proteins, fibrinogen-like lectins, and convertase-like factors. In the case of *Ixodes ricinus*, C3-like molecules facilitate yeast phagocytosis (Aguilar-Díaz and Cossío-Bayúgar 2018). On the other hand, encapsulation is a process that involves the accumulation of hemocytes around the pathogen, opsonizing and forming nodules. This mechanism occurs when hemocytes express lectins on their surface, which are involved in recognizing pathogens. These lectins can bind to lipopolysaccharides (LPS) present on the surface of pathogens. So far, several lectins related to the immune response have been identified in tick hemocytes. In this regard, a protein called Dorin-M has been discovered, a lectin with high hemagglutinating activity found in hemocytes and hemolymph plasma. Furthermore, Ixoderin A, another lectin present in the midgut and hemocytes, has been described in *I. ricinus*. The interaction between these proteins and carbohydrates confers the ability of hemocytes to form aggregates, resulting in the capture and opsonization of pathogens (Aguilar-Díaz and Cossío-Bayúgar 2018). On the other hand, the encapsulation process has been studied using artificial implants inoculated in ticks; however, it remains to be determined if this process is also activated against microorganisms (Aguilar-Díaz et al. 2021a).

### 10.3.2 Humoral Immune Response

The humoral immune response is a fundamental part of the tick immune system, focusing on producing soluble small molecules of 3 to 20 kDa. These peptides are known as AMPs and are the basis of the humoral response due to their ability to combat various pathogens effectively, quickly, and at very low concentrations. Its function is based on its ability to bind to the membrane or cell wall of pathogens, causing structural alterations that result in the loss of membrane potential and, ultimately, the death of the pathogen (Aguilar-Díaz et al. 2021a). The fat body and hemocytes secrete AMPs, although the midgut can produce some. Several AMPs have been identified in ticks, such as defensins, microplusin, hebraein, ixodicin, and even some derivatives of the host's hemoglobin (Aguilar-Díaz and Cossío-Bayúgar 2018). On the other hand, it has been suggested that lysozymes have digestive and antimicrobial functions. Its antimicrobial activity lies in its ability to break down bacterial cell walls. In ticks, a significant increase in type C lysozyme has been observed in the hemolymph after exposure to bacteria, suggesting a possible role in immune defense. Additionally, differential expression of lysozymes has been reported in different tick tissues, such as fat body, midgut, ovaries, and hemolymph, supporting the idea that in ticks, lysozymes have both metabolic and immune functions, acting in synergy with other antimicrobial peptides (Aguilar-Díaz and Cossío-Bayúgar 2018).

### 10.3.3 Oxidative Stress

To date, hemocytes can generate reactive oxygen species (ROS) in response to the presence of pathogens, which are eliminated by respiratory bursts mediated by protein kinase C. In *R. microplus* hemocytes, the production of hydrogen peroxide ($H_2O_2$) has been observed in response to microbial challenges with the bacteria

*Micrococcus luteum*, zymosan, and phorbol 12-myristate 13-acetate (PMA). Additionally, it is reported that tick hemocytes generate ROS during phagocytosis, similar to phagocytes from other invertebrates. Finally, it has been suggested that ROS could be involved in cellular signaling mechanisms related to the activation of ETosis (Extracellular Traps) in response to pathogens (Aguilar-Díaz and Cossío-Bayúgar 2018).

## 10.4 Arthropod Endocrine System

The endocrine system in arthropods plays a fundamental role in the regulation of a wide range of physiological processes, such as development and reproduction, growth, molting and metamorphosis, metabolism, immune response, and even the response to environmental stimuli (Roe et al. 2008). Although less understood than vertebrates, the endocrine system of invertebrates has been the subject of increasing attention due to its importance in the adaptation and survival of these ectoparasites. The most detailed understanding of the arthropod endocrine system and the crucial role hormones play have been elucidated mainly in the context of crustaceans and insects (Knigge et al. 2021). In this regard, it has been shown that estradiol (E2) causes a significant increase in cytosolic $Ca^{2+}$ in hemocytes of *Mytilus galloprovincialis*, suggesting that the mechanisms of action of estradiol can trigger immunoendocrine interactions in invertebrates (Canesi et al. 2004). Additionally, it has been shown that E2 is one of the main factors controlling vitellogenesis in the oyster *Crassostrea gigas* (Li et al. 1998).

On the other hand, it has been shown that a variant of crustacean hyperglycemic hormones (CHHs) is closely involved in the osmoregulation of the white shrimp *Litopenaeus vannamei*, during hypo-regulation by modulating NKA at the transcriptional level (Ponce-Rivas et al. 2021), which suggests that this hormone plays a direct role in the regulation of osmo-ionic mechanisms in most crustaceans. In the case of insects, it is known that juvenile hormone (JH) actively participates in molting and development. In addition, some reports have identified an overexpression of adipokinetic hormone II (AKH II) in the brains of *Anopheles albimanus* mosquitoes previously infected with the malaria parasite (Alvarado-Delgado et al. 2021).

### 10.4.1 Hormones as Regulators of the Endocrine System

The hormonal action mechanism initiates the specific interaction between the hormone and its receptor, which can be in the cell membrane or in the cytoplasm of the target cells where the hormone exerts its physiological function. This interaction is characterized by a constant dynamic of binding and dissociation, determined by the association and dissociation rates between the hormone and the receptor (Pérez-Rivero et al. 2005). Once the hormone-receptor complex is formed, a signaling cascade culminates, regulating various biological processes (Ayres 2019). It is known that steroid hormones cross the cell membrane by passive diffusion through the lipid bilayer or with the help of transport proteins that bind to classic steroid receptors in the cytosol.

Hormone receptors are classified into membrane receptors and nuclear receptors. The former are predominantly linked to peptide hormones and small molecules unable to cross the plasma membrane. On the other hand, nuclear receptors bind to small lipid-soluble molecules, which can diffuse or be transported across the cell membrane (Leblebicioglu et al. 2013).

Currently, we know that hormones play a primary role in regulating all endocrine mechanisms. In turn, hormones function as ligands for nuclear and membrane receptors, and through genomic and non-genomic effects, they control crucial processes, such as growth, differentiation, and reproduction (Fig. 10.3) (Aguilar-Díaz et al. 2023; Escobedo et al. 2005). The genomic mechanisms are triggered by the binding of the hormone to a nuclear receptor in the cell's cytoplasm. Once the receptor is bound to its ligand, the complex migrates to the nucleus, binding to hormone response elements in the DNA, functioning as a factor that activates and regulates gene transcription (genomic mechanism). This mechanism may involve a considerable time between the arrival of the hormone/receptor complex and the significant accumulation of the newly formed protein (Fig. 10.3) (Lösel and Wehling 2003). In contrast, non-genomic mechanisms are rapid and less susceptible to inhibitors of transcription and protein synthesis, manifesting in milliseconds, and are mainly activated in response to the interaction of the hormone with membrane receptors. These mechanisms generally activate signaling cascades mediated by MAP kinases, cAMP, and increased intracellular $Ca^{2+}$, among others (Fig. 10.3). Interestingly, it has been observed that both effects depend on the type of hormone, cell, tissue, and species involved (Falkenstein et al. 2000).

### 10.4.2 Hormones in Ticks

In arthropods, the two most studied hormones are juvenile hormone (JH) and ecdysteroid hormone. These hormones have been identified in ticks and are involved in molting, development, and reproduction (vitellogenesis) (Aguilar-Díaz et al. 2023; Ponnusamy et al. 2021; Schooley et al. 2012). In *Rhipicephalus haemaphysaloides*, after engorgement, ecdysteroid hormones trigger salivary gland degeneration (Lu et al. 2021). Additionally, there are reports in *Dermacentor variabilis* that propose that the tick microbiome responds to the hormone 20-hydroxydecdysone and then regulates vitellogenesis and egg development, highlighting that this species has been the most investigated for its hormonal response (Ponnusamy et al. 2021).

### 10.4.3 Steroid Receptors in Ticks

In arthropods, the presence of different types of receptors with the ability to bind steroid hormones has recently been demonstrated, such as estrogen receptors (ER) and estrogen-related receptors (ERR), whose function is related to various

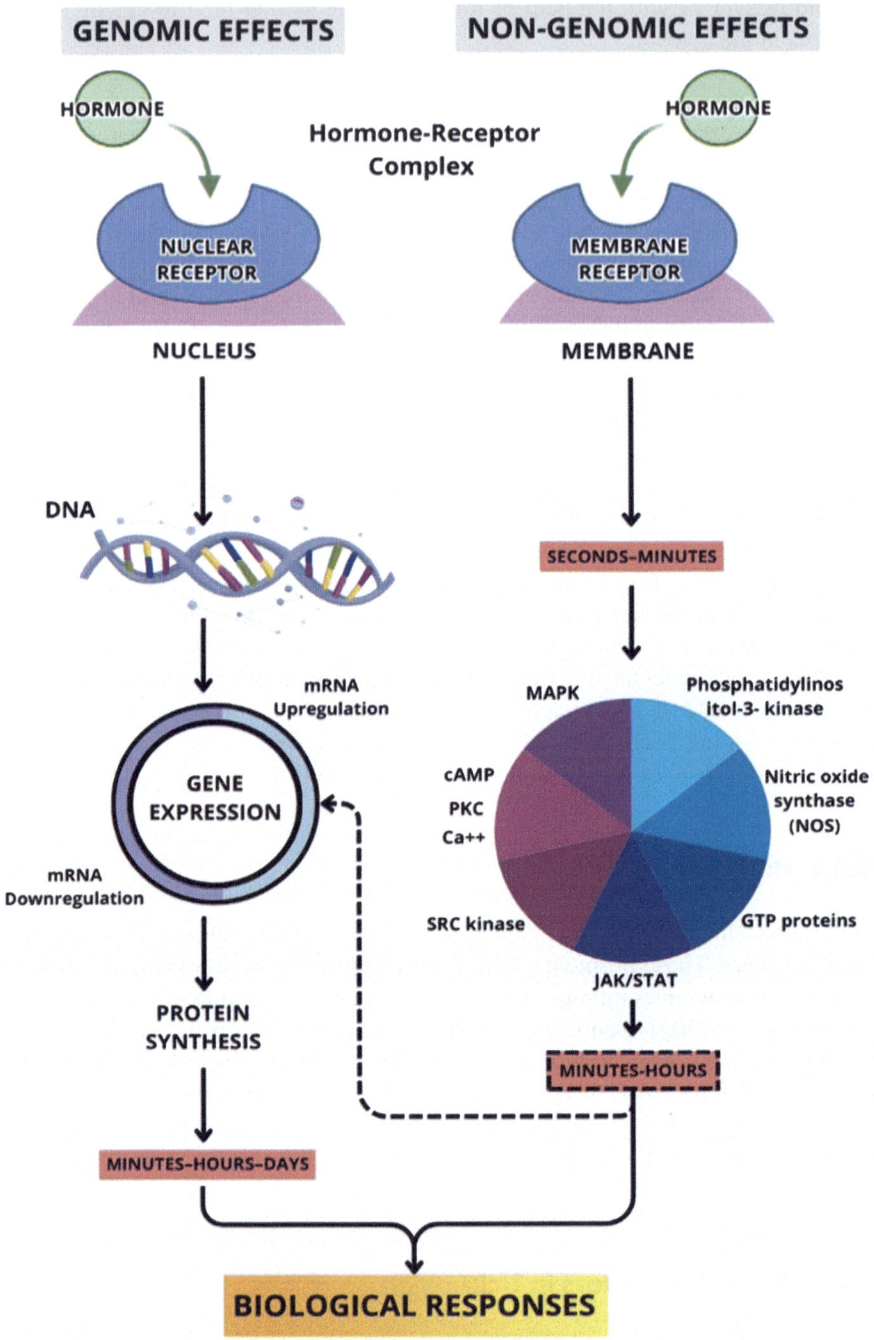


**Fig. 10.3** Genomic and non-genomic effects produced by steroid hormones. These effects trigger when hormone binds to nuclear and/or membrane receptors present on the target cell. Each type of effect presents different characteristics at the time and molecular participant level. (Fig. created in Canva https://www.canva.com/)

physiological and reproductive processes, through the regulation of the expression of steroidogenic genes. In this regard, recent studies have demonstrated the presence and expression of the estrogen-related receptor (ERRrm) gene in ovarian tissue, embryonic cells, and hemolymph of *R. microplus*. Additionally, the in silico analysis demonstrated that the ERRrm presents a molecular coupling to natural estrogens, estrone (E1), estradiol (E2), and estriol (E3), to estrogenic antagonists, tamoxifen, 4-hydrotamoxifen, and the endocrine disruptor bisphenol A (BPA) (Aguilar-Díaz et al. 2023). On the other hand, there is a wide variety of membrane receptors capable of binding to the steroid hormone progesterone (P4). Among the main receptors of this type are mPRα, mPRβ, and mPRγ, as well as those of the MAPR family, such as the membrane component associated with the progesterone receptor (PGRMC), a receptor associated with the cell surface capable of binding P4 (Kimura et al. 2012; Mifsud and Bateman 2002). Analysis in various tissues of *R. microplus* demonstrated the expression of the membrane-associated progesterone receptor (RmMAPRC) and the molecular coupling with different derivative estrogenic components, including P4, desogestrel, medroxyprogesterone, mifepristone, even a P4 antagonist.

## 10.5 Immunoendocrine Network

Various studies have proposed that biological regulation mechanisms are associated with systemic networks that contribute to maintaining the organism's homeostasis. Likewise, parasitic infections have a direct relationship between the immune and endocrine systems and the eventual elimination or establishment of the pathogen in the host, as well as the role of estrogens in regulating Th1 and Th2 immune responses has been demonstrated during an infection. On the other hand, it has been determined, based on sexual dimorphism, that males have greater susceptibility to parasitic infections than females, placing T4 as a hormone associated with host immunosuppression. These findings suggest a strong relationship between the immune system and the endocrine system, considering it a macrosystem or immunoendocrine network that works in a coordinated manner. This network is regulated by immune molecules such as interleukins, chemokines, and cytokines, as well as endocrine components such as steroids and metabolic and sexual hormones. Together, these molecules are responsible for bidirectional regulation in both systems (Fig. 10.4).

## 10.6 Omics Approaches in the Study of Pathogens

Omics approaches, such as metagenomics, transcriptomics, proteomics, and metabolomics, offer a powerful tool for *R. microplus* control. These techniques allow a comprehensive exploration of the tick microbiome and its interactions with the host and pathogens, providing critical information on the microbial diversity, gene expression, proteins, and metabolites involved, which can contribute to the

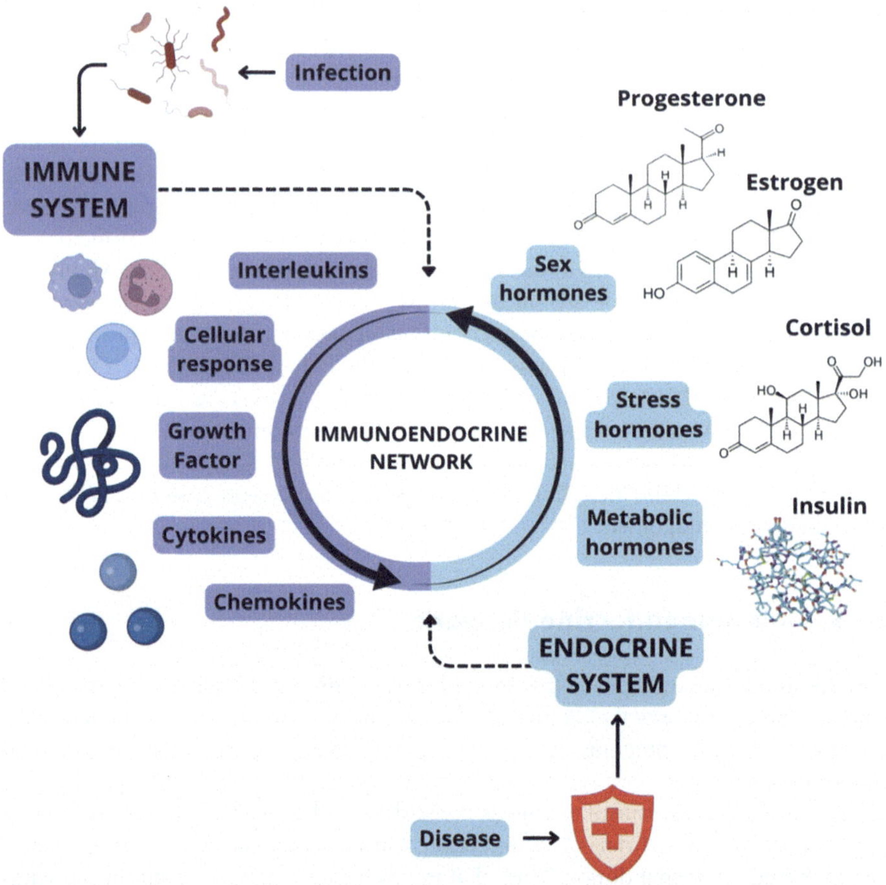


**Fig. 10.4** Immunoendocrine network. Diverse molecules associated with immune response and endocrine regulation are shown bidirectionally in response to an infection or disease development. (Fig. created in Canva https://www.canva.com/)

development of more specific and effective control strategies, including the identification of therapeutic targets, the design of vaccines, and the optimization of acaricidal treatments. In this regard, metagenomic studies and metatranscriptomics have allowed the characterization of different strains of pathogens and the microbiota associated with their hosts, including some arthropod vectors (Greay et al. 2018). Likewise, metaproteomics and metabolomics have emerged as powerful tools in investigating the biological processes involved in the interactions between host, vector, pathogen, and microbiome (Fig. 10.5) (Lou et al. 2017).

In the case of ticks, integrative approaches to metagenomic studies have provided a detailed characterization of the *Ixodes ricinus* microbiota, identifying more than 100 taxa of commensal bacteria, endosymbionts, and pathogens (Hernández-Jarguín et al. 2018). Furthermore, using microarrays and RNAseq technology has

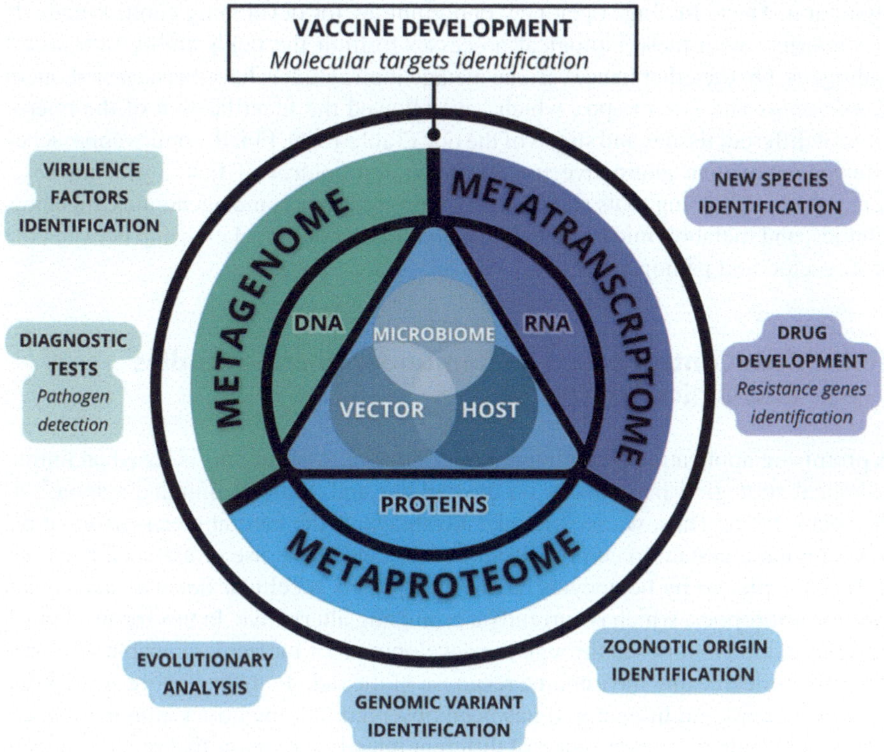


**Fig. 10.5** Omics approaches in the study of pathogens of medical-veterinary importance. The vision of understanding the metagenome, metatranscriptome, and metaproteome allows us to have a scenario of options for the development of vaccines and other analyses. (Fig. created in Canva https://www.canva.com/)

allowed us to examine the expression patterns of the microbiome in ticks, evaluating its variability under various conditions (Rodriguez-Valle et al. 2018). On the other hand, recent progress in genomics, transcriptomics, and proteomics has allowed the exploration of new approaches in the endocrine and molecular interactions between the host-vector-pathogen triad (Aguilar-Díaz et al. 2023). In this context, the analysis of the ganglionic transcriptome of *Ixodes scapularis* has shown the presence of numerous neuropeptides, hormonal receptors, and steroidogenesis regulatory proteins (Egekwu et al. 2014). Additionally, the use of metagenomics based on the 16S rRNA gene has generated new knowledge about pathogens associated with ticks, contributing to the detection of bacteria such as *Ralstonia*, *staphylococci* and *Francisella* spp. in the ticks *R. microplus*, *Hyalomma anatolicum*, and *Haemaphysalis montgomery*. Therefore, these analyses demonstrate the wide biodiversity in these ectoparasites and their relationship with the pathogens they transmit (Aguilar-Díaz et al. 2021b; Karim et al. 2017). Transcriptomic studies of different organs of *R. microplus* have revealed expression patterns that suggest the involvement of hormones and neuropeptides in crucial processes such as molting and hormonal regulation. These findings open new opportunities for developing control methods that interfere with these biological processes to limit the tick's ability to transmit pathogens. On the other hand, various metagenomic studies have been carried out in *R. microplus* and *Ixodes* spp., which have allowed the identification of the microbiota of different tissues and stages of the tick (Table 10.1). Finally, omics approaches offer an innovative alternative for the integrated control of ticks by using next-generation sequencing tools and omics techniques, such as metagenomics, metaproteomics, and metabolomics, allowing the elucidation of the relationship between the host, vector, and pathogen.

## 10.7 Tick Control Based on Immunoendocrine Studies and Omics Approaches

A promising application in the integrated control of *R. microplus* is based on immunological strategies, particularly on the cellular and humoral immune response of the vector itself. Thus, we seek to take advantage of the natural mechanisms of the tick's immune system to combat its spread. Recently, the use of extracellular traps (ETosis) mediated by hemocytes has been explored, a cellular defense mechanism in some arthropods, which is currently a promising alternative. In this regard, immunosuppression is proposed through the development of molecules capable of blocking ETosis, decreasing the immune response of the tick, to make it more susceptible to its pathogens. Additionally, it has been observed that the host's immune mechanisms can result in the expression of different intestinal proteins that modify the tick microbiome's composition, affecting biofilms' formation. This strategy has been proposed as a microbial defense mechanism that protects the tick against the host's

**Table 10.1** Omics approaches in ticks

| Tick | Approach | Reference |
|---|---|---|
| *R. microplus* | Metagenomics of the microbiome in male and female adults | Rojas-Jaimes et al. (2021) |
| *R. microplus* | Hemolymph proteomics | Aguilar-Díaz et al. (2018) |
| *Ixodes ricinus* | Metatranscriptomics and metaproteomics of salivary glands and internal tissue | Hernández-Jarguín et al. (2018) |
| *Ixodes holocyclus* | Transcriptomics in microbiome expression patterns | Rodriguez-Valle et al. (2018) |
| *Dermacentor nuttalli* and *Ixodes persulcatus* | Metagenomics in the identification of pathogens in livestock | Jiao et al. (2021) |
| *Ixodes ovatus*, *Ixodes persulcatus*, *Amblyomma variegatum* | Metagenomics of the microbiota in male and female adults | Obregón et al. (2019) |
| *R. microplus*, *Hyalomma anatolicum*, *Haemaphysalis montgomery* | Metagenomics determines microbiome and pathobionts diversity | Karim et al. (2017) |

immune response (Estrada-Peña et al. 2020). The strategies are based on treatment with different antibiotics that alter the microbial composition within the tick, resulting in increased sensitivity against the immune mechanisms of the bovine, thus reducing the population density, including the diseases it transmits.

On the other hand, some of the data reported suggest that parasites take advantage of the endocrine mechanisms developed by the host for their benefit through trans-regulation mechanism (Escobedo et al. 2005). This mechanism suggests that the parasite can synthesize molecules and receptors like those of the host to maximize the benefit that it obtains from the host. Therefore, in the search for innovative solutions for an integrated control of *R. microplus,* it is necessary to consider the trans-regulation mechanism. Whereby the tick directly or indirectly uses the hormones or growth factors of the host to facilitate its establishment and an increase in growth and reproduction rates, thus ensuring the availability of nutrients necessary for its development (Escobedo et al. 2005). In this context, identifying and characterizing steroid hormone receptors in embryonic cells and ovarian tissue of the tick represents a promising strategy. Some potential nuclear receptors include r-AR, r-prl, ERRrm, and the membrane receptor RmMAPRC. This variety of receptors could provide potential intervention points for developing more effective control strategies. For example, vaccines based on the peptide sequences of r-AR, r-prl and ERRrm that induce the production of antibodies that neutralize the functions of these receptors, affecting the development and reproduction of ticks. Additionally, the use of hormonal antagonists has been proposed, such as tamoxifen and diethylstilbestrol, compounds that couple with ERRrm, preventing binding with its ligand and blocking the hormonal signaling necessary for the reproductive functions and development of the pathogen. Another strategy is based on in silico studies, which, combined with experimental validation, open the possibility to design new compounds for coupling to the hormone receptors of *R. microplus*, inhibiting the interaction with their ligands.

## 10.8 Concluding Remarks

The economic impact generated by *R. microplus* in the livestock industry is considerable and multifaceted. In addition to the significant decrease in livestock products due to skin lesions and anemia in livestock, infestation by *R. microplus* can cause the death of the animal due to the pathogens it transmits (Estrada-Peña et al. 2013). Likewise, the economic impacts are exacerbated by the high costs associated with control based on chemical acaricides. However, the excessive use of these compounds has resulted in the development of resistant populations, and the additional environmental impact (Rodríguez-Vivas et al. 2012). Given this scenario, the need to explore new alternatives and more sustainable approaches for controlling *R. microplus* becomes evident. So, studying the immunoendocrine system is a promising and sustainable strategy. This approach includes understanding and manipulating the interactions between the different actors: the tick as a vector, the pathogens it transmits, the host, and even the associated microbiota. In this regard, tick immunosuppression and endocrine regulation based on a trans-regulation mechanism are viable alternatives in the search for new control targets. Additionally, the strategies based on immune mechanisms that reduce the ability of ticks to defend themselves against their natural enemies have been proposed. Also, from an endocrine approach, the development of vaccines is proposed to generate an immune response against specific hormonal receptors of ticks to interfere with the hormonal signaling necessary for the development and reproduction of ticks.

Additionally, novel approaches propose the manipulation of the tick microbiota to reduce its vector capacity (anti-microbiota vaccines). Other strategies, like omics approaches offer an innovative perspective for the control of *R. microplus*. These approaches allow for characterizing the microbiome, revealing the bacterial diversity of ticks, and identifying potential associated pathogens, as well as the elucidation of the genetic mechanisms involved in the interaction with the host. Finally, it is crucial to consider that combining immunological, endocrine and omics approaches offer a wide range of potential strategies for controlling *R. microplus* in the livestock industry. These strategies can potentially reduce the pest damage to public health and increase the economic impact while promoting more sustainable and environmentally friendly control practices.

**Acknowledgments** This research was funded by INIFAP Fondos Fiscales 2023, grant number 13232936047.

## References

Aguilar-Díaz H, Cossío-Bayúgar R (2018) Immune system and its relationships with pathogens: structure, physiology, and molecular biology. In: Farm animals diseases, recent omic trends and new strategies of treatment, p 21

Aguilar-Díaz H, Esquivel-Velázquez M, Quiroz-Castañeda RE, Miranda-Miranda E, Conde-Baeye RJP, Cobaxín-Cárdenas M, Ostoa-Saloma P, Cossío-Bayúgar R (2018) Comparative hemolymph proteomic and enzymatic analyses of two strains of *Rhipicephalus (Boophilus) microplus* ticks resistant and susceptible to Ixodicides. Biomed Res Int 2018:1. https://doi.org/10.1155/2018/9451547

Aguilar-Díaz H, Quiroz-Castañeda RE, Cobaxin-Cárdenas M, Salinas-Estrella E, Amaro-Estrada I (2021a) Advances in the study of the tick cattle microbiota and the influence on vectorial capacity. Front Vet Sci 8:710352. https://doi.org/10.3389/fvets.2021.710352

Aguilar-Díaz H, Quiroz-Castañeda RE, Salazar-Morales K, Cossío-Bayúgar R, Miranda-Miranda E (2021b) Tick immunobiology and extracellular traps: an integrative vision to control of vectors. Pathogens 10(11):1511. https://doi.org/10.3390/pathogens10111511

Aguilar-Díaz H, Quiroz-Castañeda RE, Díaz-Esquivel IG, Cossío-Bayúgar R, Miranda-Miranda E (2023) A novel *Rhipicephalus microplus* estrogen related receptor (*RmERR*), a molecular and *in silico* characterization of a potential protein binding estrogen. Microorganisms 11(9):2294. https://doi.org/10.3390/microorganisms11092294

Alvarado-Delgado A, Martínez-Barnetche J, Téllez-Sosa J, Rodríguez MH, Gutiérrez-Millán E, Zumaya-Estrada FA, Saldaña-Navor V, Rodríguez MC, Tello-López A, Lanz-Mendoza H (2021) Prediction of neuropeptide precursors and differential expression of adipokinetic hormone/corazonin-related peptide, hugin and corazonin in the brain of malaria vector *Nyssorhynchus albimanus* during a *Plasmodium berghei* infection. Curr Res Insect Sci 1:100014. https://doi.org/10.1016/j.cris.2021.100014

Antón-Marín Y (2009) El sistema inmune de los invertebrados-The immune system of the invertebrates. REDVET Rev Electrón Vet 10(9):467–481
Ayres KL (2019) Endocrinology and behavior: methods. In: Encyclopedia of animal behavior, vol 3, 2nd edn, pp 1–5. https://doi.org/10.1016/B978-0-12-809633-8.90087-6
Brayton KA (2012) Transmisión de *Anaplasma marginale* por garrapatas. Revista Mexicana de Ciencias Pecuarias 3:41–50
Canesi L, Ciacci C, Betti M, Lorusso LC, Marchi B, Burattini S, Falcieri E, Gallo G (2004) Rapid effects of 17β-estradiol on cell signaling and function of *Mytilus hemocytes*. Gen Comp Endocrinol 136(1):58. https://doi.org/10.1016/j.ygcen.2003.12.003
Chevillon C, de Garine-Wichatitsky M, Barré N, Ducornez S, de Meeûs T (2013) Understanding the genetic, demographical and/or ecological processes at play in invasions: lessons from the southern cattle tick *Rhipicephalus microplus* (Acari: Ixodidae). Exp Appl Acarol 59(1–2):203. https://doi.org/10.1007/s10493-012-9602-5
Egekwu N, Sonenshine DE, Bissinger BW, Michael Roe R (2014) Transcriptome of the female synganglion of the black-legged tick *Ixodes scapularis* (Acari: Ixodidae) with comparison between Illumina and 454 systems. PLoS One 9(7):e102667. https://doi.org/10.1371/journal.pone.0102667
Escobedo G, Roberts CW, Carrero JC, Morales-Montor J (2005) Parasite regulation by host hormones: an old mechanism of host exploitation? Trends Parasitol 21(12):588–593
Estrada-Peña A (1999) Geostatistics and remote sensing using NOAA-AVHRR satellite imagery as predictive tools in tick distribution and habitat suitability estimations for *Boophilus microplus* (Acari: Ixodidae) in South America. Vet Parasitol 81(1):73. https://doi.org/10.1016/S0304-4017(98)00238-6
Estrada-Peña A (2001) Climate warming and changes in habitat suitability for *Boophilus microplus* (Acari: Ixodidae) in Central America. J Parasitol 87(5):978. https://doi.org/10.2307/3285219
Estrada-Peña A, de la Fuente J (2014) The ecology of ticks and epidemiology of tick-borne viral diseases. Antiviral Res 108:104–128
Estrada-Peña A, Sánchez Acedo C, Quílez J, Del Cacho E (2005) A retrospective study of climatic suitability for the tick *Rhipicephalus (Boophilus) microplus* in the Americas. Glob Ecol Biogeogr 14(6):565. https://doi.org/10.1111/j.1466-822X.2005.00185.x
Estrada-Peña A, Gray JS, Kahl O, Lane RS, Nijhof AM (2013) Research on the ecology of ticks and tick-borne pathogens-methodological principles and caveats. Front Cell Infect Microbiol 3:29. https://doi.org/10.3389/fcimb.2013.00029
Estrada-Peña A, Cabezas-Cruz A, Obregón D (2020) Resistance of tick gut microbiome to anti-tick vaccines, pathogen infection and antimicrobial peptides. Pathogens 9(4). https://doi.org/10.3390/pathogens9040309
Falkenstein E, Tillmann HC, Christ M, Feuring M, Wehling M (2000) Multiple actions of steroid hormones—a focus on rapid, nongenomic effects. In. Pharmacol Rev 52(4):513
FAO (2004) Management and integrated parasite control in ruminants guidelines, module 1. Ticks: Acaricide resistance: diagnosis, management and prevention, food and agriculture organization. In: Animal production and health division. FAO, Rome
Greay TL, Gofton AW, Paparini A, Ryan UM, Oskam CL, Irwin PJ (2018) Recent insights into the tick microbiome gained through next-generation sequencing. Parasit Vectors 11(1):12. https://doi.org/10.1186/s13071-017-2550-5
Hernández-Jarguín A, Díaz-Sánchez S, Villar M, De La Fuente J (2018) Integrated metatranscriptomics and metaproteomics for the characterization of bacterial microbiota in unfed *Ixodes ricinus*. Ticks Tick Borne Dis 9(5):1241–1251. https://doi.org/10.1016/j.ttbdis.2018.04.020
Jiao J, Lu Z, Yu Y, Ou Y, Fu M, Zhao Y, Wu N, Zhao M, Liu Y, Sun Y, Wen B, Zhou D, Yuan Q, Xiong X (2021) Identification of tick-borne pathogens by metagenomic next-generation sequencing in *Dermacentor nuttalli* and *Ixodes persulcatus* in Inner Mongolia, China. Parasit Vectors 14(1):287. https://doi.org/10.1186/s13071-021-04740-3
Karim S, Budachetri K, Mukherjee N, Williams J, Kausar A, Hassan MJ, Adamson S, Dowd SE, Apanskevich D, Arijo A, Sindhu ZU, Kakar MA, Khan RMD, Ullah S, Sajid MS, Ali A, Iqbal

Z (2017) A study of ticks and tick-borne livestock pathogens in Pakistan. PLoS Negl Trop Dis 11(6):e0005681. https://doi.org/10.1371/journal.pntd.0005681

Kimura I, Nakayama Y, Konishi M, Terasawa K, Ohta M, Itoh N, Fujimoto M (2012) Functions of MAPR (membrane-associated progesterone receptor) family members as Heme/steroid-binding proteins. Curr Protein Pept Sci 13(7):687. https://doi.org/10.2174/138920312804142110

Knigge T, LeBlanc GA, Ford AT (2021) A crab is not a fish: unique aspects of the crustacean endocrine system and considerations for endocrine toxicology. Front Endocrinol 12:587608. https://doi.org/10.3389/fendo.2021.587608

Leblebicioglu B, Connors J, Mariotti A (2013) Principles of endocrinology. Periodontol 2000 61(1):54. https://doi.org/10.1111/j.1600-0757.2011.00440.x

Lew-Tabor AE, Valle MR (2016) A review of reverse vaccinology approaches for the development of vaccines against ticks and tick borne diseases. Ticks Tick Borne Dis 7(4):573–585

Li Q, Osada M, Suzuki T, Mori K (1998) Changes in vitellin during oogenesis and effect of estradiol-17β on vitellogenesis in the pacific oyster *Crassostrea gigas*. Invertebr Reprod Dev 33(1):87. https://doi.org/10.1080/07924259.1998.9652345

Lösel R, Wehling M (2003) Nongenomic actions of steroid hormones. Nat Rev Mol Cell Biol 4(1):46–55

Lou Y, Liu L, Gao D (2017) Modeling co-infection of *Ixodes* tick-borne pathogens. Math Biosci Eng 14(5–6):1301–1316. https://doi.org/10.3934/mbe.2017067

Lu X, Zhang Z, Yuan D, Zhou Y, Cao J, Zhang H, da Silva Vaz I, Zhou J (2021) The ecdysteroid receptor regulates salivary gland degeneration through apoptosis in *Rhipicephalus haemaphysaloides*. Parasit Vectors 14(1):612. https://doi.org/10.1186/s13071-021-05052-2

Marín YA, Salazar-Lugo R (2009) El sistema inmune de los invertebrados. REDVET Rev Electrón Vet 10(9)

Mifsud W, Bateman A (2002) Membrane-bound progesterone receptors contain a cytochrome b5-like ligand-binding domain. Genome Biol 3(12):RESEARCH0068. https://doi.org/10.1186/gb-2002-3-12-research0068

Minard G, Tran FH, Van VT, Goubert C, Bellet C, Lambert G, Kim KLH, Thuy THT, Mavingui P, Valiente Moro C (2015) French invasive Asian tiger mosquito populations harbor reduced bacterial microbiota and genetic diversity compared to Vietnamese autochthonous relatives. Front Microbiol 6(SEP):970. https://doi.org/10.3389/fmicb.2015.00970

Obregón D, Bard E, Abrial D, Estrada-Peña A, Cabezas-Cruz A (2019) Sex-specific linkages between taxonomic and functional profiles of tick gut microbiomes. Front Cell Infect Microbiol 9:298. https://doi.org/10.3389/fcimb.2019.00298

Pérez-Rivero JJ, Aguilar-Setién Á, Villa-Godoy A, Serrano H (2005) Relación entre estructura y función de receptores para hormonas esteroidales: Receptores estrogénicos. Vet Méx 36(4):437–452

Ponce-Rivas E, Camacho-Jiménez L, Diaz F, Sánchez-Castrejón E, Montiel-Arzate A (2021) Dose-dependent effect of recombinant CHH-B1 on osmoregulatory capacity and $Na^+/K^+$-ATPase expression in bilaterally eyestalk-ablated shrimp *Litopenaeus vannamei*. Biotecnia 23(3). https://doi.org/10.18633/biotecnia.v23i3.1441

Ponnusamy L, Sutton H, Mitchell RD, Sonenshine DE, Apperson CS, Roe RM (2021) Tick ecdysteroid hormone, global microbiota/rickettsia signaling in the ovary versus carcass during vitellogenesis in part-fed (virgin) american dog ticks, *Dermacentor variabilis*. Microorganisms 9(6):1242. https://doi.org/10.3390/microorganisms9061242

Rodriguez-Valle M, Moolhuijzen P, Barrero RA, Ong CT, Busch G, Karbanowicz T, Booth M, Clark R, Koehbach J, Ijaz H, Broady K, Agnew K, Knowles AG, Bellgard MI, Tabor AE (2018) Transcriptome and toxin family analysis of the paralysis tick, *Ixodes holocyclus*. Int J Parasitol 48(1):71–82. https://doi.org/10.1016/j.ijpara.2017.07.007

Rodriguez-Vivas RI, Jonsson NN, Bhushan C (2018) Strategies for the control of *Rhipicephalus microplus* ticks in a world of conventional acaricide and macrocyclic lactone resistance. Parasitology research, 117: 3–29. https://doi.org/10.1007/s00436-017-5677-6

Rodríguez-Vivas IR, Hodgkinson JE, Trees AJ (2012) Resistencia a los acaricidas en *Rhipicephalus (Boophilus) microplus*: situación actual y mecanismos de resistencia. Revista Mexicana De Ciencias Pecuarias 3(SUPPL. 1)

Rodríguez-Vivas RI, Grisi L, De León AAP, Villela HS, De Jesús Torres-Acostaa JF, Sánchez HF, Salas DR, Cruz RR, Saldierna F, Carrasco DG (2017) Potential economic impact assessment for cattle parasites in Mexico. Review. Revista Mexicana De Ciencias Pecuarias 8(1):61. https://doi.org/10.22319/rmcp.v8i1.4305

Roe RM, Donohue KV, Khalil SMS, Sonenshine DE (2008) Hormonal regulation of metamorphosis and reproduction in ticks. Front Biosci 13(18):7250. https://doi.org/10.2741/3226

Rojas-Jaimes J, Lindo-Seminario D, Correa-Núñez G, Diringer B (2021) Characterization of the bacterial microbiome of *Rhipicephalus (Boophilus) microplus* collected from *Pecari tajacu* "Sajino" Madre de Dios, Peru. Sci Rep 11(1):6661. https://doi.org/10.1038/s41598-021-86177-3

Schooley DA, Horodyski FM, Coast GM (2012) Hormones controlling homeostasis in insects. In: Insect endocrinology. Elsevier, Amsterdam, pp 366–429

Strand MR (2008) The insect cellular immune response. Insect Sci 15(1):1–14

Ulvedal C, Bertolotti MA, Cagnolo SR, Almirón WR (2017) Ensayos de sensibilidad de larvas de *Aedes aegypti* y *Culex quinquefasciatus* frente al nematodo *Heterorhabditis bacteriophora* en condiciones de laboratorio. Biomedica 37:67–76

# Exploring the Potential of Plant Extracts as Novel Bioacaricides

# 11

Nosheen Malak, Sadaf Niaz, Bader S. Alotaibi, Shakir Ullah, Afshan Khan, Imtiaz Ahmad, and Adil Khan

**Abstract**

In tropical and subtropical regions of the world, ticks and mites are among the most common and successful pests that cause considerable economic losses. Bioacaricides are effective botanical extracts that provide natural and safe substitutes for synthetic pesticides for pest control because the chemicals present in the plant drastically affect pest physiology without affecting nontarget organisms or the environment. An innovative approach to enhancing the precision and effectiveness of bioacaricides is to merge nanotechnology with plant extracts and their bioactive constituents. Nanotechnology-based platforms enable the encapsulation and regulated release of various chemicals at the desired site of action, resulting in improved stability and sustained effectiveness and decreased dispersion of these chemicals in the environment. In this chapter, we reviewed some of the interesting studies that have used nanotechnology-associated bioacaricides for pest management and control.

**Keywords**

Ticks · Mites · Bioacaricides · Plant extracts · Nanoparticles

N. Malak · S. Niaz · S. Ullah · A. Khan
Department of Zoology, Abdul Wali Khan University Mardan, Mardan, Pakistan

B. S. Alotaibi
Department of Clinical Laboratory Sciences, College of Applied Medical Sciences, Al-Quwayiyah, Shaqra University, Riyadh, Saudi Arabia

I. Ahmad · A. Khan (✉)
Department of Botany and Zoology, Bacha Khan University, Charsadda, Pakistan
e-mail: dradilkhan@bkuc.edu.pk


S. Kumar et al. (eds.), *Acaricides Resistance in Ticks*,
https://doi.org/10.1007/978-981-97-7411-1_11

## 11.1 Introduction

In the contemporary landscape of livestock production, the imperative contributions of animals to the global economy and food security are universally acknowledged. Central to the productivity of animals is their ability to maintain optimal health conditions. However, the multifaceted challenges in livestock production include various factors, with infestations by both endo- and ectoparasites emerging as significant impediments to animal health and performance (Jadhao et al. 2022). Ticks are ranked second as the most successful pest after mosquitoes, and they act as vectors of numerous infectious diseases for both human and animal populations globally (Singh and Rath 2013). Infestation by ticks induces physiological stresses in animals, leading to anemia, immunosuppression and consequential impacts on behavior, productivity, and overall welfare (Hurtado and Giraldo-Ríos 2018). Among livestock, cattle are susceptible to various tick-borne protozoan diseases, such as babesiosis, theileriosis, anaplasmosis, and heart water disease, further exacerbating this challenge (Ghosh et al. 2007). Although the host mortality rates that are directly attributed to tick infestations are relatively low, the economic repercussions stemming from reduced growth rates and productivity losses are substantial, especially for small-scale dairy farmers (Marcelino et al. 2012). Globally, ticks are recognized as one of the most economically detrimental pests in livestock management, with more than 931 species identified (Nava et al. 2017). Economic losses incurred due to tick infestations include decreased weight gain; diminished production yields of meat, milk, fur, and skin; and decreased expenses associated with control measures (Rodriguez-Vivas et al. 2018). For decades, synthetic acaricides have been considered the traditional and most successful approach for controlling ticks (De Meneghi et al. 2016; Higa et al. 2019). Among the conventional acaricides that are frequently used for this purpose are pyrethroids, carbamates, organophosphates, formamidine, neonicotinoids, phenylpyrazolebenzoylphenyl ureas (BPUs) and macrocyclic lactones (MLs) (De Meneghi et al. 2016; Rajput et al. 2006; Sharma et al. 2018). The excessive use of these chemicals, especially above the recommended doses, has been linked to resistance development among pests, and their residues are found in treated livestock's milk and meat (De Meneghi et al. 2016). The quest for a more effective, environmentally acceptable, and tick-host friendly substitute has been prompted by the drawbacks of these synthetic acaricides. The use of botanicals has recently attracted much interest as a potentially effective tick control strategy, and they have significant economic and welfare implications (Kiss et al. 2012).

A diverse array of mite species, numbering more than 10, is known to affect both human and animal health. Among them, notable varieties include *Psoroptes cuniculi* (*P. cuniculi*), *Sarcoptes scabiei* (*S. scabiei*), *Dermanyssus gallinae* (*D. gallinae*), and *Demodex* mites. *Dermanyssus gallinae*, commonly known as the chicken mite, inflicts significant challenges to poultry farms worldwide. Its presence leads to diminished food intake, compromised immune responses and mortality among chickens in severe cases (Kim et al. 2018). Additionally, *D. gallinae* infestations are correlated with decreased egg production and reduced egg weight (Sleeckx et al.

2019). The ability of mites to spread several illnesses, such as pullorum disease, Newcastle disease virus, poultry spirochetosis, and poultry plague, further compounds this threat, resulting in substantial economic losses and animal health concerns within the poultry industry (Sparagano 2020; Valiente Moro et al. 2009). *Psoroptes cuniculi*, which targets the auditory canal outside the body of rabbits, poses a significant threat to the rabbit farming industry due to its rapid transmission and spread, and effective control measures are needed to mitigate its adverse effects (Ma et al. 2019). *Sarcopetes scabiei*, which causes sarcoptic mange, a highly contagious skin disease in humans and various mammals, manifests as severe itching, baldness, hyperkeratosis, inflammation, and irritation (Bernigaud et al. 2020; Richards 2021). Global prevalence estimates suggest a considerable burden of scabies annually (Karimkhani et al. 2017). *Sarcoptic* infestations substantially impact animal health and production, resulting in decreased growth rates, decreased feed efficiency, and weakened immune systems, increasing moral and financial issues (Li et al. 2023). *Demodex* mites, long-standing commensal ectoparasites of various mammalian species, including humans, have been associated with ocular manifestations and inflammatory conditions (Fromstein et al. 2018; Lee et al. 2022; Palopoli et al. 2015). Mite control traditionally relies on synthetic acaricides, but concerns about resistance development and chemical residues have underscored the necessity of using different tactics (Baran et al. 2020). Varying degrees of acaricide resistance have been observed in populations of *D. gallinae*, emphasizing the necessity of exploring alternative control measures (Lee et al. 2017). Acaricide resistance can originate from target site mutations or from the overexpression of genes encoding detoxifying enzymes (Al Khoury et al. 2020). Concerns have been raised about the presence of ivermectin residues in animal milk, which is a potential risk to human consumers (Romero et al. 2016).

The pursuit of novel bioactive agents with efficacy, selectivity, and safety has led to growing interest in natural products for acaricide development (Zhu et al. 2020). With their potential for ecological compatibility and effectiveness, botanicals have emerged as promising alternatives for tick and mite control (Adenubi et al. 2016; Benelli and Pavela 2018; Benelli et al. 2016; Pavela 2016). In this chapter, we present a comprehensive update on the present knowledge and utilization status of botanical acaricides and repellents for managing ticks and mites predominantly affecting production animals. Our focus is on exploring the current landscape of botanicals for tick and mite control, along with addressing the associated challenges and prospects for future advancements in this field. Our goal is to provide insightful information for the advancement of innovative integrated parasite control strategies.

### 11.1.1 Contemporary Overview

Plants produce secondary metabolites to guard against pests and diseases, and many of these substances also possess antioxidative, fungicidal, and bactericidal properties (Cowan 1999; Dubey 2011; Scartezzini and Speroni 2000). These substances have been utilized historically for pest control, such as the application of finely powdered chrysanthemum flowers to repel fleas and lice (Benelli et al. 2015a, b; Karunamoorthi et al. 2009). Pyrethrins and nicotine from plants serve as models for synthetic pesticides (El-Wakeil 2013). Currently, extracts from certain plant species are incorporated into commercial botanical pesticides or products for agricultural and veterinary use, including tick control (Benelli 2016; Benelli et al. 2015a, b; Davidović et al. 2011; El-Wakeil 2013; Isman 2006; Isman 2015; Marchand 2015). Despite the limited use of plant species for botanical pesticides, plant substances hold promise for the creation of novel plant insecticides intended for commercial use (Dubey 2011; Isman 2015).

Globally, a significant number of plant species, exceeding 200, are recognized for their tick-repellent or acaricidal properties (Adenubi et al. 2016). The majority of these species belong to the Lamiaceae family, which is renowned for hosting a diverse array of antiparasitic secondary metabolites that are frequently explored in ethnomedicinal studies (Wink 2012). Leaves have emerged as the most utilized plant part for extraction, owing to their rich content of bioactive constituents crucial for photosynthesis, coupled with the minimal impact on the plant's life cycle upon collection (Alamgeer et al. 2018; Tangjitman et al. 2015). The main plant-based compounds evaluated in tick tests are essential oils, extracts, or pure allelochemicals. Many extraction techniques, including hydrodistillation and steam distillation (Gomes et al. 2012), spilanthol and methanolic extraction (Cruz et al. 2016), ethanolic and aqueous extraction (Costa-Júnior et al. 2016), and hexane, ethyl, and acetate extractions (Souza Conceição et al. 2017), have been employed to obtain these bioactive substances. Numerous studies have demonstrated that secondary plant metabolites are harmful to a variety of arthropod species, including mites, and have repellent, antiovipositional, antifeedant, and growth-inhibiting properties (Benelli et al. 2015a, b; Martinez-Velazquez et al. 2011; Pavela 2016; Pavela and Herda 2007; Pavela et al. 2014; Regnault-Roger et al. 2012; Santos and Vogel 2012).

The most employed tick species for assessing the acaricidal and repellent properties of botanicals is *Rhipicephalus microplus*, primarily because of its notable influence on the bovine industry and tolerance to a wide range of acaricides (Coles and Dryden 2014; Malak et al. 2022). Most of the related research has focused predominantly on females, particularly engorged or semiengorged individuals, owing to their pivotal role in tick management attributed to their reproductive potential (fecundity) (Sarli et al. 2023). Diverse extracts derived from various plant parts dissolved in different solvents have been evaluated for their acaricidal activity against different mite species. For instance, crude extracts of *Onobrychis ptolemaica* (Shahatha 2020), *Annona squamosa* (Roy et al. 2005), *Vitex negundo* (Khan et al. 2012), *Tecomella undulata* (Khan et al. 2013), *Ligularia virgaurea* (Luo et al. 2015), and *Acalypha indica* (Astuti et al. 2019) have been examined for their effects on various mite species.

## 11.2 Acaricidal and Repellent Effects on Ticks

Several extracts and essential oils from plants have been tested for their ability to kill ticks (Table 11.1, Fig. 11.1). Among the methods used for assessing efficacy, the adult immersion test (AIT) is widely used in the evaluation of the efficacy of botanical acaricides against adult ticks (Adenubi et al. 2016; Ravindran et al. 2011). Here, we focused on AIT predominantly in female *R. microplus* ticks due to their reproductive potential. For instance, immersion of *R. microplus* females for 2 min in *Piper nigrum* methanolic extracts at 1.1% wt/vol (11 mg/mL) resulted in a mortality rate of 95.8% ($LC_{50}$ = 0.48% wt/vol), and a 96.9% reduction in oviposition 14 days postimmersion. However, *Piper longum* methanolic extracts need a 5% weight/volume concentration (50 mg/mL) to reach a mortality of 87.5% ($LC_{50}$ = 2.13%), and oviposition decreases by 89.3% (Godara et al. 2018). Treating *R. microplus* with 100 mg/mL *C. cyminum* essential oils (EOs) for 5 min completely killed the engorged females and suppressed their reproductive system after 14 days of immersion (Villarreal et al. 2017). Furthermore, after immersion of *R. microplus* for 2 min in a mixture of 10% ethanol and 2% tween 20, which included an extract from the aerial portions of *Ageratum conyzoides*, 90.7% of the oviposition was inhibited, and deformed oocytes were observed after 14 days ($LC_{90}$ = 8.91% wt/vol) (Ajith Kumar et al. 2019). The average $LC_{50}$ values were 115.21, 161.02, and 61.82 mg/mL for adults of the tick *Rhipicephalus turanicus* when they were immersed in acetone

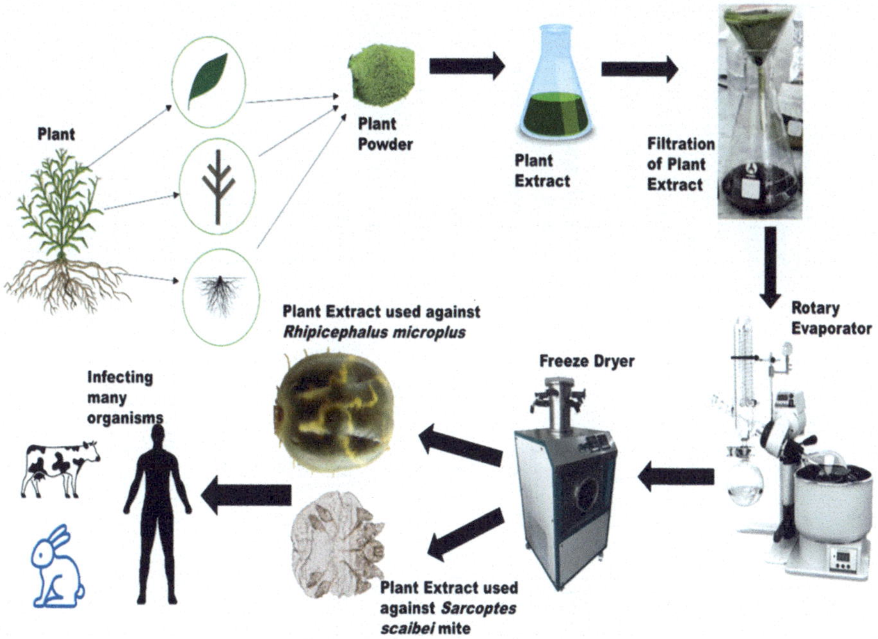


**Fig. 11.1** This paper provides an overview of the production of plant extracts and their application as acaricides against larval and adult ticks to prevent diseases in humans and animals

**Table 11.1** Various plant extracts used against different tick species in in vitro, in vivo, and in silico experiments

| Source plant | Family | Extract | Assessment mode | Targeted tick | Reference |
|---|---|---|---|---|---|
| *Tithonia diversifolia* | Asteraceae | Acetone and ethanol extracts | In vitro | *Rhipicephalus microplus* | (Aimée et al. 2017) |
| *Conyza dioscoridis* | Asteraceae | Essential oil | In vitro | *Ixodes Ricinus* | (El-Seedi et al. 2017) |
| *Artemisia herba-alba* | Asteraceae | Essential oil | In vitro | *Ixodes Ricinus* | (El-Seedi et al. 2017) |
| *Calendula officinalis* | Asteraceae | Essential oil | In vitro | *Ixodes Ricinus* | (El-Seedi et al. 2017) |
| *Piper longum* | Piperaceae | Alcoholic and aqueous extracts | In vitro | *Hyalomma anatolicum* | (Singh et al. 2017) |
| *Piper nigrum* | Piperaceae | Alcoholic and aqueous extracts | In vitro | *Hyalomma anatolicum* | (Singh et al. 2017) |
| *Zingiber officinale* | Zingiberaceae | Alcoholic and aqueous extracts | In vitro | *Hyalomma anatolicum* | (Singh et al. 2017) |
| *Allium sativum* | Amaryllidaceae | Ethanolic and aqueous extracts | In vitro | *Rhipicephalus decoloratus*<br>*Rhipicephalus microplus* | (Mgocheki 2017) |
| *Ocimum basilicum* | Lamiaceae | Ethanolic and aqueous extracts | In vitro | *Dermacentor reticulatus* | (Štefanidesová et al. 2017) |
| *Citrus bergamia* | Rutaceae | Essential oil | In vitro | *Dermacentor reticulatus* | (Štefanidesová et al. 2017) |
| *Syzygium aromaticum* | Myrtaceae | Essential oil | In vitro | *Dermacentor reticulatus* | (Štefanidesová et al. 2017) |
| *Cymbopogon winterianus* | Poaceae | Essential oil | In vitro | *Dermacentor reticulatus* | (Štefanidesová et al. 2017) |
| *Thymus serpyllum)* | Lamiaceae | Essential oil | In vitro | *Dermacentor reticulatus* | (Štefanidesová et al. 2017) |
| *Thymus vulgaris* | Lamiaceae | Essential oil | In vitro | *Dermacentor reticulatus* | (Štefanidesová et al. 2017) |

| Source plant | Family | Extract | Assessment mode | Targeted tick | Reference |
|---|---|---|---|---|---|
| *Menipemaceae* | Antizoma angustifolia | Ethanolic | In vitro | *Rhipicephalus microplus* *Rhipicephalus turanicus* | (Fouche et al. 2017) |
| *Calpurnia aurea* | Fabaceae | Acetone extract | In vitro | *Rhipicephalus turanicus* | (Fouche et al. 2017) |
| *Senna italica subsp. arachoides* | Fabaceae | Acetone extract | In vitro | *Rhipicephalus turanicus* | (Fouche et al. 2017) |
| *Schkuhria pinnata* | Asteraceae | Acetone extract | In vitro | *Rhipicephalus turanicus* | (Fouche et al. 2017) |
| *Ficus sycomorus* | Moraceae | Acetone extract | In vitro | *Rhipicephalus turanicus* | (Fouche et al. 2017) |
| *Monsonia angustifolia* | Sapindaceae | Ethanolic | In vitro | *Rhipicephalus turanicus* | (Fouche et al. 2017) |
| *Cleome gynandra* | | Ethanolic | In vitro | *Rhipicephalus turanicus* | (Fouche et al. 2017) |
| *Ageratum conyzoides L* | Asteraceae | Ethanolic | In vitro | *Rhipicephalus annulatus* | (Nair et al. 2017) |
| *A. olerace* | Brassicaceae | Ethanolic | In vitro | *Amblyomma cajennens* | (Anholeto et al. 2018) |
| *Jatropha curcas* | Euphorbiaceae | Ethanolic | In vitro | *Ripichephalus microplus* | (Anholeto et al. 2018) |
| *Anonna muricata* | Annonaceae | Ethanolic | In vitro | *Ripichephalus microplus* | (Anholeto et al. 2018) |
| *Aloe vera* | Asphodelaceae | Ethanolic | In vitro | *Ripichephalus microplus* | (Anholeto et al. 2018) |
| *Cissus quadrangularis* | Vitaceae | Ethanolic | In vitro | *Ripichephalus microplus* | (Anholeto et al. 2018) |
| *Maerua edulis* | Capparaceae | Ethanolic | In vitro | *Ripichephalus microplus* | (Anholeto et al. 2018) |
| *Ocotea aciphylla* | Lauraceae | Ethanolic | In vitro | *Ripichephalus microplus* | (Conceicao et al. 2017) |
| *Crescentia cujete* | Bignoniaceae | Ethanolic | In vitro | *Rhipicephalus microplus* | (Pereira et al. 2017) |
| *Callistemon viminalis* | Myrtaceae | Essential oil | In vitro | *Amblyomma variegatum* | (Kouam et al. 2017) |
| *Cupressus lusitanica* | | Essential oil | In vitro | *Amblyomma variegatum* | |
| *Morus nigra* | Moraceae | Methanolic extract | In vitro | *Rhipicephalus microplus* | (Dantas et al. 2017) |
| *Havardia albicans* | Fabaceae | Methanolic | In vitro | *Rhipicephalus microplus* | (Rosado-Aguilar et al. 2017) |
| *Caesalpinia gaumeri* | Fabaceae | Methanolic | In vitro | *Rhipicephalus microplus* | |

(continued)

**Table 11.1** (continued)

| Source plant | Family | Extract | Assessment mode | Targeted tick | Reference |
|---|---|---|---|---|---|
| *Ricinus communis* | Euphorbiaceae | Methanolic | In vitro | *Rhipicephalus microplus* | (Islam et al. 2018) |
| *Borago officinalis* | Boraginaceae | Ethanolic | In vitro | *Rhipicephalus sanguineus* | (El Haddad et al. 2018) |
| *Schinopsis brasiliensis* | Anacardiaceae | Methanolic and ethanolic extract | In vitro | *Dermacentor nitens* | (Vasconcelos et al. 2018) |
| *Piptadenia viridiflora* | Fabaceae | Methanolic and ethanolic extract | In vitro | *Dermacentor nitens* | |
| *Ximenia americana* | Olacaceae | Methanolic and ethanolic extract | In vitro | *Dermacentor nitens* | |
| *Serjania lethalis* | | Methanolic and ethanolic extract | In vitro | *Dermacentor nitens* | |
| *Piper longum* | Piperaceae | Methanolic and ethanolic extract | In vitro | *Rhipicephalus microplus* | (Godara et al. 2018) |
| *Piper nigrum* | Piperaceae | Methanolic and ethanolic extract | In vitro | *Rhipicephalus microplus* | |
| *Gallesia integrifolia Spren* | Phytolaccaceae | Ethanolic | In vitro | *Rhipicephalus microplus* | (Dias et al. 2018) |

| Source plant | Family | Extract | Assessment mode | Targeted tick | Reference |
|---|---|---|---|---|---|
| *Azadirachta indicae* | Meliaceae | Ethanolic | In vitro | *Amblyomma testudinarium*<br>*Dermacentor auratus*<br>*Haemaphysalis bispinosa* | (Adenubi et al. 2018a) |
| *Ynandropsis gynandra* | Cleomaceae | Ethanolic | In vitro | *Amblyomma testudinarium*<br>*Dermacentor auratus*<br>*Haemaphysalis bispinosa* | |
| *Avandula angustifolia* | Lamiaceae | Ethanolic | In vitro | *Amblyomma testudinarium*<br>*Dermacentor auratus*<br>*Haemaphysalis bispinosa* | |
| *Pelargonium roseum* | Geraniaceae | Ethanolic | In vitro | *Amblyomma testudinarium*<br>*Dermacentor auratus*<br>*Haemaphysalis bispinosa* | |
| *Cymbopogon* | Poaceae | Ethanolic | In vitro | *Amblyomma testudinarium*,<br>*Dermacentor auratus*,<br>*Haemaphysalis bispinosa* | |
| *Matricaria chamomilla* | Asteraceae | Methanolic and ethanolic extract | In vitro | *Argas persicus* | (Tavassoli et al. 2018) |
| *Acmella oleracea* | Asteraceae | Ethanolic and distilled water | In vitro | *Rhipicephalus sanguineus* | (de Oliveira et al. 2018) |
| *Acmella oleracea* | Asteraceae | Essential oil | In vitro | *Hyalomma aegyptium* | (Laghzaoui et al. 2018) |
| *Acmella oleracea* | Asteraceae | Ethanolic extract | In vitro | *Amblyomma cajennens* | (Anholeto et al. 2018) |
| *Clausena anisata* | Rutaceae | Ethanolic extract | In vitro | *Amblyomma variegatum*,<br>*Rhipicephalus decoloratus*<br>*Rhipicephalus microplus* | (Mollong et al. 2018) |
| *Ylang-ylang* | Annonaceae | Essential oil | In vitro | *Ixodes ricinus* | (Elmhalli et al. 2018) |
| *Cananga odorata* | Annonaceae | Essential oil | In vitro | *Ixodes ricinus* | |

(continued)

**Table 11.1** (continued)

| Source plant | Family | Extract | Assessment mode | Targeted tick | Reference |
|---|---|---|---|---|---|
| *Schinus molle* | Anacardiaceae | Essential oil | In vitro | *Rhipicephalus sanguineus* | (Rey-Valeirón et al. 2018) |
| *Andrographis echioides* | Acanthaceae | Methanolic | In vitro | *Rhipicephalus microplus* | (Mathivanan et al. 2018) |
| *Artocapus lakoocha* | Moraceae | Ethanolic | In vitro | *Rhipicephalus microplus* | (Srisanyong et al. 2021) |
| *Gallesia integrifolia Sprenge* | Phytolaccaceae | Acetone and ethanolic extract | In vitro | *Rhipicephalus microplus* | (Dias et al. 2018) |
| *Nicotiana glutinosa* | Solanaceae | Acetone and ethanolic extract | In vitro | *Rhipicephalus microplus* | |
| *Nicotiana glauca* | Solanaceae | Acetone and crude ethanol extract | In vitro | *Rhipicephalus microplus* | |
| *Nicotiana tabacum* | Solanaceae | Methanolic | In vitro | *Rhipicephalus sanguineus* | (Weber et al. 2019) |
| *Tabernaemontana elegans* | Solanaceae | Methanolic | In vitro | *Rhipicephalus turanicus* | |
| *Calpurnia aurea* | Fabaceae | Methanolic | In vitro | *Rhipicephalus turanicus* | |
| *Schkuhria pinnata* | Asteraceae | Methanolic | In vitro | *Rhipicephalus turanicus* | |
| *Aloe rupestris* | Asphodelaceae | Hydroethanolic | In vitro | *Rhipicephalus turanicus* | (Adenubi et al. 2019) |
| *Calotropis procera* | Apocynaceae | Ethanolic | In vitro and in silico | *Rhipicephalus microplus* | (Khan et al. 2019) |
| *Taraxacum officinale* | Asteraceae | Ethanolic | In vitro and in silico | *Rhipicephalus microplus* | |
| *Tephrosia vogelii* | Fabaceae | Ethanolic | In vitro | *Rhipicephalus appendiculatus, Rhipicephalus microplus, Amblyomma variegatum* | (Siame et al. 2019) |
| *Protium spruceanum* | Burseraceae | Ethanolic | In vitro | *Rhipicephalus microplus* | (Figueiredo et al. 2019) |

| Source plant | Family | Extract | Assessment mode | Targeted tick | Reference |
|---|---|---|---|---|---|
| *Tabernaemontana elegans* | Apocynaceae | Ethanolic | In vitro and in silico | *Rhipicephalus turanicus* | (Adenubi et al. 2019) |
| *Calpurnia aurea* | Fabaceae | Ethanolic | In vitro and in silico | *Rhipicephalus turanicus* | |
| *Schkuhria pinnata* | Asteraceae | Ethanolic | In vitro and in silico | *Rhipicephalus turanicus* | |
| *Aloe rupestris* | Asphodelaceae | Ethanolic | In vitro and in silico | *Rhipicephalus turanicus* | |
| *Nicotiana tabacum* | Solanaceae | Methanolic | In vitro and in silico | *Rhipicephalus sanguineus* | (Oyagbemi, Ashafa, Adejinmi, et al., 2019) |
| *Calpurnia aurea* | Fabaceae | Ethanolic | In vitro | *Amblyomma variegatum* | (Amante et al. 2019) |
| *Allium sativum, Zingiber officinale* | Amaryllidaceae | Aqueous extract | In vitro | *Rhipicephalus sanguineus* | (Jeyathilakan et al. 2019) |
| *Zingiber officinale* | Zingiberaceae | Aqueous extract | In vitro | *Rhipicephalus sanguineus* | |
| *Aloe vera* | Asphodelaceae | Aqueous extract | In vitro | *Rhipicephalus sanguineus* | |
| *Ficus exasperata* | Moraceae | Ethanolic | In vitro | *Rhipicephalus sanguineus* | (Oyagbemi, Ashafa, & Adejinmi, 2019) |
| *Nicotiana tabacum* | Solanaceae | Aqueous extract | In vitro | *Rhipicephalus sanguineus* | (Jeyathilakan et al. 2019) |
| *Ageratum conyzoide* | Asteraceae | Ethanolic | In vitro | *Rhipicephalus microplus* | (Ajith Kumar et al. 2019) |
| *Acmella oleracea* | Asteraceae | Ethanolic | In vitro and in silico | *Rhipicephalus sanguineus* | (de Oliveira et al. 2019) |

(continued)

**Table 11.1** (continued)

| Source plant | Family | Extract | Assessment mode | Targeted tick | Reference |
|---|---|---|---|---|---|
| *Salvadora persica* | Salvadoraceae | Essential oil | In vitro | *Ixodes Ricinus* | (Elmhalli et al. 2019) |
| *Rosmarinus ofcinalis* | Lamiaceae | Essential oil | In vitro | *Ixodes Ricinus* | |
| *Momordica charantia* | Cucurbitaceae | Essential oil | In vitro | *Ixodes Ricinus* | |
| *Megaskepasma erythrochlamys* | Acanthaceae | Essential oil | In vitro | *Ixodes Ricinus* | |
| *Gliricidia sepium* | Fabaceae | Essential oil | In vitro | *Ixodes Ricinus* | |
| *Allium sativum* | Amaryllidaceae | Essential oil | In vitro | *Rhipicephalus microplus* | |
| *Carica papaya* | Amaryllidaceae | Essential oil | In vitro | *Rhipicephalus microplus* | |
| *Cissus quadrangularis* | Vitaceae | Essential oil | In vitro | *Rhipicephalus evertsi evertsi* | |
| *Gomphocarpus physocarpus* | Apocynaceae | Essential oil | In vitro | *Rhipicephalus evertsi evertsi* | |
| *Consolida orientalis* | Ranunculaceae | Ethanolic | In vitro | *Argas persicus* | (Ghanbarpour et al. 2019) |
| *Datura metel leaves* | Solanaceae | Ethanolic | In vitro | *Hyalomma schulzei* | (Al-Hasnawi and Wathah 2019) |
| *Maerua edulis* | Capparaceae | Ethanolic | In vitro | *Boophilus decoloratus* | (Nyahangare et al. 2019) |
| *Cissus quadrangulari* | Vitaceae | Ethanolic | In vitro | *Boophilus decoloratus* | |
| *Aloe vera* | Asphodelaceae | Ethanolic | In vitro | *Boophilus decoloratus* | |
| *Datura stramonium* | Solanaceae | Ethanolic | In vitro | *Boophilus decoloratus* | |
| *Phytolacca dodecandra* | Phytolaccaceae | Ethanolic | In vitro | *Boophilus decoloratus* | (Onyango et al. 2019) |
| *Cissus quadrangularis* | Vitaceae | Ethanolic | In vitro | *Boophilus decoloratus* | |

| Source plant | Family | Extract | Assessment mode | Targeted tick | Reference |
|---|---|---|---|---|---|
| *Trichilia pallida* | Sapindaceae | Essential oil | In vitro | *Rhipicephalus sanguineus* | (Amaro et al. 2019) |
| *Sesamum indicum Linn* | Pedaliaceae | Essential oil | In vitro | *Rhipicephalus sanguineus* | |
| *Lamiales* | Lamiaceae | Essential oil | In vitro | *Rhipicephalus sanguineus* | |
| *Pedaliaceae* | Pedaliaceae | Essential oil | In vitro | *Rhipicephalus sanguineus* | |
| *Ananas comosus* | Bromeliaceae | Essential oil | In vitro | *Rhipicephalus sanguineus* | |
| *Ananas comosus* | Bromeliaceae | Acetone extract | In vitro | *Rhipicephalus appendiculatus* | (Mawela et al. 2019) |
| *Clerodendrum glabrum* | Verbenaceae | Acetone extract | In vitro | *Rhipicephalus appendiculatus* | |
| *Zingiber officinalis* | Zingiberaceae | Essential oil | In vitro | *Rhipicephalus bursa* | (Madreseh-Ghahfarokhi et al. 2019) |
| *Eucalyptus globulus* | Myrtaceae | Essential oil | In vitro | *Rhipicephalus bursa* | |
| *Tagetes patula* | Asteraceae | Essential oil | In vitro | *Rhipicephalus microplus* | (Politi et al. 2019) |
| *Chrysanthenum cinerariaefolium* | Asteraceae | Essential oil | In vitro | *Rhipicephalus microplus* | (Khare et al. 2019) |
| *Azadiracta indica* | Meliaceae | Aqueous extract | In vitro | *Rhipicephalus microplus* | (Varadharajan and Gnanasekar 2019) |
| *Mangifera indica* | Anacardiaceae | Aqueous extract | In vitro | *Rhipicephalus microplus* | |
| *Polyalthia longifolia* | Annonaceae | Aqueous extract | In vitro | *Rhipicephalus microplus* | |
| *Annona squamosa* | Annonaceae | Aqueous extract | In vitro | *Rhipicephalus microplus* | |
| *Ficus benghalensis* | Ficus benghalensis | Aqueous extract | In vitro | *Rhipicephalus microplus* | |
| *Peperomia borbonensis* | | Aqueous extract | In vitro | *Rhipicephalus microplus* | (Dorla et al. 2019) |
| *Zanthoxylum heterophyllum* | Rutaceae | Aqueous extract | In vitro | *Rhipicephalus microplus* | |
| *Citrullus colocynthis* | Cucurbitaceae | Aqueous extract | In vitro | *Rhipicephalus microplus* | (Loach et al. 2019) |

(continued)

**Table 11.1** (continued)

| Source plant | Family | Extract | Assessment mode | Targeted tick | Reference |
|---|---|---|---|---|---|
| *Allium sativum* | Amaryllidaceae | Aqueous extract | In vitro and in silico | *Rhipicephalus microplus* | (Nasreen et al. 2020) |
| *Cannabis sativa* | Cannabaceae | Aqueous extract | In vitro and in silico | *Rhipicephalus microplus* | |
| *Vernonia amygdalina* | Asteraceae | Ethanolic | In vitro | *Rhipicephalus decoloratus*<br>*Rhipicephalus pulchellus* | (Kemal et al. 2020b) |
| *Calpurnia aurea* | Anacardiaceae | Ethanolic | In vitro | *Rhipicephalus decoloratus*<br>*Rhipicephalus pulchellus* | |
| *Schinus molle* | Anacardiaceae | Ethanolic | In vitro | *Rhipicephalus decoloratus*<br>*Rhipicephalus pulchellus* | |
| *Ricinus communis* | Euphorbiaceae | Ethanolic | In vitro | *Rhipicephalus decoloratus*<br>*Rhipicephalus pulchellus* | |
| *Croton macrostachyus* | Euphorbiaceae | Ethanolic | In vitro | *Rhipicephalus decoloratus*<br>*Rhipicephalus pulchellus* | |
| *Nicotiana tabacum* | Solanaceae | Ethanolic | In vitro | *Rhipicephalus decoloratus*<br>*Rhipicephalus pulchellus* | |
| *Curcuma longa* | Zingiberaceae | Ethanolic | In vitro | *Ornithodoros savignyi* | (Abdel-Shafy et al. 2020) |
| *Argemone mexicana* | Papaveraceae | Ethanolic | In vitro | *Rhipicephalus microplus* | (Upadhaya et al. 2020) |
| *Datura metel* | Papaveraceae | Ethanolic | In vitro | *Rhipicephalus microplus* | |
| *Ocimum americanum* | Lamiaceae | Ethanolic | In vitro | *Rhipicephalus microplus* | (Coulibaly et al. 2020) |
| *Ocimum gratissimum* | Lamiaceae | Ethanolic | In vitro | *Rhipicephalus microplus* | |
| *Laggera oloptera* | Asteraceae | Ethanolic | In vitro | *Rhipicephalus microplus* | |

| Source plant | Family | Extract | Assessment mode | Targeted tick | Reference |
|---|---|---|---|---|---|
| *Calpurnia aurea* | Fabaceae | Methanolic | In vitro | *Amblyomma variegatum, A. gemma, R. decoloratus* | (Kemal et al. 2020a) |
| *Otostegia integrifolia* | Lamiaceae | Methanolic | In vitro | *R. evertsi evertsi R. pulchellus* | |
| *A. Nilagirica* | Muridae | Ethanolic | In vitro | *Rhipicephalus annulatus* | (Udayan et al. 2020) |
| *Citrullus colocynthis* | Cucurbitaceae | Ethanolic | In vitro | *Hyalomma dromedarii* | (Mahran et al. 2020) |
| *Azadirachta indica* | Meliaceae | Ethanolic | In vitro | *Hyalomma dromedarii* | |
| *Haemonchus contortus* | Trichostrongylidae | Ethanolic | In vitro | *Rhipicephalus microplus* | (Minho et al. 2020) |
| *L. inermis leaves* | Lythraceae | Ethanolic | In vitro | *Hyalomma marginatum* | (Shnawa et al. 2023) |
| *Aizoon canariensis* | Aizoaceae | Ethanolic | In vitro | *Rhipicephalus annulatus* | |
| *Origanum compactum* | Lamiaceae | Ethanolic | In vitro | *Rhipicephaluspp* | (Salman et al. 2020) |
| *Coriandrum sativum* | Apiaceae | Ethanolic | In vitro | *Rhipicephaluspp* | |
| *Beauveria bassiana* | Cordycipitaceae | Acetone extract | In vitro | *Rhipicephalus appendiculatus* | (Staffa et al. 2020) |
| *Tulbaghia violacea* | Amaryllidaceae | Acetone extract | In vitro | *Rhipicephalus appendiculatus* | |
| *Cymbopogon citratus* | Poaceae | Essential oil | In vitro | *Haemaphysalis longicornis* | (Nwanade et al. 2021) |
| *Adhatoda vasica* | Acanthaceae | Chloroform extract | In vitro | *Rhipicephalus microplus* | (Jadhav et al. 2021) |
| *Citrus hystrix* | Rutaceae | Chloroform extract | In vitro | *Rhipicephalus microplus* | |
| *Cymbopogon citratus* | Poaceae | Essential oil | In vitro | *Rhipicephalus microplus* | (Shezryna et al. 2020) |
| *Prosopis juliflora* | Fabaceae | Methanolic extract | In vitro and in silico | *Rhipicephalus microplus* | (Lima et al. 2020) |
| *Citrus hystrix* | Rutaceae | Methanolic extract | In vitro | *Rhipicephalus microplus* | (Marchesini et al. 2020) |
| *Cymbopogon citratus* | Poaceae | Methanolic extract | In vitro | *Rhipicephalus microplus* | |
| *Gallesia integrifolia* | Petiveriaceae | Ethanolic | In vitro | *Rhipicephalus microplus* | (Maddikontla et al. 2023) |
| *Nicotiana tabacum* | Solanaceae | Ethanolic | In vitro | *Rhipicephalus microplus* | (Anshu et al. 2020) |

(continued)

**Table 11.1** (continued)

| Source plant | Family | Extract | Assessment mode | Targeted tick | Reference |
|---|---|---|---|---|---|
| *Psidium rufum* | Myrtaceae | Essential oil | In vitro | *Rhipicephalus microplus* | (Branco et al. 2020) |
| *Adiantum capillus-veneris* | Pteridaceae | Essential oil | In vitro | *Argas persicus* | |
| *Funaria hygrometric* | Funariaceae | Alcoholic extracts | In vitro | *Argas persicus* | (Taha and Baioumy Ali 2020) |
| *Cymbopogon citratus* | Poaceae | Ethanolic | In vitro | *Haemaphysalis longicornis* | (Agwunobi et al. 2020) |
| *Cymbopogon citratus* | Poaceae | Essential oil | In vitro | *Rhipicephalus microplus* | (da Silva et al. 2020) |
| *Cymbopogon nardus* | Poaceae | Essential oil | In vitro | *Rhipicephalus microplus* | |
| *Mentha arvensis* | Lamiaceae | Essential oil | In vitro | *Rhipicephalus microplus* | |
| *Glaucium flavum* | Papaveraceae | Methanolic extract | In vitro | *Rhipicephalus* sp. | (Kebbi et al. 2020) |
| *Peganum harmala* | Nitrariaceae | Methanolic extract | In vitro | *Rhipicephalus* sp. | |
| *Cannabis sativa* | Cannabaceae | Essential oil | In vitro | *Hyalomma dromedarii* | (Tabari et al. 2020a) |
| *Dermanyssus gallinae* | Animalia | Essential oil | In vitro | *Hyalomma dromedarii* | |
| *Punica granatum* | Lythraceae | Ethanol extracts | In vitro | *Rhipicephalus annulatus* | (Guneidy et al. 2021) |
| *Acacia saligna* | Fabaceae | Ethanol extracts | In vitro | *Rhipicephalus annulatus* | |
| *Randia aculeata* | Rubiaceae | Phenolic | In vitro | *Rhipicephalus microplus* | (Bravo-Ramos et al. 2021) |
| *Moringa oleifera* | Moringaceae | Phenolic | In vitro | *Rhipicephalus microplus* | |
| *Carica papaya* | Caricaceae | Phenolic | In vitro | *Rhipicephalus microplus* | |
| *Artocapus lakoocha* | Moraceae | Phenolic | In vitro | *Rhipicephalus microplus* | (Srisanyong et al. 2021) |
| *Artocapus lakoocha* | Meliaceae | Phenolic | In vitro | *Hyalomma dromedarii* | (Abdel-Ghany et al. 2021b) |
| *Artemisia herba-alba* | Asteraceae | Phenolic | In vitro | *Hyalomma dromedarii* | |
| *Citrus limetta* | Rutaceae | Essential oil | In vitro | *Rhipicephalus microplus* | (Jain et al. 2021) |
| *Curcuma longa* | Zingiberaceae | Acetone, chloroform, and ethanol | In vitro | *Rhipicephalus microplus* | (Nazim et al. 2021b) |
| *Laurus nobilis* | Lauraceae | Acetone and ethanol | In vitro | *Hyalomma scupense* | (Alimi et al. 2021) |

| Source plant | Family | Extract | Assessment mode | Targeted tick | Reference |
|---|---|---|---|---|---|
| *Artemisia herba alba* | Asteraceae | Ethanol extracts | In vitro | *Ixodes ricinus* | (Elmhalli et al. 2021) |
| *Origanum majorana* | Lamiaceae | Ethanol extracts | In vitro | *Ixodes ricinus* | |
| *Juniperus phoenicea* | Cupressaceae | Ethanol extracts | In vitro | *Ixodes ricinus* | |
| *Furcraea foetida* | Juglandaceae | Aacetone, chloroform, and ethanol | In vitro | *Rhipicephalus microplus* | (Nazim et al. 2021a) |
| *Cinnamomum cassia* | Asparagaceae | Aacetone, chloroform, and ethanol | In vitro | *Rhipicephalus microplus* | |
| *Capsicum frutescens* | Lauraceae | Essential oil | In vitro | *Haemaphysalis longicornis* | (Nwanade et al. 2021) |
| *Allium cepa L* | Acanthaceae | Chloroform extract | In vitro | *Rhipicephalusmicroplus* | (Jadhav et al. 2021) |
| *Cinnamomum cassia* | Amaryllidaceae | Methanol extracts | | *Rhipicephalus annulatus* | (Oyewusi et al. 2021) |
| *Jatropha curcas* | Lauraceae | Essential oil | In vitro | *H. longicornis, R. haemaphysaloides, and H. asiaticum* | (Zhou et al. 2023) |
| *Artemisia herba* | Colchicaceae | Essential oil | In vitro | *Hyalomma spp* | (Norouzi et al. 2021) |
| *Melia azedarach* | Asteraceae | Essential oil | In vitro | *Hyalomma dromedarii* | (Abdel-Ghany et al. 2021a) |
| *Thymus mongolicus* | Asteraceae | Essential oil | In vitro | *Hyalomma dromedarii* | |
| *Cinnamomum verum* | Lamiaceae | Essential oil | In vitro | *Haemaphysalis longicornis* | (Qiao et al. 2021) |
| *Origanum vulgare* | Lauraceae | Essential oil | In vitro | *Haemaphysalis longicornis* | |
| *Eptospermum scoparium* | Lamiaceae | Essential oil | In vitro | *Haemaphysalis longicornis* | |
| *Origanum vulgare* | Myrtaceae | Essential oil | In vitro | *Rhipicephalus microplus* | (Duque et al. 2021) |
| *Litsea cubeba* | Lamiaceae | Essential oil | In vitro | *Rhipicephalus microplus* | |
| *Annona squamosa* | Lauraceae | Essential oil | In vitro | *Rhipicephalus microplus* | |
| *Datura innoxia* | Cucurbitaceae | Fruit extract | In vitro | *Hyalomma dromedarii* | (Mohamed et al. 2022) |
| *Tephrosia vogelii* | Solanaceae | Ethanol extracts | In vitro | *Rhipicephalus microplus* | (Saman et al. 2022) |
| *Juniperus communis* | Fabaceae | Ethanol extracts | In vitro | *Rhipicephalus microplus* | (Jerjero 2022) |

(continued)

**Table 11.1** (continued)

| Source plant | Family | Extract | Assessment mode | Targeted tick | Reference |
|---|---|---|---|---|---|
| *Tephrosia vogelii* | Cupressaceae | Ethanol extracts | In vitro | *Hyalomma scupense* | (Alimi et al. 2022) |
| *Calotropis procera* | Fabaceae | Ethanol extracts | In vitro | *Hyalomma scupense* | |
| *Syzygium cumini* | Apocynaceae | Methanolic extract | In vitro | *Rhipicephalus microplus* | (Nawaz et al. 2022) |
| *Ziziphus jujube* | Myrtaceae | Methanolic extract | In vitro | *Rhipicephalus microplus* | |
| *Nepeta cataria* | Rhamnaceae | Methanolic extract | In vitro | *Rhipicephalus microplus* | |
| *Pelargonium graveolen* | Lamiaceae | Ethanol extracts | In vitro | *Ixodes scapularis and Haemaphysalis longicornis* | (González et al. 2022) |
| *Piper nigrum* | Eraniaceae | | In vitro | *Rhipicephalus annulatus* | (Ibrahium et al. 2022a) |
| *Saussurea costus* | Piperaceae | Fruit extracts | In vitro | *Rhipicephalus australis* | (Toussirot et al. 2022) |
| *Melaleuca alternifoli* | Asteraceae | Methanol extract | In vitro | *Hyalomma dromedari*<br>*Rhipicephalus annulatus* | (Hegazy et al. 2022) |
| *Citrus Limon* | Myrtaceae | Essential oil | In vitro | *Rhipicephalus annulatus* | (Ibrahium et al. 2022b) |
| *Azadirachta indica* | Rutaceae | Essential oil | In vitro | *Rhipicephalus annulatus* | |
| *Melia azedarach* | Meliaceae | Ethanol extracts | In vitro | *Haylomma anatolicum* | (Hatzade et al. 2022) |
| *Azadirachta indica* | Meliaceae | Ethanol extracts | In vitro | *Haylomma anatolicum* | |
| *Piper longum* | Meliaceae | Ethanol extracts | In vitro | *Rhipicephalus microplus* | (Dalei et al. 2022) |
| *Azadirachta indica* | Piperaceae | Ethanol extracts | In vitro | *Rhipicephalus microplus* | (Saini et al. 2022) |
| *Syzygium aromaticum* | Meliaceae | Ethanol extracts | In vitro | *Hyalomma dromedari* | (Gareh et al. 2022) |
| *Protium spruceanum* | Myrtaceae | Essential oil | In vitro | *Haemaphysalis longicornis* | (Gao et al. 2022) |
| *Azadirachta indica* | Burseraceae | Essential oil | In vitro | *Rhipicephalus microplus* | (Silva et al. 2022) |

| Source plant | Family | Extract | Assessment mode | Targeted tick | Reference |
|---|---|---|---|---|---|
| *Allium sativum* | Meliaceae | Aqueous extract | In vitro | *Rhipicephalus microplus* | (Luns et al. 2022) |
| *Capsicum chinense* | Amaryllidaceae | Aqueous extract | In vitro | *Rhipicephalus microplus* | |
| *Nicotiana tabacum* | Solanaceae | Aqueous extract | In vitro | *Rhipicephalus microplus* | |
| *Dysphania ambrosioides* | Solanaceae | Aqueous extract | In vitro | *Rhipicephalus microplus* | |
| *Momordica charantia* | Dysphania ambrosioides | Aqueous extract | In vitro | *Rhipicephalus microplus* | |
| *Ricinus communis* | Meliaceae | Ethanol extracts | In vitro | *Rhipicephalus microplus* | (Singh et al. 2022) |
| *Cymbopogon flexuosus* | Euphorbiaceae | Ethanol extracts | In vitro | *Rhipicephalus microplus* | |
| *Eucalyptus globulus* | Poaceae | Ethanol extracts | In vitro | *Rhipicephalus microplus* | |
| *Murraya koenigii* | Myrtaceae | Ethanol extracts | In vitro | *Rhipicephalus microplus* | |
| *Allium sativum* | Rutaceae | Ethanol extracts | In vitro | *Rhipicephalus microplus* | |
| *Salvia officinalis* | Amaryllidaceae | Ethanol extracts | In vitro | *Rhipicephalus microplus* | |
| *Rosmarinus officinalis* | Lamiaceae | Ethanol extracts | In vitro | *Rhipicephalus microplus* | |
| *Ocimum basilicum* | Lamiaceae | Ethanol extracts | In vitro | *Rhipicephalus microplus* | |
| *Ambrosia peruviana* | Meliaceae | Aqueous extract | In vitro | *Hyalomma dromedarii* | (Abdel-Ghany et al. 2022) |
| *Lepechinia mutica* | Asteraceae | Essential oil | In vitro | *Rhipicephalus microplus* | (Guzmán et al. 2022) |
| *Randia aculeata* | Meliaceae | Essential oil | In vitro | *Rhipicephalus microplus* | |
| *Ferula asafoetida* | Rubiaceae | Ethanol extracts | In vitro | *Rhipicephalus microplus* | (Bravo-Ramos et al. 2023) |
| *Trachyspermum ammi* | | Methanolic extracts | In vitro | *Hyalomma dromedarii* | (Moudgil et al. 2023) |
| *Azadirachta indica* | Apiaceae | Methanolic extracts | In vitro | *Hyalomma dromedarii* | |
| *Vitex negundo* | Meliaceae | Aqueous extract | In vitro | *Rhipicephalus microplus* | (Tiwari et al. 2023) |
| *Piper nigrum* | Lamiaceae | Aqueous extract | In vitro | *Rhipicephalus microplus* | |

(continued)

**Table 11.1** (continued)

| Source plant | Family | Extract | Assessment mode | Targeted tick | Reference |
|---|---|---|---|---|---|
| *Annona muricata* | Piperaceae | Ethyl acetate extract and the methanolic extract | In vitro | *Rhipicephalus australis* | (Toussirot et al. 2023) |
| *Jatropha curcas* | Annonaceae | Ethanolic extract | In vitro | *Rhipicephalus species* | (Zakari et al. 2023) |
| *Laurus nobilis* | Uphorbiaceae | Methanol extract | In vitro | *Rhipicephalus decoloratus* | (Ijoh et al. 2023) |
| *Nigella sativa* | Pteridaceae | Methanolic extracts | In vitro | *Argas species* | (Ali and Taha 2023) |
| *Egletes viscosa* | Ranunculaceae | Essential oil | In vitro | *Rhipicephalus microplus* | (Al-Hoshani et al. 2023) |
| *Thymus vulgaris* | Asteraceae | Essential oil | In vitro | *Rhipicephalus sanguineus* | (Pereira et al. 2023) |
| *Plumbago zeylanica* | Lamiaceae | Essential oil | In vitro | *Rhipicephalus sanguineus* | (Alibeigi et al. 2023) |
| *Moringa oleifera* | Myrtaceae | | In vitro | *Rhipicephalus microplus* | (Reis et al. 2023) |
| *Ailanthus altissima* | Asteraceae | Ethanolic extract | In vitro | *Hyalomma anatolicum* | (Noaman and Bahreininejad 2024) |
| *Rosmarinus officinalis* | Simaroubaceae | Ethanolic extract | In vitro | *Hyalomma anatolicum* | |
| *Eucalyptus camaldulensi* | Lamiaceae | Ethanolic extract | In vitro | *Hyalomma anatolicum* | |
| *Lavandula angustifolia* | Myrtaceae | Ethanolic extract | In vitro | *Hyalomma anatolicum* | |
| *Mentha piperita* | Lamiaceae | Ethanolic extract | In vitro | *Hyalomma anatolicum* | |
| *Nicotiana tobacum* | Lamiaceae | Ethanolic extract | In vitro | *Hyalomma anatolicum* | |
| *Allium sativum* | Solanaceae | Ethanolic extract | In vitro | *Hyalomma anatolicum* | |
| *Thymbra sintenisii* | Amaryllidaceae | Ethanolic extract | In vitro | *Hyalomma anatolicum* | |

extracts of *Senna italica*, *Calpurnia aurea*, and *Schkuhria pinnata, respectively,* for 1 min (Fouche et al. 2017). Discrepancies in acaricidal activities may arise from differences in immersion time, concentration, and the active substances that these plants contain. The heightened acaricidal activity of *C. cyminum* EOs may be attributed to longer immersion times and higher concentrations, while active compounds such as o-cymene, γ-terpinene, β-pinene, and cuminaldehyde, which are found in *C. cyminum* EOs, could contribute to its efficacy (Villarreal et al. 2017).

Plant essential oils (EOs) and extracts are also known for their acaricidal effects on tick larvae. The larval packet test (LPT) is the recommended method for determining the larvicidal activity of such materials. Usually, at least 100 larvae are employed in the LPT, and the death rate is noted 24 h after treatment. When applied topically to *R. microplus* ticks, ethanol extracts of *S. italica* from the fruit, roots, and leaves; ethanol extracts from the leaves and flowers of *C. aurea;* and acetone and ethanol extracts from *C. quadrangularis* stem demonstrated efficacy (> 96% mortality) against larvae at 10 mg/mL at 1% weight/vol (Wellington et al. 2017). In a related study, *Bursera graveolens* and *Schinus molle* EOs showed 100% efficacy against the same larvae at a concentration of 5% wt/vol (50 mg/mL) (Rey-Valeirón et al. 2017). The $LC_{50}$ value for *Aloe yavellana* leaf latex applied to *Amblyomma variegatum* larvae was 35.82 mg/mL, and 62.5% mortality was observed (Hailesillassie et al. 2018). However, an $LC_{50}$ of 5.9% wt/vol (59 mg/mL) and 100% mortality of *R. microplus* larvae were reported following their exposure to a 10% (100 mg/mL) ethyl acetate fraction of the ethanol extract of *Crescentia cujete* (Pereira et al. 2017). When *Hyalomma lusitanicum* larvae were exposed to 20 mg/mL *Geranium macrorrhizum*, $LC_{50}$ values of 6.97 mg/mL and 1.37 mg/mL were recorded for resistant and wild-type larvas, respectively (Navarro-Rocha et al. 2018). The $LC_{50}$ values of *Andrographis echioides* for *R. microplus* larvae were 0.11, 0.14, 0.15, and 0.22 mg/mL for the methanolic, petroleum, ethyl acetate, and aqueous extracts, respectively (Mathivanan et al. 2018). In addition, EOs from *Cinnamomum zeylanicum*, *Cymbopogon citratus,* and *Syzygium aromaticum* had $LC_{50}$ values for the same larvae corresponding to concentrations of 0.086% wt/vol (0.86 mg/mL), 0.25% wt/vol (2.46 mg/mL), and 0.30% wt/vol (3.01 mg/mL), respectively (Jyoti et al. 2019). In Iran, eight plant-derived products were assessed for acaricidal effects on *Hyalomma anatolicum* larvae, with notable efficacy demonstrated by *Nicotiana tabacum* and *Allium sativum* extracts resulting in larval mortality rates of 100% and 65%, respectively, at the highest applied concentration (200 mg/mL) (Noaman and Bahreininejad 2024).

### 11.2.1 Plant Extracts as Repellents

In addition to their acaricidal effects, plant essential oils and extracts also exhibit repellent effects, although these effects vary depending on factors such as tick age, test duration, methodology, and concentration (Adenubi et al. 2018b, Bissinger et al. 2011). For instance, acetone extracts from *Rotheca glabrum* leaves exhibited an average repellence of 87.3% against adults of *Rhipicephalus appendiculatus*, with 100% repellent activity observed for up to 50 min (except at 20 min) at a concentration of 30% wt/vol (300 mg/mL) (Mawela et al. 2019). *Anthemis melampodina* and *Anthemis scrobicularis* essential oils showed repellent activities of 80.0% and 96.7%, respectively, against nymphs of *Amblyomma americanum* at a concentration of 2.5% (25 mg/mL) when treated for 15 min (Yusufoglu et al. 2018). On the other hand, at a concentration of 1 mg/mL, the repellent properties of the essential oils *Conyza dioscoridis*, *Artemisia* herba-alba, and *Calendula officinalis* against *I. ricinus* nymphs were 94%, 84.2%, and 82%, respectively, after 5 min of treatment (El-Seedi et al. 2017). Under field conditions, *C. dioscoridis* oil showed 61.1% repellence at a concentration of 6.5 μg/cm$^2$. By the fifth day under semifield conditions, adult *R. appendiculatus* ticks and other ticks treated with 1 g of petroleum jelly containing essential oil from *Tagetes minuta* or *Tithonia diversifolia* exhibited repellent qualities above 75% and 60%, respectively (Wanzala et al. 2018). Additionally, essential oils from *Cinnamomum cassia* and *Cinnamomum camphora* exhibited potent acaricidal activity against *Haemaphysalis longicornis*, with *C. cassia* demonstrating superior toxicity to unfed adults. Enzyme assays indicated significant inhibition of acetylcholinesterase and carboxylesterase by oils, highlighting their potential as effective alternatives to synthetic acaricides (Bai et al. 2024).

Some plant-based products can repel ticks and kill them. For example, at 25 mg/mL, the ethanolic extract and essential oil (EO) extracts of *Tagetes patula* aerial portions were 100% and 99.1% effective at repelling *R. microplus* larvae, respectively. The ethanolic extract also showed larvicidal efficacy of 98.4% ($LC_{50}$ = 3.798 mg/mL) and 99.2% ($LC_{50}$ = 18.60 mg/mL) at dosages of 100 and 200 mg/mL, respectively, on females who were engorged (Politi et al. 2019). When applied to *Ix.* for approximately 5 h at a concentration of 1 μL/cm$^2$, the essential oil (EO) of *Salvadora persica* showed nearly 100% repellent effects; however, when given to the same nymphs, the EO of *Rosmarinus officinalis* demonstrated acaricidal effects (100% mortality and 0.7 μL/cm$^2$ $LC_{50}$ value) (Elmhalli et al. 2019). In a related investigation using *R. microplus* larvae, *Ocotea elegans* EOs showed 77.4% larvicidal activity ($LC_{50}$ = 59.68 mg/mL) during a 48-h exposure at 100 mg/mL and 100% repellent action ($LC_{50}$ = 0.04 mg/mL) at 50 mg/mL. In engorged females, the EOs likewise demonstrated 100% effectiveness ($LC_{50}$ = 4.96 mg/mL) at 50 mg/mL (Figueiredo et al. 2018). Piperitone, piperitenone, and sesquirosefuran, the active chemicals found in *T. patula* and *O. elegans*, respectively, have shown encouraging insecticidal and repellent properties against mosquitoes (Aguiar et al. 2015; Tripathi et al. 2004). Additionally, the essential oils of *Origanum minutiflorum* and *Dorystoechas hastata* showed significant larvicidal activity against *R. sanguineus* s.l. The Larval Repellency Assay Test (LRAT) revealed that *O. minutiflorum* oil has a remarkable repellency of 84.14% to 100% at a 1% concentration, which is comparable to that of DEET (Koc et al. 2024).

## 11.3 Acaricidal Plants and Their Active Phytochemical Compounds

According to various studies, a diverse range of herbs and medicinal plants exhibit acaricidal activity (Attia et al. 2012; Krishna et al. 2014; Yang et al. 2014). More than 200 plant species worldwide have been identified as possessing tick-repellent or acaricidal characteristics (Adenubi et al. 2016). The separation of these molecules presents a major problem in the identification and characterization of bioactive compounds since plant extracts contain a variety of bioactive chemicals with varying polarities (Ingle et al. 2017). Biochemical tests are used in qualitative phytochemical screening to investigate several types of active compounds (tannins, glycosides, essential oils, flavonoids, alkaloids, esters, and fatty acids) that are present in the extract (Hikal et al. 2017).

Adenubi et al. (2020) extensively reviewed various isolated compounds found in different plant species with acaricidal properties, such as precocene I and precocene II in *Ageratum conyzoides*; azadirachtin in *Azadirachta indica*; elimicin, catechol, chlorogenic acid, and quercetin in *Cymbopogon citratus*; 1–8 cineole and spathulenol in *Eucalyptus globulus*; nicotine, solanesol, and 1-quinic acid in *Nicotiana* tabum; thymol, eugenol, and terpen-4-ol in *Ocimum gratissimum*; and quercetin and ellagic acid in *Ricinus communis*. Neem extracts, particularly azadirachtin, have been studied extensively for their acaricidal properties. Treatment with aqueous extracts of neem leaf at concentrations of 10% and 20% induces morphological changes during oocyte development in adult female ticks (Denardi et al. 2010). *R. microplus* egg deposition and larval hatching rates are affected by fresh and dry *Aloe arborecens* extracts, which include water-soluble tannins (De Matos et al. 2017). The egg production index (EPI) and hatching rate are considerably reduced by clove essential oil, which is primarily composed of eugenol (Ferreira et al. 2018). Acaricidal activity has been observed in root and stem extracts from *Petiveria alliacea*, which contain metabolites of BTS and BDS (benzyltrisulfide and benzyldisulfide, respectively) (Rosado-Aguilar et al. 2010). Cadina-4, 10 (15)-dien-3-one derived from Hyptis verticillata leaves and stems hinders oviposition and hatching of *Rh.* (*B.*) *microplus* eggs (Porter et al. 1995). The methanolic extract of *Calotropis procera* has acaricidal effects on *R. microplus* due to the presence of active compounds such as 3-isopropoxy-1,1,1,7,7,7-hex, naphthalene, 1,6-dimethyl-4, cyclohexane, and 2-(2′,4′,6′,8′,8′-hept (Bhaskar et al. 2021).

Herbal acaricides can exert various effects on ticks, including inhibiting the development of eggs, acting as repellants, having antifeedant properties, having antagonistic effects on hormone regulation, interfering with sexual communication and mating, and preventing the production of chitin (Khare et al. 2019). Some essential oils are neurotoxic because they compete with octopamine neurotransmitter receptors, inhibit acetylcholinesterase (AChE), or cause gamma-aminobutyric acid (GABA) to close chloride channels (Camilo et al. 2017). The essential oil components may interact with tyramine receptors, potentially affecting tick biology (Gross et al. 2017). The effect of herbal acaricidal drugs has been suggested to be caused by an increase in AChE concentration in tick synganglions or neurons; this could result in excessive salivation, paralysis, lacrimation, and finally death from ticks (Jain et al. 2020).

The alkaloid nicotine, which resembles the excitatory neurotransmitter acetylcholine, is the primary bioactive component of *Nicotiana tabacum* (Ujváry 2010). Similarly, azadirachtin, the active ingredient in Azadirachta indica, inhibits protein synthesis in a variety of tick tissues, including the midgut, which hinders the digestion of food proteins. Additionally, it inhibits the firing of phagostimulatory receptors on tick-feeding stimulatory cells and activates chemoreceptors on restriction cells (Koul 2008; Ujváry 2010). Ticks that are exposed to neem oil experience notable morphophysiological changes that compromise their reproductive systems (Remedio et al. 2015). Plant-derived monoterpenoids, including eucalyptol, linalool, and citral, function by reversibly inhibiting acetylcholinesterase (Siramon et al. 2009). *Rh.* (*B.*) *microplus* is strongly inhibited by thymol and 1,8-cineole, which are found in *O. gratissimum* (Castro et al. 2018). Further research is necessary since it is currently uncertain exactly how other plant extracts and essential oil components affect tick biology (Quadros et al. 2020).

## 11.4 Acaricidal Activity of Plant Extracts on Mites

However, concerns regarding the adverse effects of excessive chemical agent use have been limited because of issues such as drug resistance, residues, and environmental contamination. As a result, there is increasing interest in finding natural, alternative acaricides made from plants (Table 11.2). Due to their poisonous, repulsive, attractant, and growth-regulating qualities, plant secondary metabolites have been thoroughly studied for possible uses (Kim et al. 2016).

The strong acaricidal activities of Ajowan's alcoholic extract (AE) and essential oil (EO) against *Dermanyssus gallinae* were shown by Baran et al. (2020). The primary component in both the EO (42.26%) and the AE (45.8%) was thymol. Additionally, they discovered that 24 h after treatment, the spraying approach outperformed the touch method in terms of effectiveness. *A. sieberi* EO was tested for toxicity against *D. gallinae* by applying fumigant and contact assays to adult mites. Camphor (12.3%), 1,8-cineole (10.09%), α-thujone (31.5%), and β-thujone (11.92%) are present in *A. sieberi* EO. According to Tabari et al. (2017), the median lethal concentration ($LC_{50}$) of EO was 15.85 μg/cm$^3$ in a contact toxicity assay conducted on adult mites. The effectiveness of *Cnidium officinale* (*C. officinale*) methanolic extract against adult *D. gallinae* was assessed by (Kim et al. 2018). At 4000 ppm (parts per million), 100% of ME patients died after 48 h of treatment, mostly from (Z)-ligustilide. Remarkably, the C. officinale extract exhibited both contact and fumigant activities, whereas (Z)-ligustilide only showed fumigant potential. *Xylopia emarginata* (*X. emarginata*) was shown to have acaricidal activity against *D. gallinae* (Pares et al. 2021), with an $LC_{50}$ value of 331.769 μg/cm$^2$. Moreover, analysis of the metabolomic profile of *X. emarginata* revealed the presence of several compounds, such as amides, alkaloids, phenolics, and terpenoids. Following a full day of therapy, the extract from *Drimia maritima* (*D. maritima*)

**Table 11.2** Various plant extracts used against different mite species in in vitro, in vivo, and in silico experiments

| Source plant | Family | In vitro and in silico | Mites species | % Mortality | Reference |
|---|---|---|---|---|---|
| *Polygonum hydropiper* | Polygonaceae | In vitro | *Oligonychus coffeae* Nietner | 69.94% | (Al Mamun et al. 2015) |
| *Xanthium strumarium* | Asteraceae | In vitro | *Oligonychus coffeae* Nietner | 89.66% | (Al Mamun et al. 2015) |
| *Datura mete* | Solanaceae | In vitro | *Oligonychus coffeae* Nietner | 84.00% | (Al Mamun et al. 2015) |
| *Swietenia mahagoni* | Meliaceae | In vitro | *Oligonychus coffeae* Nietner | 86.21% | (Al Mamun et al. 2015) |
| *Azadirachta indica* | Meliaceae | In vitro | Oligonychus *coffeae* Nietner | 81% | (Al Mamun et al. 2015) |
| *Photinia serrulata Lindl.* | Rosaceae | In vitro | *Tetranychus cinnabarinus* | 51.97% | (Chen and Dai 2015) |
| *Ligustrum lucidum Ait.* | Oleaceae | In vitro | *Tetranychus cinnabarinus* | 56.77 | (Chen and Dai 2015) |
| *Cinnamomum camphora (L.) Presl* | Lauraceae | In vitro | *Tetranychus cinnabarinus* | 97.54% | (Chen and Dai 2015) |
| *Polygonum hydropiper L.* | Polygonum hydropiper L. | In vitro | *Tetranychus cinnabarinus* | 13.35 | (Chen and Dai 2015) |
| *Ulmus pumila L.* | Ulmaceae | In vitro | *Tetranychus cinnabarinus* | 8.92% | (Chen and Dai 2015) |
| *Pinus massoniana Larmb* | Pinaceae | In vitro | *Tetranychus cinnabarinus* | 93.93% | (Chen and Dai 2015) |
| *Dalbergia hupeana Hance* | Leguminosae | In vitro | *Tetranychus cinnabarinus* | 32.27% | (Chen and Dai 2015) |
| *Euphorbia helioscopia L* | Euphorbiaceae | In vitro | *Tetranychus cinnabarinus* | 48.10% | (Chen and Dai 2015) |
| *Leucaena glauca* | Fabaceae | In vitro | *Tetranychus urticae* Koch | 98.90% | (Auamcharoen and Chandrapatya 2015) |
| *Satureja hortensis L* | Lamiaceae | In vitro | *Tetranychus turkestani* | 96.50% | (Zandi-Sohani and Ramezani 2015) |
| *Mentha pulegium L.)* | Lamiaceae | In vitro | *Tetranychus turkestani* | 98,3% | (Zandi-Sohani and Ramezani 2015) |

(continued)

**Table 11.2** (continued)

| Source plant | Family | In vitro and in silico | Mites species | % Mortality | Reference |
|---|---|---|---|---|---|
| *Rosmarinus officinalis* | Lamiaceae | In vitro | *Tetranychus turkestani* | 99.10% | (Zandi-Sohani and Ramezani 2015) |
| *Zataria multiflora* | Lamiaceae | In vitro | *Tetranychus turkestani* | 97.10% | (Zandi-Sohani and Ramezani 2015) |
| *Mentha piperita* | Lamiaceae | In vitro | *Phytoseiulus persimilis* | 96.55% | (Abdallah et al. 2015) |
| *Syzygium aromaticum L* | Myrtaceae | In vitro | *Athias-Henrio* | 96.36% | (Abdallah et al. 2015) |
| *Culinary plants* | Apiaceae | In vitro | *Tetranychus urticae* Koch. | 90% | (Lakhdari et al. 2015) |
| *Saponaria officinalis)* | Caryophyllaceae | In vitro | *Tetranychus urticae* Koch | 90% | (Lakhdari et al. 2015) |
| *Ammi visnaga* | Apiaceae | In vitro | *Tetranychus urticae* Koch. | 90% | (Lakhdari et al. 2015) |
| *Glycyrrhiza glabra* | Fabaceae | In vitro | *Tetranychus urticae* Koch | 90% | (Lakhdari et al. 2015) |
| *Palmaria palmata* | Palmariaceae | In vitro | *Tetranychus urticae* Koch | 90% | (Lakhdari et al. 2015) |
| *Leuzea carthamoide,* | Asteraceae | In vitro | *Tetranychus urticae* Koch | 90% | (Lakhdari et al. 2015) |
| *Origanum majorana* | Lamiaceae | In vitro | *Tetranychus urticae* Koch | 90% | (Lakhdari et al. 2015) |
| *Salvia officinalis* | Lamiaceae | In vitro | *Tetranychus urticae* Koch | 90% | (Lakhdari et al. 2015) |
| *Chenopodium quinoa Willd* | Amaranthaceae | In vitro | *Tetranychus urticae* Koch | 93% | (Harder et al. 2016) |
| *Azadirachta indica* | Meliaceae | In vitro | Predatory mite | 55% | (Zahid et al. 2016) |
| *Eucalyptus* | Myrtaceae | In vitro | Predatory mite | 27.50% | (Zahid et al. 2016) |
| *Allium sativum* | Amaryllidaceae | In vitro | Predatory mite | 27.50% | (Zahid et al. 2016) |
| *Gossypium hirsutum* | Malvaceae | In vitro | Predatory mite | 22.50% | (Zahid et al. 2016) |
| *Vitex negundo L* | Lamiaceae | In vitro | *Oligonychus coffeae* | 66.71% | (Zahid et al. 2016) |
| *Clerodendrum infortunatum L* | Lamiaceae | In vitro | *Oligonychus coffeae* | 57.45% | (Zahid et al. 2016) |
| *Ziziphus joazeiro* | Rhamnaceae | In vitro | *Tetranychus ludeni* | 76.47% | (Ferraz et al. 2017) |

| Source plant | Family | In vitro and in silico | Mites species | % Mortality | Reference |
|---|---|---|---|---|---|
| *Matricaria chamomilla* | Asteraceae | In vitro | *Tetranychus urticae* Koch | 83% | (Tabet et al. 2018) |
| *Pimpinella anisum L* | Apiaceae | In vitro | *Tetranychus urticae* Koch | 75% | (Tabet et al. 2018) |
| *Origanum vulgare* | | In vitro | *Tetranychus urticae* Koch | 22% | (Tabet et al. 2018) |
| *Zingiberofficinale* | Zingiberaceae | In vitro | *Eutetranychus orientalis* seemed | 98.87% | (Ahmad et al. 2018) |
| *Nigella Sativum* | Ranunculaceae | In vitro | *Eutetranychus orientalis* | 40.25% | (Ahmad et al. 2018) |
| *Rosmarinusofficinalis* | Lamiaceae | In vitro | *Eutetranychus orientalis* | 90.44% | (Ahmad et al. 2018) |
| *Commiphoramyrrha* | | In vitro | *Eutetranychus orientalis* | 60.14% | (Ahmad et al. 2018) |
| *Salvia officinalis L* | Lamiaceae | In vitro | *Phytoseiulus persimilis* | 88.80% | (Ahmad et al. 2018) |
| *Rosmarinus officinalis L* | Lamiaceae | In vitro | *Neoseiulus californicus* | 50.10% | (Salman et al. 2018) |
| *Allium sativum* | Amaryllidaceae | In vitro | *Amblyseius andersoni* | 93.15% | (ELRoby and Darwish 2018) |
| *Origanum majorana* | Lamiaceae | In vitro | *Amblyseius andersoni* | 94.67% | (ELRoby and Darwish 2018) |
| *Peganum harmala* | Nitrariaceae | In vitro | *Amblyseius andersoni* | 94.67% | (ELRoby and Darwish 2018) |
| *Nigella sativa* | Ranunculaceae | In vitro | *Amblyseius andersoni* | 94.42% | (ELRoby and Darwish 2018) |
| *Leonotis nepetifolia* | Lamiaceae | In vitro | *Tetranychus urticae* | 69.06% | (Ogayo 2019) |
| *Ocimum gratissimum* | Lamiaceae | In vitro | *Tetranychus urticae* | 69.06% | (Ogayo 2019) |
| *Mentha longifoli* | Lamiaceae | In vitro | *Tetranychus urticae* | 99.40% | (Momen et al. 2018) |
| *Mentha longifoli* | Lamiaceae | In vitro | *Typhlodromips swirskii* | 99.40% | (Momen et al. 2018) |
| *Andrographis paniculata L* | . Acanthaceae | In vitro | *Tetranychus urticae* | 77.77% | (Premalatha et al. 2018) |
| *Achyranthes aspera L.* | Amaranthaceae | In vitro | *Tetranychus urticae* | 85.57% | (Premalatha et al. 2018) |

(continued)

**Table 11.2** (continued)

| Source plant | Family | In vitro and in silico | Mites species | % Mortality | Reference |
|---|---|---|---|---|---|
| *Anacardium occidentale L.* | Anacardiaceae | In vitro | *Tetranychus urticae* | 85.57% | (Premalatha et al. 2018) |
| *Annona squamosa L* | . Annonaceae | In vitro | *Tetranychus urticae* | 85.57% | (Premalatha et al. 2018) |
| *Leonotis nepetifolia* | Lamiaceae | In vitro | *Tetranychus urticae)* | 93.80% | (Ogayo 2019) |
| *Ocimum gratissimum* | Lamiaceae | In vitro | *Tetranychus urticae)* | 96.40% | (Ogayo 2019) |
| *Arachis hypogaea Linn* | Leguminosae | In vitro | *Tetranychus cinnabarinus* | 99.61% | (Liu et al. 2019) |
| *Perilla frutescens (L.) Britt.* | Labiatae | In vitro | *Tetranychus cinnabarinus* | 36% | (Liu et al. 2019) |
| *Lilium brownii var. viridulum baker* | Liliaceae | In vitro | *Tetranychus cinnabarinus* | 33.92% | (Liu et al. 2019) |
| *Nelumbo nucifera* | Nymphaeaceae | In vitro | *Tetranychus cinnabarinus* | 28.83% | (Liu et al. 2019) |
| *Phragmites australis* | Gramineae | In vitro | *Tetranychus cinnabarinus* | 24.40% | (Liu et al. 2019) |
| *Platycladus orientalis* | Cupressaceae | In vitro | *Tetranychus cinnabarinus* | 24.28% | (Liu et al. 2019) |
| *Zanthoxylum myriacanthum Wall* | Rutaceae | In vitro | *Tetranychus urticae* Koch | 64% | (Kruewong and Auamcharoen 2023) |
| *Zanthoxylum myriacanthum Wall* | Rutaceae | In vitro | *Tetranychus truncatus* | 64% | (Kruewong and Auamcharoen 2023) |
| *Zygophyllum album* | Zygophyllaceae | In vitro | *Tetranychus urticae* Koch | 66.66% | (Emam and Ibrahim 2020) |
| *Calotropis porcera* | Apocynaceae | In vitro | *Tetranychus urticae* Koch | 93.33% | (Emam and Ibrahim 2020) |
| *Jatropha curcas L* | Euphorbiaceae | In vitro | *Eutetranychus orientalis* | 94.12% | (Jang and Kuk 2020) |
| *Datura stramonium* | Solanaceae | In vitro | *Tetranychus urticae* | 93.30% | (Abou-Shosha 2020) |
| *Hyoscoyamus muticus* | Solanaceae | In vitro | *Tetranychus urticae* | 94.12% | (Abou-Shosha 2020) |
| *Jatropha curcas* | Euphorbiaceae | In vitro | *Tetranychus urticae* | 98.58% | (Abou-Shosha 2020) |
| *Azadirachtin indica* | Meliaceae | In vitro | *Sarcoptes scabiei* | 25% | (Pasipanodya et al. 2021) |
| *Dittrichia viscosa* | Asteraceae | In vitro | *Varroa destructo* | 27% | (Assouguem et al. 2022) |

| Source plant | Family | In vitro and in silico | Mites species | % Mortality | Reference |
|---|---|---|---|---|---|
| *Euclaptus globulus* | Myrtaceae | In vitro | *Varroa destructors* | 100% | (Assouguem et al. 2022) |
| *Calpurnia aurea* | Fabaceae | In vitro | *Varroa destructors* | 80% | (Assouguem et al. 2022) |
| *Ocimum basilicum* | Lamiaceae | In vitro | *Varroa destructors* | 100% | (Assouguem et al. 2022) |
| *Allium sativum* | Amaryllidaceae | In vitro | *Varroa destructors* | 100.00% | (Assouguem et al. 2022) |
| *Cymbopogon citratus* | Poaceae | In vitro | *Varroa destructors* | 100.00% | (Assouguem et al. 2022) |
| *Mentha piperita* | Lamiaceae | In vitro | *Varroa destructors* | 93.33% | (Assouguem et al. 2022) |
| *Ocimum gratissimum* | Lamiaceae | In vitro | *Varroa destructors* | 86.67% | (Assouguem et al. 2022) |
| *Murraya paniculata* | Rutaceae | In vitro | *Oligonychus coffeae* | 50.85% | (Assouguem et al. 2022) |
| *Senna tora* | Fabaceae | In vitro | *Oligonychus coffeae* | 53.46% | (Assouguem et al. 2022) |
| *Amphineuron opulentum* | Thelypteridaceae | In vitro | *Oligonychus coffeae* | 67.03% | (Assouguem et al. 2022) |
| *Tithonia diversifolia* | Asteraceae | In vitro | *Oligonychus coffeae* | 69.77% | (Assouguem et al. 2022) |
| *Cassia alata* | Fabaceae | In vitro | *Oligonychus coffeae* | 59.40% | (Assouguem et al. 2022) |
| *Acacia nilotica* | Fabaceae | In vitro *and* in silico | *Sarcoptes scabiei* | 100% | (Khan et al. 2022) |
| *Psidium guajava* | Myrtaceae | In vitro *and* in silico | *Sarcoptes scabiei* | 100% | (Khan et al. 2022) |
| *Foeniculum vulgare* | Apiaceae | In vitro *and* in silico | *Varroa destructor* | 68% | (Bava et al. 2022) |
| *Mentha piperita* | Lamiaceae | In vitro | *Tetranychus urticae* | 50% | (Souza et al. 2022) |
| *Passiflora edulis* | Passifloraceae | In vitro | *Raoiella indica* | 98.80% | (Cuzzuol et al. 2023) |

demonstrated remarkable acaricidal activity against *D. gallinae*, achieving a 100% death rate at 100 mg/mL. Bufadienolides were identified as the cause of the remarkable potency of the *D. maritima* extract (Rhimi et al. 2019). The contact toxicity of the essential oil (EO) extracts from the following plants was tested: *D. gallinae*, a dangerous ectoparasite in avian systems; *Clausena anisata, Litchi chinensis, Lippia alba, Heracleum sphondylium, Pimpinella anisum, Crithmum maritimum*, and *Syzygium aromaticum*, which are among the plants that belong to this group. According to (Tabari et al. 2020b), *Syzygium aromaticum* and *Litchi chinensis* are possible sources of biopesticides for effective control strategies against *D. gallinae* infestations.

The in vitro acaricidal activity of EOs and crude extracts from *Laurus nobilis* against *D. gallinae* was assessed by (Alimi et al. 2021) using a contact toxicity test. 1.8-cineole (46.56%) was the main constituent of the *L. nobilis* derivative. Furthermore, the fumigant bioassay demonstrated significant activity for the EOs from *Cinnamomum cassia* (C. cassia) and *C. camphora* var. *linalooliferum* ($LC_{50}$, $25.43 \pm 1.0423$ μg/cm$^3$), with mortality rates of 96% and 61%, respectively. Gas chromatography–mass spectrometry (GC–MS) revealed that the main component of the EO from *C. cassia* and the linalool from *C. camphora* var. *linalooliferum* were trans-cinnamaldehyde (Bordin et al. 2021). The toxicity of *Pinus sylvestris* essential oil and its components against *Hyalomma scupense* and *Dermanyssus gallinae* ticks was examined, with D-limonene being the most effective molecule. D-limonene showed potential acaricidal action with $LC_{50}$ values lower than those of the essential oil as a whole. On the other hand, δ-3-carene showed slightly reduced toxicity. Overall, *P. sylvestris* oil has promise as a greener substitute, necessitating additional in vivo testing for safe veterinary application (Alimi et al. 2024). *Pistacia lentiscus* essential oil and its constituents were tested against *Dermanyssus gallinae* to determine their acaricidal effects; spraying proved to be more successful. The most active compound was 4-terpineol, while α-pinene also showed notable activity. Furthermore, 4-terpineol has been shown to have strong anti-acetylcholinesterase effects (Alimi et al. 2023).

Several investigations have shown that certain plant extracts, including those from *Syzygium aromaticum, Eupatorium adenophorum* (*E. adenophorum*), *Azadirachta indica*, and *Adonis coerulea* are extremely toxic to *Psoroptes cuniculi* and *Sarcoptes scabiei*. *E. adenophorum* is a common weed in woods, plantations, natural ecosystems, and agricultural settings in many regions of the world, particularly in China. Interestingly, the alcoholic extract (AE) from *E. adenophorum* showed significant toxicity against mites, eliminating all *S. scabiei* at concentrations of 0.5% and 1.0% (w/v). Furthermore, the extract completely eradicated *P. cuniculi* in 4 h at a concentration of 1% (w/v). At a concentration of 0.5%, the 9-hydroxy-ageraphorone compound was found to have a greater insecticidal impact than fenvalerate and 9-oxo-ageraphorone. Furthermore, compared to 9-hydroxy-ageraphorone, 9-oxo-10,11-dehydro-ageraphorone has stronger insecticidal effects (Nong et al. 2014).

The oil derived from *Origanum vulgare* (Oregano, Labiateae family) has strong acaricidal effects on *P. cuniculi.*, with effects that were dependent on both time and dose. Its main constituents are p-cymene, thymol, and carvacrol. In vitro tests revealed that oregano oil completely eradicated *P. cuniculi* in 1 h and 6 h at doses of 0.05% and 0.02%, respectively (v/v). Furthermore, a 20-day clinical evaluation of naturally infected rabbits showed that oregano oil, at doses of 1% and 5%, completely eradicated *P. cuniculi* infection, improving the mental and physical health of the animals (Shang et al. 2016b). Strong in vitro acaricidal activity against adult *P. cuniculi* was demonstrated by essential oil (EO) extracts from the shoots and leaves of *Rhododendron nivale*, with an $LT_{50}$ value of up to 4.17 mg/mL. The ears of the *P. cuniculi*-infected rabbits were clear of scabs and secretions by day 20 because of the EO treatment. *R. nivale* essential oil (EO) has strong acaricidal effects on *P. cuniculi* in vitro and is predominantly composed of cadinene (Guo et al. 2017). The acaricidal activity of the perennial herbaceous plant *Peganum harmala* against *P. cuniculi* was assessed in vitro. At a concentration of 100 mg/mL, the microwave-assisted extract (MAE) from *Peganum harmala* demonstrated an $LT_{50}$ value of 17.322 h. Vasicine, harmaline, and harmine were found to be the primary active components in the MAE extract (Shang et al. 2016a).

*Ailanthus altissima* (*A. altissima*) bark AE has been shown to have acaricidal efficacy against *P. cuniculi* and *S. scabiei* according to Gu et al. The $LT_{50}$ values of *A. altissima* bark AE at doses of 1, 0.5, and 0.25 g/mL (w/v) against *S. scabiei* were 0.60, 0.78, and 1.48 h, respectively. At the same doses according to (Gu et al. 2014), the median lethal time ($LT_{50}$) values for *P. cuniculi* were 1.29, 3.33, and 0.74 h, respectively. Thirty-one essential oils (EOs) from various plants have been shown to have acaricidal activity against *S. scabiei*. At concentrations between 10% and 0.1% (v/v), the maximum activity was shown by EOs of *Ocimum sanctum* and *Cinnamomum zeylanicum* (Andriantsoanirina et al. 2022). Ten essential oils were tested for their ability to effectively combat *S. scabiei*; palmarosa oil and 1% (v/v) clove oil were the most effective, eliminating all mites in 50 and 20 min, respectively. Clove > palmarosa > geranium > tea tree > lavender > manuka > bitter orange > eucalyptus > Japanese cedar was the sequence in which the tested oils were found to be most effective. However, there was no effect of cabare oil on *S. scabiei* (Fang et al. 2016).

The alcoholic extract (AE) of *Ligularia virgaurea* exhibited strong acaricidal effects on *S. scabiei*. According to Luo et al. (2015), the $LC_{50}$ values against mites varied depending on the period and were as follows: 1.388 g/mL at 1 h, 0.624 g/mL at 2 h, 0.310 g/mL at 4 h, and 0.213 g/mL at 6 h. The acaricidal activity of Benthic oil toward *Elsholtzia densa* (*E. densa*) was found to be significant in in vitro studies. The $LC_{50}$ values against *S. scabiei* were 7.678 mg/mL at 1 h, 4.623 mg/mL at 2 h, 2.543 mg/mL at 4 h, 1.502 mg/mL at 8 h, 1.298 mg/mL at 16 h, and 0.981 mg/mL at 24 h. Gas chromatography–mass spectrometry (GC–MS) revealed that the principal components of the Benth oil were thymol (26.58%) and 4-pyridinol (28.16%) (Zhou et al. 2019). Lemongrass oil had strong acaricidal effects on *Sarcoptes* mites. All mites were eliminated at concentrations of 10% and 5% (v/v) in 10 and 25 min, respectively. At 1, 3, 6, 12, and 24 h, the $LC_{50}$ values were 1.37%, 1.08%, 0.91%, 0.64%, and 0.48%, respectively. Furthermore, at different doses, lemongrass oil dramatically lowered the hatching rate of *the Sarcopetes* eggs. According to mass spectrometry research, citral is the primary ingredient in LG oil (Li et al. 2020). Three aqueous neem fruit extract concentrations (5%, 10%, and 25% w/v) were contrasted in a comparison study on pigs treated with a commercial acaricide called 12.5% amitraz-based Triatix spray (which was used as the positive control). Topical use of 25% aqueous neem fruit extract resulted in greater mite-fighting efficacy than did commercial acaricides (Pasipanodya et al. 2021).

*Adonis coerulea Maxim* exhibited acaricidal activity both in vitro and in vivo. Its main constituents are isoorientin, luteolin, apigenin, ellagic acid, convallatoxin, strophanthidin, and cymarin. It also minimizes the activity of the enzymes $Na^+$-$K^+$-ATPase and acetylcholinesterase (AchE) (Shang et al. 2017, 2020). Dai et al. (2020) investigated the mechanism by which the methanolic extract (ME) of *A. coerulea* affects AchE using LC–MS/MS and molecular docking. The main components identified were silibinin, quercetin, and corilagin, which had $IC_{50}$ values of 40.11, 46.15, and 50.98 μg/mL, respectively, indicating the inhibition of AchE activity at the cellular level (Dai et al. 2020). Both in vitro and in vivo, coconut seed extract demonstrated acaricidal effects on S. scabies. After 1 day in vitro, the mortality rate of mites reached 99%, and molecular analysis revealed the inhibition of the expression of various genes. Molecular docking research revealed that 300 (1000-O-β-D-glucopyranosyl)-sucrose and gondoic acid were the primary compounds in coconut seed extract that killed mites (Zahran et al. 2022).

## 11.5 Acaricidal Activity of Plant Compounds on Mites

This section discusses some naturally occurring substances that have acaricidal properties. Cinnamaldehyde is an α,β-unsaturated aldehyde that is one of the phytochemicals present in essential oils (EOs) and is known for its exceptional antibacterial qualities and ability to increase the efficacy of antibiotics. Since cinamic acid and its esters are found in many different plants, they have garnered much interest because of their varied pharmacological properties. The acaricidal properties of trans-cinnamaldehyde and ethyl cinnamate, which are analogs of cinnamic acid, have also been documented. Due to its antibacterial effect, cinnamonaldehyde—which is particularly prevalent in essential oils derived from Cinnamomum species—finds extensive use as a food additive and is valuable for possible application in the food and medical industries (Usai and Di Sotto 2023). The acaricidal action of trans-cinnamaldehyde against *P. cuniculi* was assessed in vitro, and mite mortality rates were shown to be significantly greater at 8 μg/mL ($p < 0.01$) (Shen et al. 2012). Derivatives of ethyl cinnamate have been found to be effective and promising acaricides against *P. cuniculi*. According to a structure-activity relationship (SAR) analysis, the activity of the benzene ring considerably increased when o-$NO_2$ or m-$NO_2$ was present; however, the activity decreased when hydroxy, methoxy, acetoxy, methylenedioxy, bromo, or chloro groups were added (Zhang et al. 2015).

The acaricidal efficacy of the *Urtica fissa* leaf ethyl acetate extract against *Sarcoptes scabiei* mites was investigated, and complete mite eradication was observed within 2 h at 100 mg/mL. LC–MS analysis revealed major compounds, including schaftoside (8.259%) and carnosol (6.736%), suggesting potential new avenues for mite management in veterinary medicine (Liao et al. 2023). To assess their in vitro acaricidal properties against *P. cuniculi*, (Chen et al. 2018) synthesized derivatives of cinnamic acid and isoaromatic ring analogs. Eight of the compounds showed greater activity. Analysis of the structure-activity relationship (SAR) emphasized how important the carbonyl group is to this activity. The steric hindrance close to the ester group and the kind and length of the alkoxy group in the ester moiety also had a large impact on the activity. In contrast to acids, amides, ketones, or thiol esters, ester derivatives showed higher activity. The activity of cinnamic esters was greatly increased by substituting α-pyridyl or α-furanyl groups with phenyl groups. Eighteen coumarins were tested for their ability to prevent pruritus; of them, 4-methoxy-coumarin demonstrated the highest anti-mite activity, 34.00 μg/mL for the $LC_{50}$ value. Significantly, 4-methoxy-coumarin showed minimal to no toxicity to normal human hepatocytes and keratinocytes, with an $LC_{50}$ value above 100 μg/mL, indicating that it might be studied further and developed further, especially for the treatment of pruritus (Shang et al. 2019). Eugenol is a naturally occurring phenolic monoterpenoid that is a member of the phenylpropanoid class of natural compounds and has bioactive characteristics. It can be extracted from clove plants (*Syzygium aromaticum*) and is present in a variety of aromatic herbal plants, including pepper, tulsi, clove, cinnamon, and nutmeg. Eugenol is widely used in the food, flavoring, cosmetics, pharmaceutical, and agricultural industries, among others, renowned for having a wide range of pharmacological qualities, such as analgesic, antibacterial, antioxidant, and anticancer activities (Sharma et al. 2022).

Eugenol at 4 mg/mL for 8 h was shown by Ma et al. (2019) to be able to completely eradicate *P. cuniculi* mites. The median lethal dose ($LD_{50}$) of eugenol at 1 to 24 h after treatment ranged from 1.564 ± 0.023 to 1.039 ± 0.009 mg/mL. One study proposed that eugenol kills mites by interfering with multiple signaling pathways, such as the TNF (tumor necrosis factor), PPAR (peroxisome proliferator-activated receptor), Rap1, NF-kappa B, and Ras pathways (Ma et al. 2019). For example, eugenol binds to NADH dehydrogenase chain 2 and blocks mitochondrial respiratory chain complex I activity in the oxidative phosphorylation pathway, resulting in mite mortality (Shang et al. 2020). Five compounds were tested for their ability to suppress the growth of both naturally infected rabbit eggs and control eggs: terpine-4-ol, citral, linalool, eugenol, and geranyl. Citral, linalool, geranyl, eugenol, and terpine-4-ol were shown to have median effect concentrations ($EC_{50}$) of 0.65%, 0.66%, 0.85%, 1.47%, and 2.87%, respectively (Fang et al. 2020).

Thymol is a monoterpene that is present in many natural plant essential oils (EOs) and is very toxic to scabies mites. After 4 h of exposure, the $LC_{50}$ of thymol against scabies mites was 3.829 mg/mL in this study. As part of its acaricidal function, thymol interferes with the energy metabolism and nerve conduction of mites.

1,8-another monoterpene present in many essential oils, cineole, has the ability to alter the activity of GSTs, NOS, and SOD in the nervous system of Scabies (Hu et al. 2015). The acaricidal activity of 9-oxo-10,11-dehydroageraphorone (euptox A), a cadinane sesquiterpene derived from *E. adenophorum*, was tested against *S. scabiei* and *P. cuniculi* both in vitro and in vivo. In vitro tests carried out within 4 h of treatment revealed that euptox A was completely lethal to *P. cuniculi* at 4 mg/mL and killed all *S. scabiei* mites at 3–5 mg/mL (Liao et al. 2014). At a dose of 2 mg/mL, euptox A demonstrated greater clinical acaricidal effectiveness against *P. cuniculi* in vivo (Hu et al. 2014).

The effectiveness of various terpene combinations, such as menthol, thymol, and carvacrol, against *D. gallinae* was evaluated by (Tabari et al. 2023) at 0.5 μg/mL, and they discovered that the combination of all three compounds killed 100% of the mites, making it the most effective. Furthermore, under field conditions, this terpene-based combination showed encouraging miticidal action, producing eggs with little residue, indicating its potential for use in ecologically friendly pest management techniques (Tabari et al. 2023).

Six terpenes often found in essential oils (EOs), namely, carvacrol, eugenol, geraniol, citral, terpine-4-ol, and linalool, were tested by Li et al. (2021) for their ability to inhibit Scabies adults and eggs. Carvacrol, eugenol, geranyl, citral, terpine-4-ol, and linalool had $EC_{50}$ values of 0.5%, 0.9%, 2.0%, 4.8%, 5.1%, and 9.8%, respectively (w/v). These terpenoids might work by piercing the egg aerogen membrane. Notably, geraniol, eugenol, and carvacrol all exhibited strong ovicidal effects (Li et al. 2021). The efficacy of carvacrol, eugenol, and geraniol against *Sarcoptes* scabiei was evaluated, with carvacrol demonstrating the highest miticidal efficacy at 0.5%, followed by eugenol and geraniol. These compounds have potential as complementary or alternative agents for treating scabies and sarcoptic mange, providing a basis for essential oil-based scabicidal product development (Li et al. 2021).

Alkaloids are essential nitrogen-containing chemical molecules found in a wide range of plant species and play significant roles in various biological activities. Three bioactive alkaloids from Peganum harmala L., vasicine, harmaline, and harmine, were tested by Shang et al. (2016a) for their acaricidal effects on *P. cuniculi* in vitro. At 2.5 mg/mL, the $LT_{50}$ values for vasicine, harmaline, and harmine against *P. cuniculi* were 9.791, 10.095, and 9.273 h, respectively (Shang et al. 2016a). The Fumariaceae, Papaveraceae, and Rutaceae families of plants include the quaternary benzo[c]phenanthridine alkaloids sanguinarine and chelerythrine. By altering the C=N+ bonds of sanguinarine and chelerythrine, Miao et al. created derivatives and evaluated their in vitro acaricidal activity against *P. cuniculi*. Compared to the commercial acaricide ivermectin, one derivative, 6-alkoxy dihydrosanguinarine, showed strong acaricidal efficacy against *P. cuniculi* at 5.0 mg/mL. The acaricidal characteristics of the sanguinarine and chelerythrine derivatives were assessed by modification of the C=N+ double bond, which revealed that quaternary benzo[c]phenanthridine alkaloids have potential for use in the creation of new isoquinoline acaricidal medications (Miao et al. 2012).

## 11.6 Green Synthesis of Nanoparticles

Nanotechnology has diverse applications in veterinary medicine, including agropecuary supply traceability, monitoring, diagnosis, and treatment (Kumar 2010). NPs offer advantages in drug delivery systems, including reduced toxicity and site-specific targeting achieved through the attachment of targeted ligands on particle surfaces. These systems allow various routes of administration, such as oral, nasal, parenteral, and intraocular routes. Additionally, the limitations of antiparasitic drugs, including toxicity and resistance, are being addressed through nanobiotechnology in livestock science, particularly in treating parasitic infections and arthropod vectors (Fig. 11.2) (Benelli and Lukehart 2017; Rai and Ingle 2012; Underwood and Van Eps 2012). NPs such as silver, gold, zinc oxide, selenium oxide, and chitosan exhibit high efficacy in inhibiting vectors of parasitic infections (Sujitha et al. 2015). With their smaller size and greater surface area, formulations of liquid nanoparticles face challenges in particle aggregation (Jawahar and Meyyanathan 2012). Although limited, researchers have begun studying the *R. microplus* toxicity of several metallic nanoparticles.

Zinc oxide nanoparticles, which are produced via a wet chemical process with sodium hydroxide and zinc nitrate, are effective at exhibiting acaricidal properties. Following treatment with ZnO nanoparticles, the mortality rates of *Rhipicephalus microplus* were 43% at 1 h, 64% at 3 h, 78% at 6 h, and 100% at 12 h. One hundred percent of *R. microplus* was killed by chemically produced ZnO nanoparticles at 10 mg/L, with an $LC_{50}$ of 13.41 mg/L (Kirthi et al. 2011). Furthermore, zinc oxide nanoparticles (Ll-ZnO NPs) produced from *Lobelia leschenaultiana* leaf extract showed efficacy against *R. microplus*. After treatment with varying quantities of zinc acetate, *L. leschenaultiana* leaf extract, and Ll-ZnO NPs for 24 h, adult *R. microplus* showed mortality rates of 93.33%, 70%, and 100%, respectively, with corresponding $LC_{50}$ values of 5 mg/L, 19.2 mg/L, and 1.7 mg/L, respectively. Interestingly, compared with those of zinc acetate and leaf extracts from *L. leschenaultiana*, the mortality and $LC_{50}$ of Ll-ZnO NPs were much lower (Banumathi et al. 2016).

Marimuthu et al. (2011) investigated the antiparasitic activity of silver nanoparticles made with aqueous *Mimosa pudica* leaf extract against *R. microplus* larvae. At 20 mg/L, the greatest death rate of 89% was recorded, with an $LC_{50}$ of 8.98 mg/L. Additionally, the antiparasitic properties of *Manilkara zapota* (*M. zapota*) stem aqueous extract and aqueous leaf extract against *R. microplus* were investigated. At concentrations of 3.125, 6.25, 12.5, 25, and 50 mg/L, the aqueous leaf extracts of *M. zapota* had mortality rates of 13%, 25%, 48%, 56%, and 75%, respectively. The highest death rates (18% at 1.25 mg/L, 34% at 2.5 mg/L, 67% at 5 mg/L, 86% at 10 mg/L, and 100% at 20 mg/L) were observed for the silver nanoparticles produced from the aqueous leaf extract of *M. zapota*. The aqueous leaf extract of *M. zapota* has an $LC_{50}$ of 3.44 mg/L for silver nanoparticles, according to Rajakumar and Rahuman (2012).

Additionally, research has been conducted on the acaricidal effects of *Cissus quadrangularis* aqueous extract and silver nanoparticles made from the stem

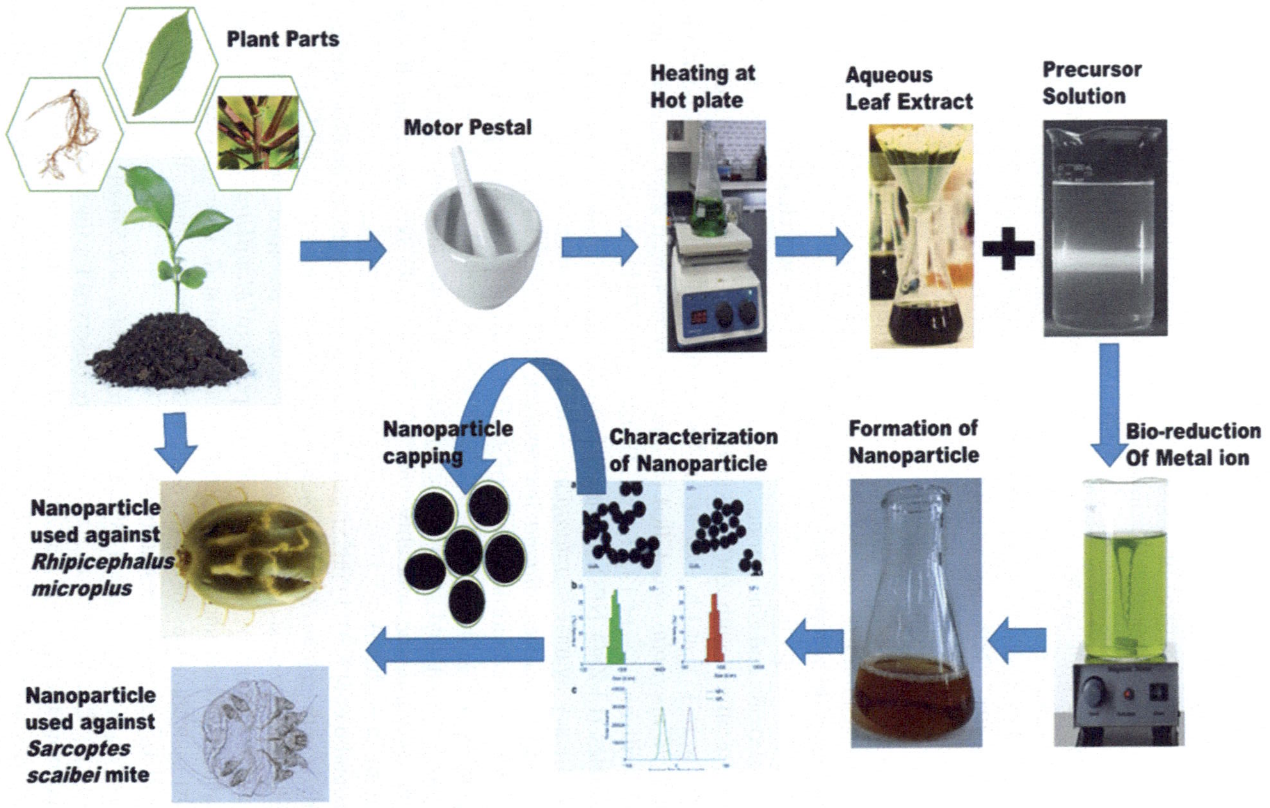


**Fig. 11.2** Green synthesis of nanoparticles that can be used as acaricides

aqueous extract of *C. quadrangularis* against *R. microplus* larvae (Santhoshkumar et al. 2012). At concentrations of 10, 20, 30, 40, and 50 mg/L, the aqueous extracts of *C. quadrangularis* resulted in mortality rates of 8%, 25%, 33%, 40%, and 59%, respectively. On the other hand, greater death rates were observed for silver nanoparticles made with *C. quadrangularis* stem aqueous extract (42% at 5 mg/L, 55% at 10 mg/L, 68% at 15 mg/L, 85% at 20 mg/L, and 100% at 25 mg/L). An aqueous stem extract of *C. quadrangularis* was used to create silver nanoparticles, which had $LC_{50}$ and $LC_{90}$ values of 7.61 mg/L and 22.68 mg/L, respectively (Santhoshkumar et al. 2012).

Metallic copper nanoparticles were synthesized through a polyol process and evaluated against *R. microplus* larvae. The mortality rates of the larvae were 36%, 47%, 69%, 88%, and 100% at concentrations of 0.5, 1.0, 2.0, 4.0, and 8.0 mg/L, respectively, with an $LC_{50}$ of 1.06 mg/L (Ramyadevi et al. 2011). The larvicidal activity against *R. microplus* was investigated using nanoparticles synthesized via a chemical route employing a solution of nickel hydrazine complexes. The mortality rates of the larvae were 25%, 45%, 69%, 80%, and 100% at concentrations of 5, 10, 15, 20, and 25 mg/L, respectively. According to Rajakumar et al. (2013), the $LC_{50}$ values of the synthesized Ni nanoparticles and the Ni–hydrazine complex solution were 10.17 mg/L and 20.35 mg/L, respectively.

Because of their stability, oxidizing capacity, and relative nontoxicity, titanium dioxide nanoparticles are recognized as possible photocatalytic materials (Murugan et al. 2016; Rajakumar et al. 2015). $TiO_2$ nanoparticles made from aqueous extracts of *Calotropis gigantea* flowers were tested against *R. microplus* larvae to determine their acaricidal activity. Following treatment with the floral extract and 50 mg/L $TiO(OH)_2$ solution, the mortality rates were 94% and 88%, respectively. At a concentration of 20 mg/L, green-synthesized $TiO_2$ nanoparticles showed 100% mortality with an $LC_{50}$ of 5.43 mg/L (Marimuthu et al. 2013). Additionally, after treatment with $TiO_2$ nanoparticles derived from the aqueous extract of *Mangifera indica*, the mortality rates of *R. microplus* were reported to be 19%, 32%, 54%, 74%, and 100% at concentrations of 5, 10, 15, 20, and 25 mg/L, respectively, with an $LC_{50}$ of 13.21 mg/L (Rajakumar et al. 2015).

In conclusion, smaller nanoparticles improve biocompatibility and have benefits for parasitology and biomedicine (Benelli et al. 2016). Further research efforts are warranted to elucidate the mechanism of action of metal and metal oxide nanoparticles as potential acaricides against *R. microplus*. Limited information is available on this topic. The small size of the nanoparticles facilitates penetration of the nuclear membrane, enabling interactions with nucleic acids and protein synthesis. Additionally, the ability of Ectoparasites to move physically may be impeded by the adherence of green-capped nanoparticles to their exoskeleton (Baun et al. 2008). Moreover, the use of phytochemical-capped nanoparticles may increase toxicity to ticks because of the large surface-to-volume ratio of the nanocarriers.

Various studies have been carried out by our laboratory to assess the therapeutic potential of different plants against ticks and mites both in vitro and in silico. These studies provided insights into the potential efficacy of plant extracts against test ticks and mites as well as the inhibitory mechanisms of action against key mite and tick proteins. For instance, Ayub et al. (2023) reported the efficacy of *Pinus roxburghii* plant extracts against *R. microplus* ticks via in vitro and in silico assays. This study revealed good interactions between catechin and myricetin pythochemicals from this plant and the active site residues of the target protein, with docking scores of −7.7 kcal/mol and −7.6 kcal/mol, respectively. Another study by Saman et al. (2022) showed that the glutathione S-transferase *R. microplus* (RmGST) was inhibited by the phytochemical extracts of *Datura innnoxia* Plants: norapoatropine and 7-hydroxyhyoscyamine strongly interacted with the active site residues of RmGST, with docking scores of −7.3 and −7.0 kcal/mol, respectively. Similarly, the triose-phosphate isomerase (RmTIM) protein showed docking scores of −8.3, − 7.7 and −6.9 kcal/mol for rutin, naringin, and myricitin, respectively, extracted from *Pleurotus ostreatus*, showing significant interactions with the active site residues of RmTIM (Alotaibi et al. 2023). Additionally, an in silico study of *Camellia sinensis* plant phytochemicals with *S. scabiei* and *R. microplus* glutathione transferase proteins SsGST and RmGST revealed a strong binding interaction between ellagic acid and the SsGST protein, with a binding energy of −7.3 kcal/mol, with respect to permethrin (−6.7 kcal/mol), whereas quercetin and RmGST resulted in a docking score of −8.6 kcal/mol compared to that of deltamethrin (−8.2 kcal/mol). Overall, this study explored the potential of *C. sinensis* as a natural alternative for controlling tick and mite infestations and provided insights into the inhibitory mechanisms of its phytochemicals (Hakami et al. 2023). The docking experiments of *Acacia nilotica* and *Psidium guajava* against *S. scabiei* aspartic protease (SsAP) revealed docking scores of −6.50993 and −6.16359, respectively, for clionasterol and mangiferin from *A. nilotica* inhibiting the targeted protein SsAP, while only beta-sitosterol from *P. guajava* interacted with the SsAP active site, with a docking score of −6.20532 (Khan et al. 2022). Seven flavonoids (methylenebisphloridzin, thearubigin, fortunellin, quercetagetin-7-O-(6-O-caffeoyl-β-D-glucopyranoside) 1, quercetagetin-7-O- (6-O-p-coumaroyl-β-glucopyranoside), rutin, and kaempferol 3-neohesperidoside) were docked against *R microplus* acetylcholinesterase (RmAChE1), confirming their strong interaction (Malak et al. 2023).

## References

Abdallah A, Abbassy M, Salem A (2015) Efficacy of two essential oil extracts and predatory mite *Phytoseiulus persimilis* in suppressing the population of the two-spotted spider mite, *Tetranychus urticae* KOCH. J Plant Protect Pathol 6(7):1123–1133

Abdel-Ghany HS, Abdel-Shafy S, Abuowarda M, El-Khateeb RM, Hoballah EM, Fahmy MM (2021a) Acaricidal activity of *Artemisia herba-alba* and *Melia azedarach* oil nanoemulsion against *Hyalomma dromedarii* and their toxicity on Swiss albino mice. Exp Appl Acarol 84:241–262

Abdel-Ghany H, Abdel-Shafy S, Abuowarda M, El-Khateeb R, Hoballah E, Fahmy M (2021b) Acaricidal activity of some medicinal plant extracts against different developmental stages of the camel tick *Hyalomma dromedarii*. Adv Anim Vet Sci 9(5):722–733

Abdel-Ghany HS, Abdel-Shafy S, Abuowarda MM, El-Khateeb RM, Hoballah EM, Fahmy MM (2022) Acaricidal efficacy of biosynthesized zinc oxide nanoparticles against *Hyalomma dromedarii* (Acari: Ixodidae) and their toxic effects on Swiss albino mice. Acta Parasitol 67(2):878–891

Abdel-Shafy S, Alanazi AD, Gabr HS, Allam AM, Abou-Zeina HA, Masoud RA, Soliman DE, Alshahrani MY (2020) Efficacy and safety of ethanolic *Curcuma longa* extract as a treatment for sand tampan ticks in a rabbit model. Vet World 13(4):812

Abou-Shosha M (2020) Field trial of three plant extracts against *Tetranychus urticae* population as a comparative with acaricidal (Abamectin) on two vegetable crops. J Plant Protect Pathol 11(9):473–476

Adenubi O, Fasina F, McGaw L, Eloff J, Naidoo V (2016) Plant extracts to control ticks of veterinary and medical importance: a review. S Afr J Bot 105:178–193

Adenubi OT, Ahmed AS, Fasina FO, McGaw LJ, Eloff JN, Naidoo V (2018a) Pesticidal plants as a possible alternative to synthetic acaricides in tick control: a systematic review and meta-analysis. Ind Crop Prod 123:779–806

Adenubi OT, McGaw LJ, Eloff JN, Naidoo V (2018b) In vitro bioassays used in evaluating plant extracts for tick repellent and acaricidal properties: a critical review. Vet Parasitol 254:160–171

Adenubi OT, Leboho T, Eloff JN, Fouche G, Naidoo V, Wellington KW, McGaw LJ (2019) Acaricidal activity of the aqueous and hydroethanolic extracts of 15 south African plants against *Rhipicephalus turanicus* and their toxicity on human liver and kidney cells. Onderstepoort J Vet Res 86(1):1–7

Adenubi O, Salihu T, Mbaoji CO, Ojogbo IA, Abdullahi M (2020) A review of ethnoveterinary botanicals used for tick control in Wukari, Taraba state, north eastern Nigeria. Egypt J Vet Sci 51(3):421–437

Aguiar RW, dos Santos SF, da Silva Morgado F, Ascencio SD, de Mendonça Lopes M, Viana KF, Didonet J, Ribeiro BM (2015) Insecticidal and repellent activity of *Siparuna guianensis* Aubl. (Negramina) against *Aedes aegypti* and *Culex quinquefasciatus*. PLoS One 10(2):e0116765. https://doi.org/10.1371/journal.pone.0116765

Agwunobi DO, Pei T, Yang J, Wang X, Lv L, Shen R, Yu Z, Liu J (2020) Expression profiles of glutathione S-transferases genes in semi-engorged *Haemaphysalis longicornis* (Acari: Ixodidae) exposed to *Cymbopogon citratus* essential oil. Syst Appl Acarol 25(5):918–930

Ahmad MS, Shawky A, Ghobashy MO, Felifel RHA (2018) Effect of some medicinal plants on life cycle of citrus Brown mites (*Eutetranychus orientalis*). Int J Pharmaceut Res Allied Sci 7(4):13–17

Aimée D, Patrick YK, Christian TDK, Alain A, Koffi K (2017) Evaluation of acaricide activity in the leaves extracts of four medicinal local plants on *Rhipicephalus* (*Boophilus*) *microplus* (Canestrini, 1888). Pharma Innov J 6(7):78–85

Ajith Kumar KG, Fular A, Chigure G, Sharma AK, Nagar G, Souza FF, Bechara GH, Ghosh S (2019) Comparative impact of coumaphos, amitraz and plant extract of *Ageratum conyzoides* on the oogenesis of *Rhipicephalus microplus*. Ticks Tick Borne Dis 10(5):1085–1095. https://doi.org/10.1016/j.ttbdis.2019.06.003

Al Khoury C, Nemer N, Nemer G, Kurban M, Bernigaud C, Fischer K, Guillot J (2020) In vitro activity of Beauvericin against all developmental stages of *Sarcoptes scabiei*. Antimicrob Agents Chemother 64(5):e02118. https://doi.org/10.1128/aac.02118-19

Al Mamun MS, Hoque MM, Ahmed M, Sarkar A, Kabir H (2015) Evaluation of some indigenous plant extracts against red spider mite, *Oligonychus coffeae* Nietner (Acari: Tetranychydae) in tea. Persian J Acarol 4(4):425

Alamgeer, Younis W, Asif H, Sharif A, Riaz H, Bukhari IA, Assiri AM (2018) Traditional medicinal plants used for respiratory disorders in Pakistan: a review of the ethno-medicinal and pharmacological evidence. Chinas Med 13:48. https://doi.org/10.1186/s13020-018-0204-y

Al-Hasnawi, M. R. A., & Wathah, E. F. (2019). Effect of temperature and different extracts of *Datura metel* leaves on some biological aspects of *Hyalomma schulzei* (Acari: Ixodidae). In J Phys Conf Ser 1294 6, 062014).

Al-Hoshani N, Zaman MA, Syaad KMA, Salman M, Rehman TU, Olmeda AS (2023) Assessment of repellency and acaricidal potential of *Nigella sativa* essential oil using *Rhipicephalus microplus* ticks. Pak Vet J 43:606–610

Ali AAB, Taha MA (2023) Controlling *Argas arboreus* and *A. Persicus* (Acari: Argasidae) by *Adiantum capillus-veneris* L. extracts with phytochemical analysis. Vet Parasitol 324:110067

Alibeigi Z, Rakhshandehroo E, Saharkhiz MJ, Alavi AM (2023) The acaricidal and repellent activity of the essential and nano essential oil of Thymus vulgaris against the brown dog tick, *Rhipicephalus sanguineus* (Acari: Ixodidae)

Alimi D, Hajri A, Jallouli S, Sebai H (2021) In vitro acaricidal activity of essential oil and crude extracts of *Laurus nobilis*,(Lauraceae) grown in Tunisia, against arthropod ectoparasites of livestock and poultry: *Hyalomma scupense* and *Dermanyssus gallinae*. Vet Parasitol 298:109507

Alimi D, Hajri A, Jallouli S, Sebai H (2022) Valorization of volatile oils and some crude extracts from the Tunisian plants *Juniperus communis* and *Origanum majorana* for the control of *Hyalomma scupense* (Acari: Ixodidae). Waste Biomass Valor 13(10):4165–4177

Alimi D, Hajri A, Jallouli S, Sebai H (2023) *Pistacia lentiscus* essential oil and its pure active components as acaricides to control *Dermanyssus gallinae* (Acari: Mesostigmata). Vet Parasitol 322:110028

Alimi D, Hajri A, Jallouli S, Sebai H (2024) Study on in vitro Acaricidal proprieties of *Pinus sylvestris* against two Ectoparasites of veterinary importance *Dermanyssus gallinae* and *Hyalomma scupense*. Waste Biomass Valor 15(1):337–347

Alotaibi BS, Malak N, Khan A, Nasreen N, Niaz S, Ahmad I, Khan A, Rodriguez-Vivas RI, Chen C-C (2023) Acaricidal assessment of the fungal extract of *Pleurotus ostreatus* against *Rhipicephalus microplus*: role of in vitro and in silico analysis. Heliyon 9(9):e19600

Amante M, Hailu Y, Terefe G, Asres K (2019) *In-vitro* louscidal and acaricidal activities of alkaloid of *Calpurnia aurea* extracts against *Linognathus ovillus* and *Amblyomma variegatum*. Int J Appl Nat Sci 10(1):431–437

Amaro NB, de Castro Junior LC, Inácio CDO, Leles R, Dalessandro W, de Freitas EF, Marques EF, Vieira PC, Fazolin M, Fernandes FF (2019) Evaluation of the potential acaricidal of the hexanic extract of *Trichilia pallida* SW.(Sapindales: Meliaceae) leaves and essential oil of *Sesamum indicum* Linn.(Lamilaes: Pedaliaceae) seeds against larval instar of *Rhipicephalus sanguineus* (Lat.)(Acari: Ixodidae). SaBios Rev Saúde e Biol 14:1–11

Andriantsoanirina V, Guillot J, Ratsimbason M, Mekhloufi G, Randriamialinoro F, Ranarivelo L, Ariey F, Durand R (2022) *In vitro* efficacy of essential oils against *Sarcoptes scabiei*. Sci Rep 12(1):7176

Anholeto LA, de Oliveira PR, Rodrigues RAF, Yamane LT, Castro KNDC, Camargo-Mathias MI (2018) Morphological alterations in the ovaries of *Amblyomma cajennense* semi-engorged ticks exposed to ethanolic extract of *Acmella oleracea*. Microsc Res Tech 81(11):1347–1357

Anshu S, Pratibha J, Sw K (2020) Efficacy of *Nicotiana tabacum* as a biocontrol agent against cattle ticks. J Entomol Zool Stud 8:220–222

Assouguem A, Kara M, Ramzi A, Annemer S, Kowalczyk A, Ali EA, Moharram BA, Lazraq A, Farah A (2022) Evaluation of the effect of four bioactive compounds in combination with chemical product against two spider mites *Tetranychus urticae* and *Eutetranychus orientalis* (Acari: Tetranychidae). Evid Based Complement Alternat Med 2022:2004623

Astuti LT, Sugihartuti R, Nagoi L, Lastuti NDR, Meles DK, Sunarso A (2019) The potential of anting–anting (Acalypha indica L.) leaf extract as anti-scabies to *Sarcoptes scabiei* var. Cuniculi in vitro. J Parasit Sci 3(2):67

Attia S, Grissa KL, Ghrabi ZG, Mailleux AC, Lognay G, Hance T (2012) Acaricidal activity of 31 essential oils extracted from plants collected in Tunisia. J Essent Oil Res 24(3):279–288

Auamcharoen W, Chandrapatya A (2015) Acaricidal and ovicidal efficacies of *Leucaena glauca* Benth. Seed crude extracts on *Tetranychus urticae* Koch (Acari: Tetranychidae). J Biopest 8(2):68

Ayub S, Malak N, Cossío-Bayúgar R, Nasreen N, Khan A, Niaz S, Khan A, Alanazi AD, Ben Said M (2023) In vitro and *in silico* protocols for the assessment of anti-tick compounds from *Pinus roxburghii* against *Rhipicephalus* (*Boophilus*) *microplus* ticks. Animals 13(8):1388

Bai L, Gao Z, Xu X, Lv W, Wang Y, Dong K, Yu Z, Yang X (2024) The acaricidal activity and enzymatic targets of the essential oils of *Cinnamomum cassia* and *Cinnamomum camphora* and their major components against *Haemaphysalis longicornis* (Acari: Ixodidae). Ind Crop Prod 209:117967

Banumathi B, Malaikozhundan B, Vaseeharan B (2016) In vitro acaricidal activity of ethnoveterinary plants and green synthesis of zinc oxide nanoparticles against *Rhipicephalus* (*Boophilus*) *microplus*. Vet Parasitol 216:93–100

Baran AI, Jahanghiri F, Hajipour N, Sparagano OAE, Norouzi R, Moharramnejad S (2020) In vitro acaricidal activity of essential oil and alcoholic extract of *Trachyspermum ammi* against *Dermanyssus gallinae*. Vet Parasitol 278:109030. https://doi.org/10.1016/j.vetpar.2020.109030

Baun A, Hartmann NB, Grieger K, Kusk KO (2008) Ecotoxicity of engineered nanoparticles to aquatic invertebrates: a brief review and recommendations for future toxicity testing. Ecotoxicology 17:387–395

Bava R, Castagna F, Palma E, Musolino V, Carresi C, Cardamone A, Lupia C, Marrelli M, Conforti F, Roncada P (2022) Phytochemical profile of *Foeniculum vulgare* subsp. *piperitum* essential oils and evaluation of acaricidal efficacy against *Varroa destructor* in Apis mellifera by in vitro and semi-field fumigation tests. Vet Sci 9(12):684

Benelli G (2016) Plant-mediated biosynthesis of nanoparticles as an emerging tool against mosquitoes of medical and veterinary importance: a review. Parasitol Res 115(1):23–34. https://doi.org/10.1007/s00436-015-4800-9

Benelli G, Lukehart CM (2017) Applications of green-synthesized nanoparticles in pharmacology, parasitology and entomology. J Clust Sci 28:1–2

Benelli G, Pavela R (2018) Repellence of essential oils and selected compounds against ticks-A systematic review. Acta Trop 179:47–54. https://doi.org/10.1016/j.actatropica.2017.12.025

Benelli G, Bedini S, Cosci F, Toniolo C, Conti B, Nicoletti M (2015a) Larvicidal and ovideterrent properties of neem oil and fractions against the filariasis vector *Aedes albopictus* (Diptera: Culicidae): a bioactivity survey across production sites. Parasitol Res 114(1):227–236. https://doi.org/10.1007/s00436-014-4183-3

Benelli G, Bedini S, Flamini G, Cosci F, Cioni PL, Amira S, Benchikh F, Laouer H, Di Giuseppe G, Conti B (2015b) Mediterranean essential oils as effective weapons against the West Nile vector *Culex pipiens* and the Echinostoma intermediate host *Physella acuta*: what happens around? An acute toxicity survey on non-target mayflies. Parasitol Res 114(3):1011–1021. https://doi.org/10.1007/s00436-014-4267-0

Benelli G, Pavela R, Canale A, Mehlhorn H (2016) Tick repellents and acaricides of botanical origin: a green roadmap to control tick-borne diseases? Parasitol Res 115(7):2545–2560. https://doi.org/10.1007/s00436-016-5095-1

Bernigaud C, Fischer K, Chosidow O (2020) The Management of *Scabies* in the 21st century: past, advances and potentials. Acta Derm Venereol 100(9):adv00112. https://doi.org/10.2340/00015555-3468

Bhaskar S, Sharma V, Rahal A (2021) Acaricidal bioefficacy of Calotropisprocera (Asclepiadaceae) of middle Gangetic region against cattle tick, *Rhipicephalus microplus* and their Gc-Ms analysis. Ann Rom Soc Cell Biol 25:1795–1809

Bissinger B, Apperson C, Watson D, Arellano C, Sonenshine D, Roe R (2011) Novel field assays and the comparative repellency of BioUD®, DEET and permethrin against *Amblyomma americanum*. Med Vet Entomol 25(2):217–226

Bordin C, Alves DS, Alves LFA, de Oliveira MS, Ascari J, Scharf DR (2021) Fumigant activity of essential oils from *Cinnamomum* and *citrus* spp. and pure compounds against *Dermanyssus gallinae* (De Geer) (Acari: Dermanyssidae) and toxicity toward the nontarget organism *Beauveria bassiana* (Vuill.). Vet Parasitol 290:109341

Branco LA, de Oliveira HLM, de Campos Bortolucci W, Fernandez CMM, Gonçalves JE, Gazim ZC, Gonçalves DD, Lourenço ELB, Borges JL, dos Santos Silva V (2020) Control of bovine tick (*Rhipicephalus microplus*) with essential oil from *Psidium rufum* DC leaves. Res Soc Dev 9(11):e409119550

Bravo-Ramos J, Flores-Primo A, Paniagua-Vega D, Sánchez-Otero M, Cruz-Romero A, Romero-Salas D (2021) Acaricidal activity of the hexanic and hydroethanolic extracts of three medicinal plants against southern cattle tick *Rhipicephalus* (*Boophilus*) *microplus* (Acari: Ixodidae). Exp Appl Acarol 85(1):113–129

Bravo-Ramos JL, Sánchez-Otero MG, Sánchez-Montes S, Ballados-Gonzalez GG, Gamboa-Prieto J, Romero-Salas D, Bonilla-Rojas S, Espín-Iturbe LT (2023) Efficacy of hydroethanolic extract of *Randia aculeata* seed against the southern cattle tick *Rhipicephalus* (*Boophilus*) *microplus* (Acari: Ixodidae) on naturally infested cattle under field conditions. Exp Appl Acarol 91(2):319–330

Camilo CJ, Alves Nonato CDF, Galvão-Rodrigues FF, Costa WD, Clemente GG, Sobreira Macedo MAC, Galvão Rodrigues FF, Da Costa JGM (2017) Acaricidal activity of essential oils: a review. Trend Phytocheml Res 1(4):183–198

Castro KNC, Canuto KM, Brito ES, Costa-Júnior LM, Andrade IM, Magalhães JA, Barros DMA (2018) In *vitro* efficacy of essential oils with different concentrations of 1,8-cineole against *Rhipicephalus* (*Boophilus*) *microplus*. Rev Bras Parasitol Vet 27(2):203–210. https://doi.org/10.1590/s1984-296120180015

Chen Y, Dai G (2015) Acaricidal activity of compounds from *Cinnamomum camphora* (L.) Presl against the carmine spider mite, *Tetranychus cinnabarinus*. Pest Manag Sci 71(11):1561–1571

Chen D-D, Zhang B-Y, Liu X-X, Li X-Q, Yang X-J, Zhou L (2018) Bioactivity and structure–activity relationship of cinnamic acid derivatives and its heteroaromatic ring analogues as potential high-efficient acaricides against *Psoroptes cuniculi*. Bioorg Med Chem Lett 28(6):1149–1153

Coles TB, Dryden MW (2014) Insecticide/acaricide resistance in fleas and ticks infesting dogs and cats. Parasit Vectors 7:8. https://doi.org/10.1186/1756-3305-7-8

Conceicao RS, Carneiro MMA, d. A., Reis, I. M. A., Branco, A., Vieira, I. J. C., Braz-Filho, R., & Botura, M. B. (2017) In vitro acaricide activity of *Ocotea aciphylla* (Nees) Mez.(Lauraceae) extracts and identification of the compounds from the active fractions. Ticks Tick Borne Dis 8(2):275–282

Costa-Júnior LM, Miller RJ, Alves PB, Blank AF, Li AY, de León AAP (2016) Acaricidal efficacies of Lippia gracilis essential oil and its phytochemicals against organophosphate-resistant and susceptible strains of *Rhipicephalus* (*Boophilus*) *microplus*. Vet Parasitol 228:60–64

Coulibaly A, Bationo RK, Koala M, Bazie VB, Biguezoton AS, Toure A, Zoungrana S, Ouedraogo JCW, Kone M, Nebie RC (2020) Acaricidal activity of three plants extracts from the central region of Burkina Faso on adult *Rhipicephalus* (*Boophilus*) *microplus* cattle ticks. Int J Biol Chem Sci 14(5):1511–1519

Cowan MM (1999) Plant products as antimicrobial agents. Clin Microbiol Rev 12(4):564–582. https://doi.org/10.1128/cmr.12.4.564

Cruz PB, Barbosa AF, Zeringóta V, Melo D, Novato T, Fidelis QC, Fabri RL, de Carvalho MG, Oliveira Sabaa-Srur AU, Daemon E, Monteiro CMO (2016) Acaricidal activity of methanol extract of *Acmella oleracea* L. (Asteraceae) and spilanthol on *Rhipicephalus microplus* (Acari: Ixodidae) and *Dermacentor nitens* (Acari: Ixodidae). Vet Parasitol 228:137–143. https://doi.org/10.1016/j.vetpar.2016.08.026

Cuzzuol TN, Piffer ABM, Holtz AM, de Paula Marchiori JJ, Holtz FG, de Carvalho JR, Aguiar RL, Fontes PSF (2023) Alternative Management of *Raoiella Indica* Hirst, 1924 (Acari: Tenuipalpidae) with passion fruit seed extract. Revista de Gestão Social e Ambiental 17(9):e04182

da Silva LC, de Souza Perinotto WM, Sá FA, de Souza MAA, de Oliveira Barbosa Bitencourt R, Sanavria A, Santos HA, Marie-Magdeleine C, da Costa Angelo I (2020) *In vitro* acaricidal activity of *Cymbopogon citratus*, *Cymbopogon nardus* and *Mentha arvensis* against *Rhipicephalus microplus* (Acari: Ixodidae). Exp Parasitol 216:107937

Dai L, Miao X, Li B, Zhang J, Pan H, Shang X (2020) The active compounds and AChE inhibitor of the methanol extract of *Adonis coerulea* maxim against *Psoroptes cuniculi*. Vet Parasitol 286:109247

Dalei MK, Dehur M, Mohanty B, Hembram A, Palai S, Kuppusamy S (2022) Phytochemical analysis of Ethanolic extract of leaf of *Azadirachta indica* and *in vitro* Acaricidal effect against *Rhipicephalus microplus*. Indian J Vet Sci Biotechnol 18(3):30–34

Dantas A, Freire D, Souza G, Almeida J, Rolim L, Castro R, Horta M (2017) Acaricidal activity of leaves of Morus nigra against the cattle tick *Rhipicephalus microplus*. Arq Bras Med Vet Zootec 69:523–528

Davidović V, Joksimović-Todorović M, Maksimović Z, Hristov S, Stanković B, Relić R (2011) A review of plants used in ethnoveterinary medicine. Macedonian J Anim Sci 1:377

De Matos AC, Ribeiro CM, Scarminio IS, Afonso S, Vidotto O (2017) Phytochemical analysis and acaricidal activity of *Aloe arborescens* mill. Extracts against *Rhipicephalus* (*Boophilus*) *microplus*. Semina: Ciências Agrárias 38(5):3113–3121

De Meneghi D, Stachurski F, Adakal H (2016) Experiences in tick control by Acaricide in the traditional cattle sector in Zambia and Burkina Faso: possible environmental and public health implications. Front Public Health 4:239. https://doi.org/10.3389/fpubh.2016.00239

de Oliveira PR, Anholeto LA, Rodrigues RAF, Bechara GH, de Carvalho Castro KN, Camargo Mathias MI (2018) The potential of *Acmella oleracea* (Jambu) extract in the control of semi-engorged *Rhipicephalus sanguineus* (Latreille, 1806) (Acari: Ixodidae) female ticks. Int J Acarol 44(4–5):192–197

de Oliveira PR, Anholeto LA, Rodrigues RAF, Arnosti A, Bechara GH, de Carvalho Castro KN, Camargo-Mathias MI (2019) Cytotoxic effects of extract of *Acmella oleracea* in the ovaries and midgut of *Rhipicephalus sanguineus* Latreille, 1806 (Acari: Ixodidae) female ticks. J MicroscUltrastruc 7(1):28–43

Denardi SE, Bechara GH, de Oliveira PR, Camargo-Mathias MI (2010) *Azadirachta indica A. Juss* (neem) induced morphological changes on oocytes of *Rhipicephalus sanguineus* (Latreille, 1806)(Acari: Ixodidae) tick females. Exp Parasitol 126(4):462–470

Dias A, Tanure A, Bertonceli R (2018) In vitro effect of extract of garlic's wood (*Gallesia integrifolia* Sprengel) harms on engorged ticks and larvae of *Ripicephalus Boophilus microplus*. Sci Electr Arch 11(5):99–103

Dorla E, Grondin I, Hue T, Clerc P, Dumas S, Gauvin-Bialecki A, Laurent P (2019) Traditional uses, antimicrobial and acaricidal activities of 20 plants selected among Reunion Island's flora. S Afr J Bot 122:447–456

Dubey NK (2011) Natural products in plant pest management. CABI, Wallingford

Duque LS, Marchesini P, Monteiro C, Gomes GA, Rodrigues THS, Mesquita DM, Teixeira ALC, da Silva FLV, Marreto LCNL, Maturano R (2021) Acaricidal activity of the essential oils from *Leptospermum scoparium*, *Origanum vulgare* and *Litsea cubeba* on *Rhipicephalus microplus*: influence of the solvents and search for fractions with higher bioactivity. Vet Parasitol 300:109606

El Haddad D, Bitam I, Bouchenak O, Toubal S, Yahiaoui K, Arab K, Boumaza S (2018) Acaricidal activity of flavonoids extract of *Borago officinalis* L.(Boraginaceae) against brown dog tick, *Rhipicephalus sanguineus* (Latreille, 1806). Trop Biomed 35(2):383–391

Elmhalli F, Pålsson K, Örberg J, Grandi G (2018) Acaricidal properties of ylang-ylang oil and star anise oil against nymphs of *Ixodes ricinus* (Acari: Ixodidae). Exp Appl Acarol 76:209–220

Elmhalli F, Garboui SS, Borg-Karlson AK, Mozūraitis R, Baldauf SL, Grandi G (2019) The repellency and toxicity effects of essential oils from the Libyan plants *Salvadora persica* and *Rosmarinus officinalis* against nymphs of *Ixodes ricinus*. Exp Appl Acarol 77(4):585–599. https://doi.org/10.1007/s10493-019-00373-5

Elmhalli F, Garboui SS, Karlson AKB, Mozūraitis R, Baldauf SL, Grandi G (2021) Acaricidal activity against *Ixodes ricinus* nymphs of essential oils from the Libyan plants *Artemisia herba alba*, *Origanum majorana* and *Juniperus phoenicea*. Vet Parasitol Reg Stud Rep 24:100575

ELRoby A, Darwish M (2018) Biological activity of certain natural products against *Varroa destructor* (Acari: Varroidae) and their selectivity against *Apis mellifera* (hymenoptera: Apidae). J Phytopathol Pest Manag 5(3):67

El-Seedi HR, Azeem M, Khalil NS, Sakr HH, Khalifa SAM, Awang K, Saeed A, Farag MA, AlAjmi MF, Pålsson K, Borg-Karlson AK (2017) Essential oils of aromatic Egyptian plants repel nymphs of the tick *Ixodes ricinus* (Acari: Ixodidae). Exp Appl Acarol 73(1):139–157. https://doi.org/10.1007/s10493-017-0165-3

El-Wakeil NE (2013) Botanical pesticides and their mode of action. Gesunde Pflanzen 65(4):125

Emam HM, Ibrahim MT (2020) Effectiveness of some plant extracts against the two-spotted spider mites, *Tetranychus urticae* Koch under laboratory and greenhouse conditions (Acari: Tetranychidae). Egypt Acad J Biol Sci B Zool 12(1):9–22

Fang F, Candy K, Melloul E, Bernigaud C, Chai L, Darmon C, Durand R, Botterel F, Chosidow O, Izri A (2016) In vitro activity of ten essential oils against *Sarcoptes scabiei*. Parasit Vectors 9:1–7

Fang F, Li M, Jiang Z, Lu X, Guillot J, Si H (2020) Comparing acaricidal and ovicidal activity of five terpenes from essential oils against *Psoroptes cuniculi*. Parasitol Res 119:4219–4223

Ferraz JCB, Matos CHC, Oliveira CRF, Rosa de Sa MG, Conceição AG (2017) Acaricidal activity of Juazeiro leaf extract against red spider mite in cotton plants. Pesq Agrop Brasileira 52:493–499

Ferreira FM, Delmonte CC, Novato TLP, Monteiro CMO, Daemon E, Vilela FMP, Amaral MPH (2018) Acaricidal activity of essential oil of *Syzygium aromaticum*, hydrolate and eugenol formulated or free on larvae and engorged females of *Rhipicephalus microplus*. Med Vet Entomol 32(1):41–47. https://doi.org/10.1111/mve.12259

Figueiredo A, Nascimento LM, Lopes LG, Giglioti R, Albuquerque R, Santos MG, Falcão DQ, Nogueira JAP, Rocha L, Chagas ACS (2018) First report of the effect of *Ocotea elegans* essential oil on *Rhipicephalus (Boophilus) microplus*. Vet Parasitol 252:131–136. https://doi.org/10.1016/j.vetpar.2018.02.018

Figueiredo JCG, Nunes YRF, de Oliveira Vasconcelos V, Arruda SR, Morais-Costa F, Santos GSC et al (2019) Effects of leaf extracts of *Protium spruceanum* against adult and larval *Rhipicephalus microplus*. Exp Appl Acarol 79:447–458

Fouche G, Sakong BM, Adenubi OT, Dzoyem JP, Naidoo V, Leboho T, Wellington KW, Eloff JN (2017) Investigation of the acaricidal activity of the acetone and ethanol extracts of 12 south African plants against the adult ticks of *Rhipicephalus turanicus*. Onderstepoort J Vet Res 84(1):e1–e6. https://doi.org/10.4102/ojvr.v84i1.1523

Fromstein SR, Harthan JS, Patel J, Opitz DL (2018) *Demodex blepharitis*: clinical perspectives. Clin Optom (Auckl) 10:57–63. https://doi.org/10.2147/opto.S142708

Gao Z, Yu Z, Qiao Y, Bai L, Song X, Shi Y, Li X, Pang B, Ayiguli M, Yang X (2022) Chemical profiles and enzyme-targeting acaricidal properties of essential oils from *Syzygium aromaticum*, *Ilex chinensis* and *Citrus Limon* against *Haemaphysalis longicornis* (Acari: Ixodidae). Ind Crop Prod 188:115697

Gareh A, Hassan D, Essa A, Kotb S, Karmi M, Mohamed AE-HH, Alkhaibari AM, Elbaz E, Elhawary NM, Hassanen EA (2022) Acaricidal properties of four neem seed extracts (*Azadirachta indica*) on the camel tick *Hyalomma dromedarii* (Acari: Ixodidae). Front Vet Sci 9:946702

Ghanbarpour K, Tavassoli M, Shamsi L (2019) Pesticide effects of *Consolida orientalis* extract on larval stage of *Argas persicus* (Acari: Argasidae). Persian J Acarol 8(3):265

Ghosh S, Azhahianambi P, Yadav MP (2007) Upcoming and future strategies of tick control: a review. J Vector Borne Dis 44(2):79–89

Godara R, Verma MK, Katoch R, Yadav A, Dutt P, Satti NK, Katoch M (2018) *In vitro* acaricidal activity of *Piper nigrum* and *Piper longum* fruit extracts and their active components against *Rhipicephalus* (*Boophilus*) *microplus* ticks. Exp Appl Acarol 75(3):333–343. https://doi.org/10.1007/s10493-018-0268-5

Gomes GA, Monteiro CM, Senra Tde O, Zeringota V, Calmon F, Matos Rda S, Daemon E, Gois RW, Santiago GM, de Carvalho MG (2012) Chemical composition and acaricidal activity of essential oil from *Lippia sidoides* on larvae of *Dermacentor nitens* (Acari: Ixodidae) and larvae and engorged females of *Rhipicephalus microplus* (Acari: Ixodidae). Parasitol Res 111:2423–2430

González J, Lockhart A, Wu Q, Simon JE, Toledo A (2022) Repellency of novel catnip (*Nepeta cataria*) cultivar extracts against *Ixodes scapularis* and *Haemaphysalis longicornis* (Acari: Ixodida: Ixodidae). Ticks Tick Borne Dis 13(6):102046

Gross AD, Temeyer KB, Day TA, de León AAP, Kimber MJ, Coats JR (2017) Interaction of plant essential oil terpenoids with the southern cattle tick tyramine receptor: a potential biopesticide target. Chem Biol Interact 263:1–6

Gu X, Fang C, Yang G, Xie Y, Nong X, Zhu J, Wang S, Peng X, Yan Q (2014) Acaricidal properties of an *Ailanthus altissima* bark extract against *Psoroptes cuniculi* and *Sarcoptes scabiei* var. *cuniculi* in vitro. Exp Appl Acarol 62:225–232

Guneidy RA, Amer MA, Hakim AEE, Abdel-Shafy S, Allam SA (2021) Effect of polyphenols extracted from *Punica granatum* and *Acacia saligna* plants on glutathione S-transferase of the cattle tick *Rhipicephalus* (*Boophilus*) *annulatus* (Acari: Ixodidae). J Parasit Dis 45:524–538

Guo X, Shang X, Li B, Zhou XZ, Wen H, Zhang J (2017) Acaricidal activities of the essential oil from *Rhododendron nivale* Hook. f. and its main compound, δ-cadinene against *Psoroptes cuniculi*. Vet Parasitol 236:51–54

Guzmán L, Malla JL, Ramírez J, Gilardoni G, Calva J, Hidalgo D, Valarezo E, Rey-Valeirón C (2022) Acaricidal efficacy of plants from Ecuador, *Ambrosia peruviana* (Asteraceae) and *Lepechinia mutica* (Lamiaceae) against larvae and engorged adult females of the common cattle tick, *Rhipicephalus microplus*. Vet Sci 9(1):23

Hailesillassie T, Bisrat D, Asres K (2018) Larvicidal effect of the leaf latex of *aloe yavellana* Reynolds and its major compounds against *Amblyomma variegatum* (Ixodidae). Vet Parasitol 263:23–26. https://doi.org/10.1016/j.vetpar.2018.09.015

Hakami MA, Malak N, Khan A, Ullah H, Cossío-Bayúgar R, Nasreen N, Niaz S, Khan A, Chen C-C (2023) *In silico* exploration and experimental validation of *Camellia sinensis* extract against *Rhipicephalus microplus* and *Sarcoptes scabiei*: an integrated approach. Life 13(10):2040

Harder M, Tello V, Giliomee J (2016) The acaricidal effect of ethanolic extracts of *Chenopodium quinoa* Willd. On *Tetranychus urticae* Koch (Acari: Tetranychidae). Afr Entomol 24(1):50–60

Hatzade HRR, Waghmare WSS, Kolte KSS, Bhikane BAA, Kuralkar KSS, Hajare HSS, Ingole IRR (2022). *In-vitro* Acaricidal efficacy of aqueous extract of *Azadirachta Indica* and *Melia Azedarach* leaves against cattle tick *Haylomma Anatolicum*

Hegazy MM, Mostafa RM, El-Sayed YA, Baz MM, Khater HF, Selim A, El-Shourbagy NM (2022) The efficacy of *Saussurea costus* extracts against hematophagous arthropods of camel and cattle. Pak Vet J. https://doi.org/10.29261/pakvetj/2022.064

Higa LDOS, Garcia MV, Rodrigues VDS, Junior PB, Barradas Pina FT, Barros JC, Andreotti R (2019) Effects of cypermethrin, chlorpyrifos and piperonyl butoxide-based pour-on and spray acaricides on controlling the tick *Rhipicephalus microplus*. Syst Appl Acarol 24(2):278–286

Hikal WM, Baeshen RS, Said-Al Ahl HA (2017) Botanical insecticide as simple extractives for pest control. Cogent Biol 3(1):1404274

Hu Y, Liao F, Hu Y, Luo B, He Y, Mo Q, Zuo Z, Ren Z, Deng J, Wei Y (2014) Clinical efficacy of 9-oxo-10, 11-dehydroageraphorone extracted from *Eupatorium adenophorum* against *Psoroptes cuniculi* in rabbits. BMC Vet Res 10:1–6

Hu Z, Chen Z, Yin Z, Jia R, Song X, Li L, Zou Y, Liang X, Li L, He C (2015) In vitro acaricidal activity of 1, 8-cineole against *Sarcoptes scabiei* var. *cuniculi* and regulating effects on enzyme activity. Parasitol Res 114:2959–2967

Hurtado OJB, Giraldo-Ríos C (2018) Economic and health impact of the ticks in production animals. Ticks Tick Borne Pathog 9:1–9

Ibrahium SM, Aboelhadid SM, Wahba AA, Farghali AA, Miller RJ, Abdel-Baki A-AS, Al-Quraishy S (2022a) Preparation of geranium oil formulations effective for control of phenotypic resistant cattle tick *Rhipicephalus annulatus*. Sci Rep 12(1):11693

Ibrahium SM, Wahba AA, Farghali AA, Abdel-Baki A-AS, Mohamed SA, Al-Quraishy S, Hassan AO, Aboelhadid SM (2022b) Acaricidal activity of tea tree and lemon oil nanoemulsions against *Rhipicephalus annulatus*. Pathogens 11(12):1506

Ijoh B, Luka J, Gimba F, George B, Chiezey N, Suleiman M, Dandam P, Inegbenosun C, Muhammad S (2023) In vitro Acaricidal effect of *Jatropha curcas* methanol extract on *Rhipicephalus* (*Boophilus*) *decoloratus* larvae. Sahel J Vet Sci 20(4):15–19

Ingle KP, Deshmukh AG, Padole DA, Dudhare MS, Moharil MP, Khelurkar VC (2017) Phytochemicals: extraction methods, identification and detection of bioactive compounds from plant extracts. J Pharmacogn Phytochem 6(1):32–36

Islam S, Talukder S, Ferdous J, Hasan M, Sarker Y, Sachi S, Alim M, Sikder M (2018) *In-vitro* efficacy of verenda (*Ricinus communis*) leaves extract against ticks in cattle, vol 16, p 81

Isman MB (2006) Botanical insecticides, deterrents, and repellents in modern agriculture and an increasingly regulated world. Annu Rev Entomol 51:45–66. https://doi.org/10.1146/annurev.ento.51.110104.151146

Isman MB (2015) A renaissance for botanical insecticides? Pest Manag Sci 71(12):1587–1590

Jadhao SG, Pal S, Borkar SD, Chigure GM, Nath S, Sanyal PK, Waghmare SS, Kumar S (2022) Molecular detection of tick-borne pathogens harbored by ticks collected from local breed (non-descript) of cattle in the Chhattisgarh state of India. Int J Trop Insect Sci 42(1):707–713

Jadhav ND, Rajurkar S, Vijay M, Narladkar B, Jadhao S, Vaidya M, Mamde C, Chigure GM (2021) Determination of in vitro efficacy of aqueous and chloroform extracts of *Adhatoda vasica* against *Rhipicephalus microplus* ticks, vol 11, p 255

Jain P, Satapathy T, Pandey RK (2020) Rhipicephalus microplus: A parasite threatening cattle health and consequences of herbal acaricides for upliftment of livelihood of cattle rearing communities in Chhattisgarh. Biocatal Agric Biotechnol 26:101611

Jain P, Satapathy T, Pandey RK (2021) Acaricidal activity and biochemical analysis of *Citrus limetta* seed oil for controlling Ixodid tick *Rhipicephalus microplus* infesting cattle. Syst Appl Acarol 26(7):1350–1360

Jang S, Kuk Y (2020) Effects of plant extracts on crop diseases, two-spotted spider mites, and weeds. J Agric Sci Technol 22(3):759–773

Jawahar N, Meyyanathan S (2012) Polymeric nanoparticles for drug delivery and targeting: a comprehensive review. Int J Health Allied Sci 1(4):217–217

Jerjero T (2022) *In-vivo* acaricidal efficacy of *Tephrosia vogelii* leaf extract against tick infestation in cattle

Jeyathilakan N, Sundar S, Sangaran A, Latha B (2019) *In vitro* acaricidal properties of aqueous extracts of *Allium sativum*, *Zingiber officinale* and *Aloe vera* on brown dog tick, *Rhipicephalus sanguineus*. J Vet Parasitol 33(1):41–46

Jyoti, Singh NK, Singh H, Mehta N, Rath SS (2019) *In vitro* assessment of synergistic combinations of essential oils against *Rhipicephalus* (*Boophilus*) *microplus* (Acari: Ixodidae). Exp Parasitol 201:42–48. https://doi.org/10.1016/j.exppara.2019.04.007

Karimkhani C, Colombara DV, Drucker AM, Norton SA, Hay R, Engelman D, Steer A, Whitfeld M, Naghavi M, Dellavalle RP (2017) The global burden of scabies: a cross-sectional analysis from the global burden of disease study 2015. Lancet Infect Dis 17(12):1247–1254. https://doi.org/10.1016/s1473-3099(17)30483-8

Karunamoorthi K, Ilango K, Endale A (2009) Ethnobotanical survey of knowledge and usage custom of traditional insect/mosquito repellent plants among the Ethiopian Oromo ethnic group. J Ethnopharmacol 125(2):224–229. https://doi.org/10.1016/j.jep.2009.07.008

Kebbi R, Besseboua O, Nait-Mouloud M, Ayad A (2020) *In-vitro* acaricidal activity of *Peganum harmala* and *Glaucium flavum* alkaloid against *Rhipicephalus* sp. of dog. Eur J Vet Sci 36(1):28

Kemal J, Alemu S, Tsegaye B, Tamerat N (2020a) Study on ruminant tick infestation, phytochemical analysis and *in vitro* acaricidal effect of *Calpurnia aurea* and *Otostegia integrifolia* extracts on *Amblyomma variegatum*. Ethiopian Vet J 24(1)

Kemal J, Zerihun T, Alemu S, Sali K, Nasir M, Abraha A, Feyera T (2020b) *In vitro* acaricidal activity of selected medicinal plants traditionally used against ticks in eastern Ethiopia. J Parasitol Res 2020:7834026

Khan M, Shah A, Maqbol A, Khan N, Rahman Z (2012) Miticidal activity of methanolic extract of *Vitex negundo-lam* against *Sarcoptes scabiei* in animals and man. J Anim Plant Sci 22:102

Khan M, Shah A, Maqbol A, Khan S, Sadique U, Idress M (2013) Study of *Tecomella undulata* G. Don. methanolic extract against *Sarcoptes scabiei* L. in vivo and in vitro. J Anim Plant Sci 23:47

Khan A, Nasreen N, Niaz S, Ayaz S, Naeem H, Muhammad I, Said F, Mitchell RD, de León AAP, Gupta S (2019) Acaricidal efficacy of *Calotropis procera* (Asclepiadaceae) and T*araxacum officinale* (Asteraceae) against *Rhipicephalus microplus* from Mardan, Pakistan. Exp Appl Acarol 78:595–608

Khan A, Sohaib M, Ullah R, Hussain I, Niaz S, Malak N, de la Fuente J, Khan A, Aguilar-Marcelino L, Alanazi AD (2022) Structure-based in silico design and in vitro acaricidal activity assessment of *Acacia nilotica* and *Psidium guajava* extracts against *Sarcoptes scabiei* var. *cuniculi*. Parasitol Res 121(10):2901–2915

Khare R, Das G, Kumar S, Bendigeri S, Sachan S, Saiyam R, Banerjee D, Khare D (2019) Herbal insecticides and acaricides: challenges and constraints. Int J Chem Stud 7(4):118–125

Kim J-R, Perumalsamy H, Lee J-H, Ahn Y-J, Lee YS, Lee S-G (2016) Acaricidal activity of A*sarum heterotropoides* root-derived compounds and hydrodistillate constitutes toward *Dermanyssus gallinae* (Mesostigmata: Dermanyssidae). Exp Appl Acarol 68:485–495

Kim HK, Lee SJ, Hwang BY, Yoon JU, Kim GH (2018) Acaricidal and repellent effects of *Cnidium officinale*-derived material against *Dermanyssus gallinae* (Acari: Dermanyssidae). Exp Appl Acarol 74(4):403–414. https://doi.org/10.1007/s10493-018-0249-8

Kirthi AV, Rahuman AA, Rajakumar G, Marimuthu S, Santhoshkumar T, Jayaseelan C, Velayutham K (2011) Acaricidal, pediculocidal and larvicidal activity of synthesized ZnO nanoparticles using wet chemical route against blood feeding parasites. Parasitol Res 109:461–472

Kiss T, Cadar D, Spînu M (2012) Tick prevention at a crossroad: new and renewed solutions. Vet Parasitol 187(3–4):357–366

Koc S, Gultekin ZN, Kahraman S, Cengiz A, Polat B, Caliskan C, Tufan-Cetin O, Cetin H (2024) Larvicidal and repellent effects of essential oils on the brown dog tick (*Rhipicephalus sanguineus* sensu lato) with description of new larval repellent activity test method. Exp Appl Acarol 92:1–11

Kouam MK, Makoulo NE, Miegoué E, Ngoula F (2017) In vitro acaricidal activity of *Callistemon viminalis* and *Cupressus lusitanica* leaf essential oil against *Amblyomma variegatum* tick. Anim Health Prod 65:509–519

Koul O (2008) Phytochemicals and insect control: an antifeedant approach. Crit Rev Plant Sci 27(1):1–24

Krishna T, Krishna T, Chithra N, Deepa P, Darsana U, Sreelekha K, Juliet S, Nair SN, Ravindran R, Ajith Kumar K (2014) Acaricidal activity of petroleum ether extract of leaves of *Tetrastigma leucostaphylum* (Dennst.) Alston against *Rhipicephalus* (*Boophilus*) *annulatus*. Sci WorldJournal 2014:715481

Kruewong W, Auamcharoen W (2023) Acaricidal and repellent activity of *Zanthoxylum myriacanthum* (Rutaceae) fruit extracts against *Tetranychus urticae* and *Tetranychus truncatus* (Acari: Tetranychidae). J Entomol Sci 58(2):119–134

Kumar S (2010) Nanotechnology and animal health. VeT World 3(12):567

Laghzaoui E-M, Kasrati A, Abbad A, Leach D, Spooner-Hart R, El Mouden EH (2018) Acaricidal properties of essential oils from Moroccan plants against immature ticks of *Hyalomma aegyptium* (Linnaeus, 1758); an external parasite of the spur-thighed tortoise (*Testudo graeca*). Int J Acarol 44(7):315–321

Lakhdari W, Dehliz A, Acheuk F, Soud A, Hammi H, Mlik R, Doumandji-Mitiche B (2015) Acaricidal activity of aqueous extracts against the mite of date palm *Oligonychus afrasiaticus* meg (Acari: Tetranychidae). J Med Plant Stud 36:113

Lee SJ, Yoon JU, Park GH, Kim HK, Kim G-H (2017) Evaluation of susceptibility of red poultry mite, *Dermanyssus gallinae* (Acari: Dermanyssidae) in five regions to 11 acaricides. Korean J Appl Entomol 56(4):427–434

Lee YI, Seo M, Cho KJ (2022) *Demodex blepharitis*: an analysis of nine patients. Korean J Parasitol 60(6):429–432. https://doi.org/10.3347/kjp.2022.60.6.429

Li M, Liu B, Bernigaud C, Fischer K, Guillot J, Fang F (2020) Lemongrass (*Cymbopogon citratus*) oil: A promising miticidal and ovicidal agent against *Sarcoptes scabiei*. PLoS Negl Trop Dis 14(4):e0008225

Li M, Liu S, Yin Z, Bernigaud C, Guillot J, Fang F (2021) Activity of terpenes derived from essential oils against *Sarcoptes scabiei* eggs. Parasit Vectors 14(1):600

Li M, Feng S, Huang S, Guillot J, Fang F (2023) In vitro efficacy of terpenes from essential oils against *Sarcoptes scabiei*. Molecules 28(8). https://doi.org/10.3390/molecules28083361

Liao F, Hu Y, Tan H, Wu L, Wang Y, Huang Y, Mo Q, Wei Y (2014) Acaricidal activity of 9-oxo-10, 11-dehydroageraphorone extracted from *Eupatorium adenophorum* in vitro. Exp Parasitol 140:8–11

Liao F, Bao T, Tao G, Hu Y, Han C (2023) *In vitro* evaluation of the composition and acaricidal efficacy of *Urtica fissa* leaf ethyl acetate extract against *Sarcoptes scabiei* mites. Vet Med 68(5):200

Lima HGD, Santos FO, Santos ACV, Silva GD, Santos RJ, Carneiro KO, Reis IMA, Estrela IO, Freitas HF, Bahiense TC (2020) Anti-tick effect and cholinesterase inhibition caused by *Prosopis juliflora* alkaloids: *in vitro* and *in silico* studies. Rev Bras Parasitol Vet 29:e019819

Liu YY, Liu J, Gao Y, Yao J, Zhao J, Dai G (2019) Effect of acaricidal compound extracted from *Arachis hypogaea* Linn against *Tetranychus cinnabarinus*. J Appl Entomol 143(9):948–956

Loach N, Kishore V, Gupta S, Srivastava C, Mohan L (2019) Acaricidal properties of *Citrullus colocynthis* roots against *Rhipicephalus microplus*. J Entomol Res 43(3):359–366

Luns DAR, Soares LDS, Guedes NA, Martins IVF, Severi JA, Costa AV, Morais PAB, de Queiroz VT (2022) Bioactivity of Meliaceae, Amaryllidaceae, Solanaceae and Amaranthaceae plant aqueous extracts against the cattle tick *Rhipicephalus microplus*. Nat Prod Res 36(22):5778–5782

Luo B, Liao F, Hu Y, Liu XI, He Y, Wu L, Tan H, Luo L, Zhou Y, Mo Q, Deng J, Wei Y (2015) Acaricidal activity of extracts from *Ligularia virgaurea* against the *Sarcoptes scabiei* mite *in vitro*. Exp Ther Med 10(1):247–250. https://doi.org/10.3892/etm.2015.2503

Ma W, Fan Y, Liu Z, Hao Y, Mou Y, Liu Y, Zhang W, Song X (2019) The acaricidal activity and mechanism of eugenol on *Psoroptes cuniculi*. Vet Parasitol 266:56–62. https://doi.org/10.1016/j.vetpar.2018.12.012

Maddikontla S, Malakondaiah P, Venu R, Kumar NV (2023) In vitro evaluation of acaricidal activity of different plant extracts against *Rhipicephalus* (*Boophilus*) *microplus*, vol 12, p 4138

Madreseh-Ghahfarokhi S, Dehghani-Samani A, Pirali Y, Dehghani-Samani A (2019) *Zingiber officinalis* and *Eucalyptus globulus*, potent lethal/repellent agents against *Rhipicephalus bursa*, probable carrier for zoonosis. J Arthropod Borne Dis 13(2):214

Mahran MO, Wahba A, Mansour KM (2020) In vitro acaricidal effect of neem leaves (*Azadirachta indica*) and *Citrullus Colocynthis* extracts against the camel ticks, *Hyalomma dromedarii* (Acari: Ixodidae). J Ecosyst Ecogr 10(1):264

Malak N, Niaz S, Wadood A, Nasreen N, Ali I, Iqbal J, Swelum AA, Alkahtani MA, Zając Z, Khan A (2022) In silico approaches to develop herbal acaricides against *R.*(*Boophilus*) *microplus* and in vitro anti-tick activities of selected medicinal plants. Saudi J Biol Sci 29(6):103302

Malak N, Alotaibi BS, Khan A, Khan A, Ullah S, Nasreen N, Niaz S, Chen C-C (2023) Density functional theory calculations and molecular docking analyses of flavonoids for their possible application against the acetylcholinesterase and triose-phosphate isomerase proteins of *Rhipicephalus microplus*. Molecules 28(8):3606

Marcelino I, de Almeida AM, Ventosa M, Pruneau L, Meyer DF, Martinez D, Lefrançois T, Vachiéry N, Coelho AV (2012) Tick-borne diseases in cattle: applications of proteomics to develop new generation vaccines. J Proteomics 75(14):4232–4250. https://doi.org/10.1016/j.jprot.2012.03.026

Marchand PA (2015) Basic substances: an opportunity for approval of low-concern substances under EU pesticide regulation. Pest Manag Sci 71(9):1197–1200. https://doi.org/10.1002/ps.3997

Marchesini P, Barbosa AF, Sanches MNG, do Nascimento RM, Vale FL, Fabri RL, Maturano R, de Carvalho MG, Monteiro C (2020) Acaricidal activity of *Acmella oleracea* (Asteraceae) extract against *Rhipicephalus microplus*: what is the influence of spilanthol? Vet Parasitol 283:109170

Marimuthu S, Rahuman AA, Rajakumar G, Santhoshkumar T, Kirthi AV, Jayaseelan C, Bagavan A, Zahir AA, Elango G, Kamaraj C (2011) Evaluation of green synthesized silver nanoparticles against parasites. Parasitol Res 108:1541–1549

Marimuthu S, Rahuman AA, Jayaseelan C, Kirthi AV, Santhoshkumar T, Velayutham K, Bagavan A, Kamaraj C, Elango G, Iyappan M (2013) Acaricidal activity of synthesized titanium dioxide nanoparticles using *Calotropis gigantea* against *Rhipicephalus microplus* and *Haemaphysalis bispinosa*. Asian Pac J Trop Med 6(9):682–688

Martinez-Velazquez M, Castillo-Herrera GA, Rosario-Cruz R, Flores-Fernandez JM, Lopez-Ramirez J, Hernandez-Gutierrez R, Lugo-Cervantes Edel C (2011) Acaricidal effect and chemical composition of essential oils extracted from *Cuminum cyminum*, *Pimenta dioica* and *Ocimum basilicum* against the cattle tick *Rhipicephalus (Boophilus) microplus* (Acari: Ixodidae). Parasitol Res 108(2):481–487. https://doi.org/10.1007/s00436-010-2069-6

Mathivanan D, Gandhi PR, Mary RR, Suseem S (2018) Larvicidal and acaricidal efficacy of different solvent extracts of *Andrographis echioides* against blood-sucking parasites. Physiol Mol Plant Pathol 101:187–196

Mawela KG, Luseba D, Magano S, Eloff JN (2019) Repellent properties of *Rotheca glabrum* plant extracts against adults of *Rhipicephalus appendiculatus*. BMC Vet Res 15:1–11

Mgocheki N (2017) Management of cattle ticks, *Rhipicephalus* spp (*decoloratus* and *microplus*) (Acarina: Ixodidae) with aqueous garlic extract. Int J Acarol 43(6):430–434

Miao F, Yang X-J, Ma Y-N, Zheng F, Song X-P, Zhou L (2012) Structural modification of sanguinarine and chelerythrine and their *in vitro* acaricidal activity against *Psoroptes cuniculi*. Chem Pharm Bull 60(12):1508–1513

Minho AP, Domingues LF, Gainza YA, Figueiredo A, Boligon AA, Domingues R, Chagas AC (2020) *In vitro* screening of plant extract on *Haemonchus contortus* and *Rhipicephalus (Boophilus) microplus*. J Essent Oil Res 32(3):269–278

Mohamed SNA, Montasser AA, Ali AAB (2022) Acaricidal effect of *Citrullus colocynthis* fruit extract on the camel tick *Hyalomma dromedarii* (Koch, 1844). Ticks Tick Borne Dis 13(5):101995

Mollong E, Yaovi N, Kasseney DB, Gomina M (2018) Acaricidal effect of essential oil of *Clausena anisata* (Rutaceae) on larvae of three tick species: *Amblyomma variegatum*, *Rhipicephalus (Boophilus) decoloratus* and *Rhipicephalus (Boophilus) microplus*. J Entomol Nematol 10(4):23–32

Momen F, Abdelkader M, Fahim S (2018) Composition, repellent and fumigant toxicity of *Mentha longifolia* essential oil on *Tetranychus urticae* and three predatory mites of the family phytoseiidae (Acari: Tetranychidae: Phytoseiidae). Acta Phytopathol Entomol Hungarica 53(2):221–232

Moudgil AD, Daundkar PS, Nehra AK, Vohra S, Gupta S, Sharma D (2023) Molecular characterization of *Hyalomma dromedarii* and evaluation of acaricidal potential of herbal methanolic extracts against *H. Dromedarii* larvae in comparison to synthetic acaricides. Exp Appl Acarol 89(1):141–156

Murugan K, Dinesh D, Kavithaa K, Paulpandi M, Ponraj T, Alsalhi MS, Devanesan S, Subramaniam J, Rajaganesh R, Wei H (2016) Hydrothermal synthesis of titanium dioxide nanoparticles: mosquitocidal potential and anticancer activity on human breast cancer cells (MCF-7). Parasitol Res 115:1085–1096

Nair SN, Juliet S, Amithamol KK, Sunil AR, Palayullaparambil AKT, Sreelekha K, Divya TM, Udayan D, Kumar KGA, Ghosh S (2017) *In vitro* acaricidal effects of ethanolic extract and its fractions of *Ageratum conyzoides* L. against common cattle tick, *Rhipicephalus (Boophilus) annulatus*. Ann Phytomed 6(2):162–168

Nasreen N, Niaz S, Khan A, Zaman MA, Ayaz S, Naeem H, Khan N, Elgorban AM (2020) The potential of *Allium sativum* and *Cannabis sativa* extracts for anti-tick activities against *Rhipicephalus (Boophilus) microplus*. Exp Appl Acarol 82:281–294

Nava S, Venzal JM, Acuña DG, Martins TF, Guglielmone AA (2017) Ticks of the southern cone of America: diagnosis, distribution, and hosts with taxonomy, ecology and sanitary importance. Academic Press, New York

Navarro-Rocha J, Barrero AF, Burillo J, Olmeda AS, González-Coloma A (2018) Valorization of essential oils from two populations (wild and commercial) of geranium macrorrhizum L. Ind Crop Prod 116:41–45

Nawaz M, Zhou JI, Shamim A, Ahmed Z, Waqas M, Ahmed I, Khalid I, Hussain A, Malik MI (2022) Antiparasitic activity of plants extract against gastrointestinal nematodes and *Rhipicephalus microplus*. Int J Vet Sci 11:474

Nazim K, Godara R, Katoch R, Yadav A, Sofi OMUD, Rafiqi S, Verma P (2021a) Acaricidal activity of *Juglans regia* hull extracts against unfed larvae of *Rhipicephalus microplus* ticks. J Entomol Zool Stud 9:651–654

Nazim K, Godara R, Katoch R, Yadav A, Sofi OMU, Kumar A, Katoch M, Verma PK, Singh NK (2021b) *In vitro* assessment of turmeric (*Curcuma longa*; family: Zingiberaceae) extracts against *Rhipicephalus microplus* (Acari: Ixodidae) ticks. Int J Acarol 47(5):456–460

Noaman V, Bahreininejad B (2024) Evaluation of the acaricide activity of extracts from eight species of medicinal plants on larvae of *Hyalomma anatolicum* (Acari: Ixodidae) ticks. J Asia Pac Entomol 27(2):102231

Nong X, Li S-H, Chen F-Z, Wang J-H, Xie Y, Fang C-L, Liu T-F, He R, Gu X-B, Peng X-R (2014) Isolation and identification of acaricidal compounds in *Eupatorium adenophorum* petroleum ether extract and determination of their acaricidal activity against *Psoroptes cuniculi*. Vet Parasitol 203(1–2):197–202

Norouzi R, Hejazy M, Armin S, Arman S (2021) Acaricidal activity of *Colchicum autumnale* (autumn crocus) extract against *Hyalomma* spp. Archiv Razi Inst 76(2):293

Nwanade CF, Wang M, Wang T, Zhang X, Wang C, Yu Z, Liu J (2021) Acaricidal activity of *Cinnamomum cassia* (Chinese cinnamon) against the tick *Haemaphysalis longicornis* is linked to its content of (E)-cinnamaldehyde. Parasit Vectors 14(1):330

Nyahangare ET, Mvumi BM, McGaw LJ, Eloff JN (2019) Addition of a surfactant to water increases the acaricidal activity of extracts of some plant species used to control ticks by Zimbabwean smallholder farmers. BMC Vet Res 15:1–7

Ogayo KO (2019) Bioefficacy of lion's ear (*leonotis nepetifolia*) and African basil (*ocimum gratissimum*) extracts against two-spotted spider mite (*tetranychus urticae*) on french beans (*phaseolus vulgaris* l), Egerton University

Onyango AO, Kokwaro JO, Onyango DW, Yusuf AO (2019) Study on ethnobotany, phytochemistry, toxicity and effectiveness of herbal remedies against *Boophilus decoloratus* in Suba, Kenya. Asian J Ethnobiol 2(1):38

Oyewusi A, Eniseyin F, Abolaji A, Salihu T, Akande F, Adenubi O (2021) In vitro acaricidal activity of extracts of red cultivar *Allium cepa* L. on engorged female *Rhipicephalus* (*Boophilus*) *annulatus* from naturally infested cattle. Savannah Vet J 4:22

Palopoli MF, Fergus DJ, Minot S, Pei DT, Simison WB, Fernandez-Silva I, Thoemmes MS, Dunn RR, Trautwein M (2015) Global divergence of the human follicle mite *Demodex folliculorum*: persistent associations between host ancestry and mite lineages. Proc Natl Acad Sci U S A 112(52):15958–15963. https://doi.org/10.1073/pnas.1512609112

Pares RB, Alves DS, Alves LFA, Godinho CC, Gobbo Neto L, Ferreira TT, Nascimento MM, Ascari J, Oliveira DF (2021) Acaricidal activity of Annonaceae plants for *Dermanyssus gallinae* (Acari: Dermanyssidae) and metabolomic profile by HPLC-MS/MS. Neotrop Entomol 50:662–672

Pasipanodya CN, Tekedza TT, Chatiza FP, Gororo E (2021) Efficacy of neem (*Azadirachta indica*) aqueous fruit extracts against *Sarcoptes scabiei* var. *suis* in grower pigs. Tropl Anim Health Prod 53:1–7

Pavela R (2016) Acaricidal properties of extracts of some medicinal and culinary plants against *Tetranychus urticae* Koch. Plant Prot Sci 52(1):54

Pavela R, Herda G (2007) Repellent effects of pongam oil on settlement and oviposition of the common greenhouse whitefly *Trialeurodes vaporariorum* on chrysanthemum. Insect Sci 14(3):219–224

Pavela R, Kaffkova K, Kumšta M (2014) Chemical composition and larvicidal activity of essential oils from different *Mentha* L. and *Pulegium* species against *Culex quinquefasciatus* say (Diptera: Culicidae). Plant Prot Sci 50(1):36

Pereira SG, de Araújo SA, Guilhon G, Santos LS, Junior LMC (2017) *In vitro* acaricidal activity of *Crescentia cujete* L. fruit pulp against *Rhipicephalus microplus*. Parasitol Res 116(5):1487–1493. https://doi.org/10.1007/s00436-017-5425-y

Pereira MC, Anholeto LA, Kasa GG, de Carvalho Castro KN, Canuto KM, de Queiroz Souza AS, Camargo-Mathias MI (2023) Efficacy of essential oils of *Egletes viscosa* and *Lippia schaueriana* on the reproductive biology of *Rhipicephalus sanguineus* sensu lato engorged females. Exp Parasitol 244:108423

Politi FAS, Fantatto RR, da Silva AA, Moro IJ, Sampieri BR, Camargo-Mathias MI, Figueiredo A, de Souza Chagas AC, Furlan M (2019) Evaluation of *Tagetes patula* (Asteraceae) as an ecological alternative in the search for natural control of the cattle tick *Rhipicephalus* (*Boophilus*) *microplus* (Acari: Ixodidae). Exp Appl Acarol 77(4):601–618. https://doi.org/10.1007/s10493-019-00368-2

Porter RB, Reese PB, Williams LA (1995) Williams DJ (1995) Acaricidal and insecticidal activities of cadina-4, 10 (15)-dien-3-one. Phytochemistry 40:735–738

Premalatha K, Nelson S, Vishnupriya R, Balakrishnan S, Santhana Krishnan V (2018) Acaricidal activity of plant extracts on two spotted spider mite, *Tetranychus urticae* Koch (Acari: Tetranychidae). J Entomol Zool Stud 6(1):1622–1625

Qiao Y, Yu Z, Bai L, Li H, Zhang S, Liu J, Gao Z, Yang X (2021) Chemical composition of essential oils from *Thymus mongolicus*, *Cinnamomum verum*, and *Origanum vulgare* and their acaricidal effects on *Haemaphysalis longicornis* (Acari: Ixodidae). Ecotoxicol Environ Saf 224:112672

Quadros DG, Johnson TL, Whitney TR, Oliver JD, Oliva Chávez AS (2020) Plant-derived natural compounds for tick pest control in livestock and wildlife: pragmatism or utopia? Insects 11(8):490

Rai M, Ingle A (2012) Role of nanotechnology in agriculture with special reference to management of insect pests. Appl Microbiol Biotechnol 94:287–293

Rajakumar G, Rahuman AA (2012) Acaricidal activity of aqueous extract and synthesized silver nanoparticles from *Manilkara zapota* against *Rhipicephalus* (*Boophilus*) *microplus*. Res Vet Sci 93(1):303–309

Rajakumar G, Rahuman AA, Roopan SM, Chung I-M, Anbarasan K, Karthikeyan V (2015) Efficacy of larvicidal activity of green synthesized titanium dioxide nanoparticles using *Mangifera indica* extract against blood-feeding parasites. Parasitol Res 114:571–581

Rajput ZI, Hu SH, Chen WJ, Arijo AG, Xiao CW (2006) Importance of ticks and their chemical and immunological control in livestock. J Zhejiang Univ Sci B 7(11):912–921. https://doi.org/10.1631/jzus.2006.B0912

Ramyadevi J, Jeyasubramanian K, Marikani A, Rajakumar G, Rahuman AA, Santhoshkumar T, Kirthi AV, Jayaseelan C, Marimuthu S (2011) Copper nanoparticles synthesized by polyol process used to control hematophagous parasites. Parasitol Res 109:1403–1415

Ravindran R, Juliet S, Kumar KG, Sunil AR, Nair SN, Amithamol KK, Rawat AK, Ghosh S (2011) Toxic effects of various solvents against *Rhipicephalus* (*Boophilus*) *annulatus*. Ticks Tick Borne Dis 2(3):160–162. https://doi.org/10.1016/j.ttbdis.2011.04.001

Regnault-Roger C, Vincent C, Arnason JT (2012) Essential oils in insect control: low-risk products in a high-stakes world. Annu Rev Entomol 57:405–424. https://doi.org/10.1146/annurev-ento-120710-100554

Reis AC, Konig IFM, Mendonça GHA, Lunguinho ADS, Cardoso MG, Remedio RN (2023) Toxic effect of *Callistemon viminalis* essential oil on the ovary of engorged *Rhipicephalus microplus* female ticks (Acari: Ixodidae). Exp Appl Acarol 90(1):99–117

Remedio R, Nunes P, Anholeto L, Oliveira P, Camargo-Mathias M (2015) Morphological effects of neem (*Azadirachta indica A. Juss*) seed oil with known azadirachtin concentrations on the oocytes of semi-engorged *Rhipicephalus sanguineus* ticks (Acari: Ixodidae). Parasitol Res 114:431–444

Rey-Valeirón C, Guzmán L, Saa LR, López-Vargas J, Valarezo E (2017) Acaricidal activity of essential oils of *Bursera graveolens* (Kunth) Triana & Planch and Schinus molle L. on unengorged larvae of cattle tick *Rhipicephalus* (*Boophilus*) *microplus* (Acari: Ixodidae). J Essent Oil Res 29(4):344–350

Rey-Valeirón C, Pérez K, Guzmán L, López-Vargas J, Valarezo E (2018) Acaricidal effect of *Schinus molle* (Anacardiaceae) essential oil on unengorged larvae and engorged adult females of *Rhipicephalus sanguineus* (Acari: Ixodidae). Exp Appl Acarol 76:399–411

Rhimi W, Camarda A, Saidi M, Boulila A, Otranto D, Cafarchia C (2019) Chemical characterization and acaricidal activity of *Drimia maritima* (L) bulbs and *Dittrichia viscosa* leaves against *Dermanyssus gallinae*. Vet Parasitol 268:61–66

Richards RN (2021) Scabies: diagnostic and therapeutic update. J Cutan Med Surg 25(1):95–101. https://doi.org/10.1177/1203475420960446

Rodriguez-Vivas RI, Jonsson NN, Bhushan C (2018) Strategies for the control of *Rhipicephalus microplus* ticks in a world of conventional acaricide and macrocyclic lactone resistance. Parasitol Res 117:3–29

Romero T, Moya VJ, Fernández N, Althaus R, Reybroeck W, Molina MP (2016) Interferences on microbial inhibitor tests related to ivermectin treatment in lactating dairy goats. J Dairy Res 83(3):341–344. https://doi.org/10.1017/s0022029916000443

Rosado-Aguilar JA, Aguilar-Caballero A, Rodriguez-Vivas RI, Borges-Argaez R, Garcia-Vazquez Z, Mendez-Gonzalez M (2010) Acaricidal activity of extracts from *Petiveria alliacea* (Phytolaccaceae) against the cattle tick, *Rhipicephalus* (*Boophilus*) *microplus* (Acari: ixodidae). Vet Parasitol 168(3–4):299–303. https://doi.org/10.1016/j.vetpar.2009.11.022

Rosado-Aguilar JA, Rodríguez-Vivas RI, Borges-Argaez R, Arjona-Cambranes KA (2017) Acaricidal activity of *Havardia albicans* and *Caesalpinia gaumeri* methanolic leaf extracts on *Rhipicephalus microplus* and its toxicity to laboratory animals. Exp Appl Acarol 71:345–354

Roy S, Jogi S, Roy M, Ali S, Sagar A (2005) Therapeutic management with crude extract of indigenous plant against sarcoptic mange in dogs. Intas Polivet 6:352

Saini S, Singh H, Rath S, Singh NK (2022) In vitro acaricidal activity of *Piper longum* L. against amitraz resistant *Rhipicephalus microplus* (Acari: Ixodidae). Exp Parasitol 241:108356

Salman SY, Özdemir SN, Sevim S (2018) Toxicity and repellency of sage (*Salvia officinalis* L.) (Lamiaceae) and rosemary (*Rosmarinus officinalis* L.) (Lamiaceae) extracts to *Neoseiulus californicus* (McGregor, 1954) and *Phytoseiulus persimilis* Athias-Henriot, 1957 (Acari: Phytoseiidae). Turk J Entomol 42(3):151–160

Salman M, Abbas RZ, Israr M, Abbas A, Mehmood K, Khan MK, Hussain R, Saleemi MK, Shah S (2020) Repellent and acaricidal activity of essential oils and their components against *Rhipicephalus* ticks in cattle. Vet Parasitol 283:109178

Saman S, Chen C-C, Malak N, Khan A, Nasreen N, Khan A, Niaz S, Rehman G, Rodriguez-Vivas RI, Cossío-Bayúgar R (2022) Ethanolic extracts of *Datura innoxia* have promising Acaricidal activity against *Rhipicephalus microplus* as it blocks the glutathione S-transferase activity of the target tick. Gene 14(1):118

Santhoshkumar T, Rahuman A, Bagavan A et al (2012) Evaluation of ste m aqueous extract and synthesized silver nanoparticle s using *Cissus quadrangularis* against *Hippobosca maculat* a and *Rhipicephalus* (*Boophilus*) *microplus*. Exp Parasitol 132(2):156–165

Santos F, Vogel F (2012) Avaliação in vitro da ação do óleo essencial de capim limão (*Cymbopogon citratus*) sobre o carrapato bovino *Rhipicephalus* (*Boophilus*) *microplus*. Rev Bras Plant Med 14:712–716

Sarli M, Morel N, Nava S (2023) Applicability of three indices to evaluate the reproductive capacity of *Rhipicephalus microplus* engorged female ticks in acaricide efficacy trials. Exp Parasitol 255:108640

Scartezzini P, Speroni E (2000) Review on some plants of Indian traditional medicine with antioxidant activity. J Ethnopharmacol 71(1–2):23–43. https://doi.org/10.1016/s0378-8741(00)00213-0

Shahatha SS (2020) Epidemiological, diagnostic and therapeutic study for mange in sheep of Anbar province-Iraq. Iraq J Vet Sci 34(1):1–7

Shang X, Guo X, Li B, Pan H, Zhang J, Zhang Y, Miao X (2016a) Microwave-assisted extraction of three bioactive alkaloids from *Peganum harmala* L. and their acaricidal activity against *Psoroptes cuniculi in vitro*. J Ethnopharmacol 192:350–361

Shang X, Wang Y, Zhou X, Guo X, Dong S, Wang D, Zhang J, Pan H, Zhang Y, Miao X (2016b) Acaricidal activity of oregano oil and its major component, carvacrol, thymol and p-cymene against *Psoroptes cuniculi in vitro* and *in vivo*. Vet Parasitol 226:93–96

Shang X, Guo X, Yang F, Li B, Pan H, Miao X, Zhang J (2017) The toxicity and the acaricidal mechanism against Psoroptes cuniculi of the methanol extract of *Adonis coerulea maxim*. Vet Parasitol 240:17–23

Shang X-F, Dai L-X, Liu Y-Q, Zhao Z-M, Li J-C, Yang G-Z, Yang C-J (2019) Acaricidal activity and enzyme inhibitory activity of active compounds of essential oils against *Psoroptes cuniculi*. Vet Parasitol 267:54–59

Shang X-F, Miao X-L, Dai L-X, Guo X, Li B, Pan H, Zhang J-Y (2020) The acaricidal mechanism and active compounds against *Psoroptes cuniculi* of the methanol extract of *Adonis coerulea* maxim II: integrated proteomics and SPR analysis. Vet Parasitol 287:109267

Sharma N, Singh V, Shyma KP, Solanki V, Gupta JP (2018) Comparative resistance status of *Hyalomma anatolicum* and *Rhipicephalus* (*Boophilus*) *microplus* ticks against synthetic Pyrethroids (deltamethrin and cypermethrin) from Banaskantha, Gujarat, India. Int J Acarol 44(6):268–275

Sharma A, Bhardwaj G, Sohal H, Gohain A (2022) Chapter 9—Eugenol. In: Kour J, Nayik GA (eds) Nutraceuticals and Health Care, Academic Press, Pages 177-198, ISBN 9780323897792, https://doi.org/10.1016/B978-0-323-89779-2.00007-7.

Shen F, Xing M, Liu L, Tang X, Wang W, Wang X, Wu X, Wang X, Wang X, Wang G (2012) Efficacy of trans-cinnamaldehyde against *Psoroptes cuniculi* in vitro. Parasitol Res 110:1321–1326

Shezryna S, Anisah N, Saleh I, Syamsa R (2020) Acaricidal activity of the essential oils from *Citrus hystrix* (Rutaceae) and *Cymbopogon citratus* (Poaceae) on the cattle tick *Rhipicephalus* (*Boophilus*) *microplus* larvae (Acari: Ixodidae). Trop Med 37:433

Shnawa BH, Mhammedsharif RM, Jalil PJ, Hamadamin SI, Ahmad SF, Abdulrahman KM, Ahmed MH (2023) Antimicrobial activity of plant-extract-mediated synthesis of silver-zinc oxide nanocomposites and their acaricidal efficacy on *Hyalomma marginatum* ticks. Biocatal Agric Biotechnol 51:102765

Siame CP, Chitambo H, Muma JB, Choongo K, Moonga E (2019) Field assessment of the efficacy of *Tephrosia vogelii* leaf extracts for control of ticks on naturally infested cattle in the field condition. J Parasit Dis 43:624–632

Silva FG, Cruz JP, Júnior VSM, Figueiredo JCG, Duarte ER, de Oliveira Vasconcelos V (2022) Efficacy of resin and ethanol extract from leaves of *Protium spruceanum* (bent) Engl. combined with Cypermethrin to control *Rhipicephalus* (*Boophilus*) *microplus* (Canestrini, 1887). Res Soc Dev 11(12):e75111234252

Singh NK, Rath SS (2013) Epidemiology of ixodid ticks in cattle population of various agro-climatic zones of Punjab, India. Asian Pac J Trop Med 6(12):947–951. https://doi.org/10.1016/s1995-7645(13)60169-8

Singh NK, Saini S, Singh H, Jyoti SS, Rath S (2017) In vitro assessment of the acaricidal activity of *Piper longum*, *Piper nigrum*, and *Zingiber officinale* extracts against *Hyalomma anatolicum* ticks. Exp Appl Acarol 71:303–317

Singh K, Sharma AK, Kumar S, Sankar M, Ghosh S (2022) Synergistic properties of essential oils of eucalyptus (*Eucalyptus globulus*) and lemon grass (*Cymbopogon flexuosus*) against cattle tick, *Rhipicephalus microplus*. Int J Acarol 48(4–5):338–343

Siramon P, Ohtani Y, Ichiura H (2009) Biological performance of *Eucalyptus* camaldulensis leaf oils from Thailand against the subterranean termite *Coptotermes formosanus* Shiraki. J Wood Sci 55:41–46

Sleeckx N, Van Gorp S, Koopman R, Kempen I, Van Hoye K, De Baere K, Zoons J, De Herdt P (2019) Production losses in laying hens during infestation with the poultry red mite *Dermanyssus gallinae*. Avian Pathol 48(sup1):S17–s21. https://doi.org/10.1080/03079457.2019.1641179

Souza Conceição R, de Carneiro MM, Alves Reis IM, Branco A, Curcino Vieira IJ, Braz-Filho R, Borges Botura M (2017) *In vitro* acaricide activity of *Ocotea aciphylla* (Nees) Mez. (Lauraceae) extracts and identification of the compounds from the active fractions. Ticks Tick Borne Dis 8(2):275–282. https://doi.org/10.1016/j.ttbdis.2016.11.013

Souza LPD, Zuim V, Stinguel P, Pinheiro PF, Zago HB (2022) Toxicity of essential oil of *Mentha piperita* (Lamiaceae) and its monoterpenoid menthol against *Tetranychus urticae* Kogan 1836 (Acari: Tetranychidae). An Acad Bras Cienc 94(suppl 4):e20200427

Sparagano O (2020) A nonexhaustive overview on potential impacts of the poultry red mite (*Dermanyssus gallinae*) on poultry production systems. J Anim Sci 98(Suppl 1):S58–s62. https://doi.org/10.1093/jas/skaa136

Srisanyong W, Bunyaluk D, Srinontong P, Chitsanoor S (2021) Acaricidal activity of phenolic crude extract from *Artocapus lakoocha* leaves against cattle tick *Rhipicephalus* (*Boophilus*) *microplus*. Int J Vet Sci 10:307

Staffa P, Nyangiwe N, Msalya G, Nagagi YP, Nchu F (2020) The effect of *Beauveria bassiana* inoculation on plant growth, volatile constituents, and tick (*Rhipicephalus appendiculatus*) repellency of acetone extracts of Tulbaghia violacea. Vet World 13(6):1159

Štefanidesová K, Škultéty Ľ, Sparagano OA, Špitalská E (2017) The repellent efficacy of eleven essential oils against adult *Dermacentor reticulatus* ticks. Ticks Tick Borne Dis 8(5):780–786

Sujitha V, Murugan K, Paulpandi M, Panneerselvam C, Suresh U, Roni M, Nicoletti M, Higuchi A, Madhiyazhagan P, Subramaniam J (2015) Green-synthesized silver nanoparticles as a novel control tool against dengue virus (DEN-2) and its primary vector *Aedes aegypti*. Parasitol Res 114:3315–3325

Tabari MA, Youssefi MR, Benelli G (2017) Eco-friendly control of the poultry red mite, *Dermanyssus gallinae* (Dermanyssidae), using the α-thujone-rich essential oil of *Artemisia sieberi* (Asteraceae): toxic and repellent potential. Parasitol Res 116(5):1545–1551. https://doi.org/10.1007/s00436-017-5431-0

Tabari MA, Khodashenas A, Jafari M, Petrelli R, Cappellacci L, Nabissi M, Maggi F, Pavela R, Youssefi MR (2020a) Acaricidal properties of hemp (*Cannabis sativa* L.) essential oil against *Dermanyssus gallinae* and *Hyalomma dromedarii*. Ind Crop Prod 147:112238

Tabari MA, Rostami A, Khodashenas A, Maggi F, Petrelli R, Giordani C, Tapondjou LA, Papa F, Zuo Y, Cianfaglione K (2020b) Acaricidal activity, mode of action, and persistent efficacy of selected essential oils on the poultry red mite (*Dermanyssus gallinae*). Food Chem Toxicol 138:111207

Tabari MA, Jafari A, Jafari M, Youssefi MR (2023) Laboratory and field efficacy of terpene combinations (carvacrol, thymol and menthol) against the poultry red mite (*Dermanyssus gallinae*). Vet Parasitol 313:109842

Tabet VG, Vieira MR, Martins GLM, Sousa CGNM (2018) Plant extracts with potential to control of two-spotted spider mite. Arq Inst Biol 85:e0762015

Taha MA, Baioumy Ali AA (2020) The first study for the Acaricidal activity of alcoholic extracts of *Adiantum capillus-veneris* and *Funaria hygrometric* against *Argas persicus*. Egypt Acad J Biol Sci F Toxicol Pest Control 12(2):203–217

Tangjitman K, Wongsawad C, Kamwong K, Sukkho T, Trisonthi C (2015) Ethnomedicinal plants used for digestive system disorders by the Karen of northern Thailand. J Ethnobiol Ethnomed 11:27. https://doi.org/10.1186/s13002-015-0011-9

Tavassoli M, Ghanbarpoor L, Shamsi L (2018) Study the pesticide effects of *Matricaria chamomilla* extract on *Argas persicus* ticks. J Vet Res 73(2):135–139

Tiwari J, Niranjan A, Verma S, Srivastava M, Sharma B (2023) Effect of silver nanoparticles biosynthesized with poly-herbal leaf extracts of neem and Nirgundi plants against *Rhipicephalus microplus* tick. Vet Pract 24(1)

Toussirot M, Coulerie P, Hüe T, Maciuk A, Kagy V (2022) Acaricidal activity of *Piper nigrum* fruit extracts on the cattle tick, *Rhipicephalus* (*Boophilus*) *australis* (syn. R. Microplus)

Toussirot M, Coulerie P, Hüe T, Maciuk A, Kagy V (2023) Larvicidal activity of the black pepper, *Piper nigrum* (fam: Piperaceae) extracts on the cattle tick, *Rhipicephalus australis* (Acari: Ixodidae). Chem Biol Technol Agric 10(1):23

Tripathi AK, Prajapati V, Ahmad A, Aggarwal KK, Khanuja SP (2004) Piperitenone oxide as toxic, repellent, and reproduction retardant toward malarial vector *Anopheles stephensi* (Diptera: Anophelinae). J Med Entomol 41(4):691–698. https://doi.org/10.1603/0022-2585-41.4.691

Udayan D, Nair SN, Juliet S, Ravindran R, Athalathil S, Adarshkrishna TP, Ajithkumar KG, Sreelekha KP, Chandrashekar L, Ghosh S (2020) Acaricidal activity of *Artemisia nilagirica* leaves against *Rhipicephalus* (*Boophilus*) *annulatus* ticks. Planta Med 86(18):1335–1344

Ujváry I (2010) Pest control agents from natural products. In: Hayes' handbook of pesticide toxicology. Elsevier, Amsterdam, pp 119–229

Underwood C, Van Eps A (2012) Nanomedicine and veterinary science: the reality and the practicality. Vet J 193(1):12–23

Upadhaya D, Kumar B, Kumar S, Sharma AK, Fular A, Bisht N, Srivastava S, Boruah RR, Nagar G, Shakya M (2020) Characterization of acaricide resistance in *Rhipicephalus microplus* populations infesting cattle in northeastern India and assessment of local plant extracts for tick management. Vet Parasitol 277:109011

Usai F, Di Sotto A (2023) Trans-cinnamaldehyde as a novel candidate to overcome bacterial resistance: an overview of *in vitro* studies. Antibiotics 12(2):254

Valiente Moro C, De Luna CJ, Tod A, Guy JH, Sparagano OA, Zenner L (2009) The poultry red mite (*Dermanyssus gallinae*): a potential vector of pathogenic agents. Exp Appl Acarol 48(1–2):93–104. https://doi.org/10.1007/s10493-009-9248-0

Varadharajan A, Gnanasekar R (2019) Acaricidal activity of herbal extracts against cattle tick (*Rhipicephalus microplus*). Pharma Innov J 8:609–611

Vasconcelos V, Costa E, Moreira V, Morais-Costa F, Duarte E (2018) Efficacy of plants extracts from the Cerrado against adult female of *Dermacentor nitens* (Acari: Ixodidae). Exp Appl Acarol 75:419–427

Villarreal JPV, Santos PRD, Silva M, Azambuja RHM, Gonçalves CL, Escareño JJH, Santos T, Pereira CMP, Freitag RA, Nascente PDS (2017) Evaluation of phytotherapy alternatives for controlling *Rhipicephalus* (*Boophilus*) *microplus* in vitro. Rev Bras Parasitol Vet 26(3):299–306. https://doi.org/10.1590/s1984-29612017052

Wanzala W, Hassanali A, Mukabana WR, Takken W (2018) Essential oils of indigenous plants protect livestock from infestations of *Rhipicephalus appendiculatus* and other tick species in herds grazing in natural pastures in western Kenya. J Pestic Sci 91:395–404

Weber SS, Kaminski KP, Perret J-L, Leroy P, Mazurov A, Peitsch MC, Ivanov NV, Hoeng J (2019) Antiparasitic properties of leaf extracts derived from selected *Nicotiana* species and *Nicotiana tabacum* varieties. Food Chem Toxicol 132:110660

Wellington KW, Leboho T, Sakong BM, Adenubi OT, Eloff JN, Fouche G (2017) Further studies on south African plants: Acaricidal activity of organic plant extracts against *Rhipicephalus* (*Boophilus*) *microplus* (Acari: Ixodidae). Vet Parasitol 234:10–12. https://doi.org/10.1016/j.vetpar.2016.12.014

Wink M (2012) Medicinal plants: a source of anti-parasitic secondary metabolites. Molecules 17(11):12771–12791

Yang J-Y, Kim M-G, Lee S-E, Lee H-S (2014) Acaricidal activities against house dust mites of spearmint oil and its constituents. Planta Med 80(02/03):165–170

Yusufoglu HS, Tabanca N, Bernier UR, Li AY, Salkini MA, Alqasoumi SI, Demirci B (2018) Mosquito and tick repellency of two Anthemis essential oils from Saudi Arabia. Saudi Pharm J 26(6):860–864. https://doi.org/10.1016/j.jsps.2018.03.012

Zahid M, Bashir M, Shahid M, Khan B (2016) Antioxidant, hemolytic, biofilm inhibition and toxicity evaluation of some selected plant origin pesticides for predatory mite *Neoseiulus Barkeri* (Acari: Phytoseiidae). Oxid Commun 39(2):1346

Zahran EM, Abdel-Maqsoud NMR, Tammam OY, Abdel-Rahman IM, Elrehany MA, Bakhsh HT, Altemani FH, Algehainy NA, Alzubaidi MA, Abdelmohsen UR (2022) Scabicidal potential of coconut seed extract in rabbits via downregulating inflammatory/immune cross talk: a comprehensive phytochemical/GC-MS and *in silico* proof. Antibiotics 12(1):43

Zakari S, Ogbu CO, Zakari H, Agwara BC, Bayode AA, Uti DE (2023) Acaricidal potentials of Ethanolic extract of *Annona Muricata* leaves (sour sop) against *Rhipicephalus* species cattle ticks (Acari: *Ixodidae).* Available at SSRN 4454442

Zandi-Sohani N, Ramezani L (2015) Evaluation of five essential oils as botanical acaricides against the strawberry spider mite *Tetranychus turkestani* Ugarov and Nikolskii. Int Biodeter Biodegr 98:101–106

Zhang B, Lv C, Li W, Cui Z, Chen D, Cao F, Miao F, Zhou L (2015) Ethyl cinnamate derivatives as promising high-efficient acaricides against *Psoroptes cuniculi*: synthesis, bioactivity and structure–activity relationship. Chem Pharm Bull 63(4):255–262

Zhou Y, Liao F, Weng J, Mo Q, Xu R, Zhang Y, Ren Z, Zhong Z, Zuo Z, Peng G (2019) Composition and acaricidal activity of essential oil from *Elsholtzia densa* Benth against *Sarcoptes scabiei* mites in vitro. Vet Med 64(4):178

Zhou Y, Cao J, Wang Y, Battsetseg B, Battur B, Zhang H, Zhou J (2023) Repellent effects of Chinese cinnamon oil on nymphal ticks of *Haemaphysalis longicornis*, *Rhipicephalus haemaphysaloides*, and *Hyalomma asiaticum.* Exp Appl Acarol 91(3):497–507

Zhu JK, Gao JM, Yang CJ, Shang XF, Zhao ZM, Lawoe RK, Zhou R, Sun Y, Yin XD, Liu YQ (2020) Design, synthesis, and antifungal evaluation of Neocryptolepine derivatives against Phytopathogenic fungi. J Agric Food Chem 68(8):2306–2315. https://doi.org/10.1021/acs.jafc.9b06793

# Using Entomopathogenic Fungi for Tick Control

12

Naunain Mehmood, Hira Muqaddas, Nimra Shahid, Saba Kousar, and Furhan Iqbal

**Abstract**

Ticks pose significant health risks to humans and domestic animals as they are serving as vectors for a variety of pathogens resulting in huge global economic loss annually. Traditionally, acaricides are used for tick control that can have detrimental effects such as animal and human toxicity, environmental pollution, and the emergence of resistance in ticks against these chemicals. Entomopathogenic fungi, which naturally infect arthropods, have shown potential in causing high mortality among the various tick life stages and have led to their reduced egg-laying capacity during laboratory trials. However, in field applications, the effectiveness of these fungi often falls short of laboratory expectations due to adverse biotic and climatic conditions of the application sites. To enhance the performance of fungal agents in controlling ticks in natural settings, it is crucial to select highly virulent fungal isolates that are also resistant to high temperatures, ultraviolet (UV) radiation and desiccation. Factors that impact the virulence of these fungi include the role of toxic metabolites produced by the fungus in ticks as well as how ticks' immune systems respond to fungal infections. Here, we are updating the literature reporting the application of fungal biocontrol agents,

N. Mehmood
Department of Zoology, University of Sargodha, Sargodha, Pakistan

Department of Veterinary Medicine, University of Sassari, Sassari, Italy

H. Muqaddas · S. Kousar
Department of Zoology, The Women University Multan, Multan, Pakistan

N. Shahid
Department of Zoology, University of Sargodha, Sargodha, Pakistan

F. Iqbal (✉)
Institute of Zoology, Bahauddin Zakariya University, Multan, Pakistan
e-mail: furhan.iqbal@bzu.edu.pk



S. Kumar et al. (eds.), *Acaricides Resistance in Ticks*,
https://doi.org/10.1007/978-981-97-7411-1_12

refining the formulations of fungal spores for more effective tick management, and integrating entomopathogenic fungi into integrated pest management strategies for ticks.

**Keywords**

Tick borne diseases · Entomopathogenic fungi · Fungal acaricides · *Beauveria bassiana* · *Metarhizium anisopliae*

## 12.1 Tick Borne Diseases: A Global Concern

Vector-borne diseases (VBDs) are a serious health concern globally as they account for more than 17% disease burden among the infectious diseases and result in around seven lakh human deaths annually (WHO 2020). Among these, tick borne diseases (TBDs) are the most prominent having significant medical and veterinary concern. Ticks are surpassed only by mosquitoes in their ability to spread zoonotic diseases (Cafarchia et al. 2022). Anaplasmosis, borreliosis, rocky mountain spotted fever, babesiosis, Colorado tick fever, tick-borne relapsing fever, Crimean-Congo hemorrhagic fever, ehrlichiosis, lyme disease, heartland virus disease, southern tick-associated rash illness, Poswassan disease, rickettsiosis, theileriosis, and tularemia are the major diseases that are transmitted by ticks (Madison-Antenucci et al. 2020). *Ixodes*, *Rhipicephalus*, *Dermacentor*, and *Amblyomma* are the most common tick genera involved in disease transmission to humans, domesticated and wild animals (Fernandes et al. 2012). Tick infestations are more severe in animals compared to humans. Animals are usually parasitized by lot more ticks than humans which impact the host either through direct injuries or through the transmission of diseases (Ghosh and Nagar 2014). Direct injuries are very serious as they induce sweating sickness and tick paralysis in animals due to toxins contained in tick saliva, skin injuries that are prone to secondary microbial infections, anemia, and screw-worm infestations (Perveen et al. 2021). Tick bites can reduce the value of skins and hides by as much as 20–30%. Globally, ticks cost around 275.7 million US$ annually including transmission of TBDs and cost of tick control (Narladkar 2018).

## 12.2 Tick Control

Tick control is mainly based on synthetic chemicals like acaricides which target ticks either on the host or in the environment. The preferred method involves applying acaricides directly on the host to eliminate the parasitic stages (Ghosh and Nagar 2014). However, this method of vector control is not much effective in targeting the species and requires multiple and repeated applications, with increased concentration, thus resulting in the development of resistance among the ticks. Moreover, these toxic molecules negatively affect the non-target organisms and incorporate into the food chains (Benelli et al. 2016). Biological control is one of the most attractive approaches for tick management amidst these negative consequences of acaricides (Ghosh and Nagar 2014).

Entomopathogenic fungi (EPF) are the microorganisms which naturally infect and kill their hosts that are mainly arthropods and play a crucial role in the microbial management of pest populations (Sinha et al. 2016). There are more than 700 species of EPF belonging to 100 genera that possess insecticidal properties, but it is interesting to know that each fungal species/strain is highly specific in causing virulence to its respective host species (Sinha et al. 2016). Most entomogenous fungi that can infect insects belong to the order Entomophthorales (in the class Zygomycetes) and Hypocreales (Cafarchia et al. 2022). The most notable species infecting ixodid ticks in their natural habitat include *Beauveria bassiana*, *Metarhizium anisopliae* s.l., *Lecanicillium lecanii*, *Isaria fumosorosea*, and *Isaria farinose*. The hyphomycetous fungi *Beauveria* and *Metarhizium* have historically and currently been the most extensively researched genera as environmentally friendly alternative to chemical acaricides for tick control (Fernandes et al. 2012). Most of the investigations have targeted the biological control for the cattle tick *Rhipicephalus microplus* as it has the highest economic impact in tropical areas (Beys-da-Silva et al. 2020; Mesquita et al. 2020). Nonetheless, EPFs have also been evaluated for their effectiveness against other tick species, such as *Ixodes ricinus*, which is the primary vector for Lyme disease in Europe (Wassermann et al. 2016; Lorenz et al. 2020). Unlike bacteria and viruses, the fungus directly penetrates their hosts through the cuticle instead of being ingested (Islam et al. 2021). Fungal conidia (spores) penetrate their hosts through the surface due to the mechanical pressure exerted by appressoria and release enzymes which degrade the integument, enabling hyphae to enter the hemolymph and colonize other tissues leading to death of host (de Lima et al. 2022). These fungi are typically considered safe for humans and other non-target organisms (Fernandes et al. 2012). Being investigated as biological control agents for arthropod pests, EPFs are highly specific for the type of host species they infect, a certain fungal species/strain could be more effective in controlling one species of tick than the other (Sinha et al. 2016). Effective management techniques utilizing these fungi necessitate a thorough understanding of dynamicity of host-pathogen interaction, as well as the impact of environmental factors to anticipate and regulate the prevalence of the disease (Fernandes et al. 2012).

## 12.3 Entomopathogenic Fungi: The Mode of Infection

The EPFs employ different strategies to infect hosts based on the host's life stage (Ortiz-Urquiza and Keyhani 2013). The fungi act as hyper-parasites and enter the ticks through natural openings in the cuticle or by creating openings using their hydrolytic enzymes which are crucial for their pathogenicity (Fang et al. 2005; Prakash et al. 2012). Different hydrolytic enzymes, including proteases, chitinases, esterases, and lipases, along with other factors, facilitate the germination and growth of the fungus on the host's surface and enable penetration through cuticular layers (Castellanos-Moguel et al. 2007; Xiao et al. 2012; Zheng et al. 2012). Among the earlier enzymes, endoproteases (PR1 and PR2) and aminopeptidase are released on the cuticle and are associated with the development of appressoria (penetration pegs; Castellanos-Moguel et al. 2007) which are specialized infection structures assisting the growing hyphae in penetrating the host integument. These enzymes are secreted during the initial phase of contact with their host (tick) that is followed by penetration. The main aim of EPF to penetrate the cuticle is to gain access to the nutrients required for its growth and reproduction. Both mechanical force and enzymatic action are required for this. The infection begins upon contact, with the attachment of single-celled dispersive forms of fungi, such as conidia or blastospores, to the insect's cuticle (Ortiz-Urquiza and Keyhani 2013). The penetration sites on the epicuticle are dark, melanotic lesions (Qayyum et al. 2021). The amount of secretion and activity of these enzymes vary among different species/strains of EPF indicating their different virulence potential (Zibaee and Ramzi 2018). It is during the later stages of this infection process that the EPF encounters the immune system of host. Cuticle active endo-protease plays a crucial role in the penetration process, given that 70% of the cuticle is made up of protein and this enzyme cocktail varies from fungus to fungus based upon their target ticks (Islam et al. 2021). In *B. bassiana*, the degradation of cuticular lipids involves several enzymes, including eight cytochrome P450 enzymes (CYP genes), three lipases/esterases, four catalases, hydrocarbon carrier protein and long-chain aldehyde and alcohol dehydrogenases (Pedrini et al. 2010).

The cuticle is a highly composite structure, varying even within different life stages of the same insect. The outermost layer, epicuticle, provides a hydrophobic barrier rich in lipids, followed by the procuticle containing chitin and sclerotized protein, further divided into exo, meso, and endo-cuticular layers. Beneath the procuticle lies the epidermis, surrounding the insect's internal structures (Ortiz-Urquiza and Keyhani 2013). The fungal growth also leads to changes in the cuticle, most notably its hydrocarbon content (Jarrold et al. 2007). The secretion of organic acids, primarily oxalic acid, may also play a role in weakening the cuticle including lipid degradation (Kirkland et al. 2005). The hydrocarbon assimilation by infecting EPF involves a degradative pathway utilizing β-oxidation by cytochrome P450 enzymes yielding fatty acyl CoAs (Pedrini et al. 2007). The recognition and assimilation of cuticular lipids represent important metabolic adaptations which most likely trigger signaling mechanisms that aid in entomopathogenesis (Ortiz-Urquiza and Keyhani 2013). The fungus directly penetrates the insect's hemocoel, breaching the cuticle or it can gain entry through the mouthparts of insect. Once inside, the fungus spreads into the hemolymph either as blastospores or in a yeast-like form, eventually reaching the insect's respiratory system to maximize the nutrient absorption (Islam et al. 2021). The death of insect results from several factors including mechanical damage due to tissue invasion, nutrient depletion, and the production of toxins within the insect's body that leads to toxicosis (Sinha et al. 2016). Figure 12.1 depicts overall mode of pathogenesis of entomopathogenic fungi in ticks.

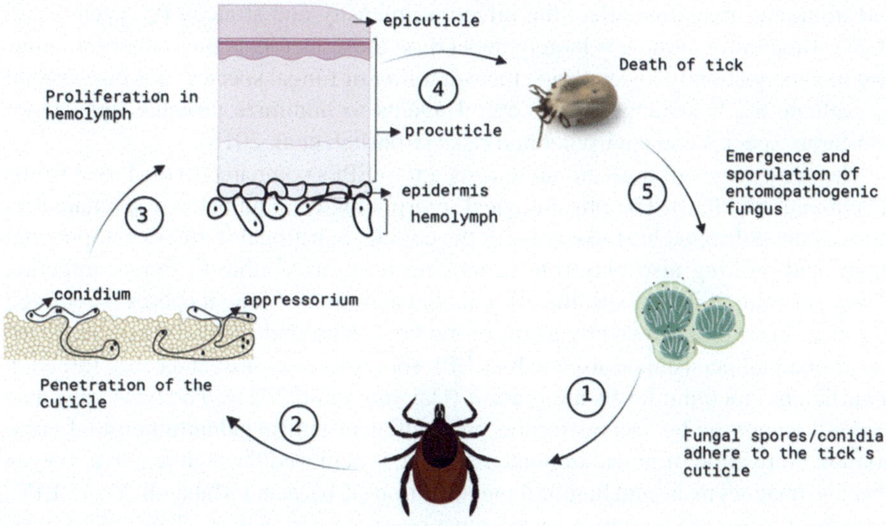


**Fig. 12.1** Mode of infection of entomopathogenic fungi. (Image created with Biorender.com)

### 12.3.1 Toxins Produced During Fungal Pathogenesis

Fungi are known to produce a number of toxins that impact the overall health of insects as they can affect different tissues in insects, with cytotoxins causing cellular disruption before fungal hyphae can even penetrate (Sinha et al. 2016). Different symptoms such as sluggishness, paralysis, and reduced irritability in insects are due to neuromuscular toxins of infecting fungal species (Sinha et al. 2016). Widely used EPF, *B. bassiana* has several toxic compounds like beauverolides, isarolides, beauvericin, and bassianolide that help in the progression of the infection (Pacheco et al. 2022). Other toxins like destruxins and cytochalasins are produced by *M. anisopliae*. Destruxin is associated with both the virulence and specificity of host (Amiri-Besheli et al. 2000). Destruxins disrupt the muscle membranes by activation of calcium channels in lepidopterans and disturb the functionality of hemocytes. The destruxins can modulate the host's cellular immune system, inhibiting phagocytosis and blocking nodule formation (Pacheco et al. 2022).

## 12.4 Virulence and Viability of Entomopathogenic Fungi

Epizootics of these infectious fungal agents mainly depend on their genetics, virulence, and host-pathogen compatibility (Herlinda 2010). Both biotic and abiotic factors influence the pathogenic mechanism. The biotic factors are usually the spore density and dispersal, host range and latency whereas, the abiotic factors include soil properties (Quesada-Moraga et al. 2007), temperature, humidity (Fernandes et al. 2012), rainfall, and sunlight (Cafarchia et al. 2022). Additionally, host biology and immunity may also affect the infection intensity and strategy (Qayyum et al. 2021). Biocontrol strategies largely depend on these factors acting either individually or synergistically to determine the suitability of fungal species. It is also crucial to evaluate the host range of biocontrol agents to minimize possible impacts on non-target species and environmental risks (Rohrlich et al. 2018).

The adult stages of ticks are more resistant to EPFs compared to the larval forms (Dannon et al. 2020). The physiological, morphological, and behavioral characteristics of the arthropod host like color of the cuticle, nutritional status, developmental stage, and molting also play role in making host susceptible to fungal infection (Qayyum et al. 2021). A specific critical concentration of fungal spores is required to cause infection followed by death of the host (Kirkland et al. 2004a). Increased environmental persistence also enables EPF spores to meet host and cause infection if sufficient inoculum levels are present (Qayyum et al. 2021). The ticks have also evolved responses by increasing the production of antifungal/antimicrobial compounds. Activation of innate immune response is achieved through reactive oxygen species, phagocytosis, and humoral melanization (Zibaee and Malagoli 2014). EPFs intended for use as biocontrol agents must possess resistance mechanisms to overcome these host immune defenses (Cafarchia et al. 2022). The resistance of entomopathogenous fungal species is imperative for tolerating the oxidative stress induced by the host. A fungal species, *Beauveria bassiana*, upregulates the production of superoxide dismutase which enhances its ability to convert superoxide ions into molecular oxygen and hydrogen peroxide thereby effectively combating oxidative stress (Zibaee and Malagoli 2014).

In environment, majority of the interactions between the host and fungus are governed by the abiotic factors. The fungal species belonging to the order Hypocreales are major pathogens of the insects in tropical and humid habitats while the Entomophthorales are prevalent in temperate areas (Islam et al. 2021). However, the two EPF species which dominate the natural habitats around the world are *B. bassiana* and *M. anisopliae* and they are affected by agricultural practices and soil tillage (Cafarchia et al. 2022). Other factors associated with greater likelihood of harboring EPF are soil acidity, heavy soil texture, and higher organic matter (Quesada-Moraga et al. 2007). Temperature plays a crucial role in influencing the viability and efficacy of EPFs. At high temperature, fungal strains of warmer regions have better infection potential, whereas those from cooler climates show optimal effectiveness at lower temperature (Qayyum et al. 2021). The dormant conidia of fungi can tolerate high temperatures due to higher amounts of saturated fatty acids, trehalose, and mannitol which decrease cellular membrane permeability and provide protection against protein denaturation (Rangel et al. 2015). The germination temperatures of individual fungal agents have a wide range, for example *B. bassiana* and *M. anisopliae* can grow between 8–37 °C but the optimum range for germination is 20–30 °C (Fernandes et al. 2008). Higher atmospheric relative humidity (>95.5%) increases the spore germination and viability of conidia. Moisture value of >96% is required for spore germination and mycelial development (Qayyum et al. 2021). The two most common EPFs, *M. anisopliae* and *B. bassiana*, can infect their hosts in low relative humidity conditions as suitable conditions are available in microhabitats (Cafarchia et al. 2022). Precipitation, on the other hand can displace conidia from the host surfaces within a short time (Qayyum et al. 2021). Despite the hydrophobic mechanisms of conidial adhesion, significant amounts of spores and conidia can be dislodged from the surface of host during rain (Cafarchia et al. 2022). Intensity and duration of exposure to solar radiation also influence conidial activation and germination, some strains of EPF are genetically more resistant to the UV radiation (Fernandes et al. 2007). The cytoplasmic membranes and organelles of conidia degrade under solar radiations: UVA (320–400 nm) and UVB (290–320 nm), most probably due to damage to DNA (Cafarchia et al. 2022). For pH, optimal growth range is 3–9, but pH of 4.4 and 6 are best for mycelium growth and spore production, respectively. A nitrogen source is not specifically required by *B. bassiana* and *Metarhizium* spp. but urea, particularly at high concentrations, greatly enhances sporulation. The concentration of sugars like sucrose, glucose, raffinose, and maltose directly affects the number of produced spores. Iron and manganese, among minerals, also affect spore production (Cafarchia et al. 2022).

## 12.5 Immune Response of Ticks Following Fungal Infection

Ticks are generally considered more resistant to EPF infection among all arthropods and exhibit differential susceptibility to different EPFs as ticks can protect themselves against mild fungal infections (Fiorotti et al. 2022). Insects, in general, have evolved several strategies besides immune responses to evade pathogens. As cuticle is the primary surface where the interaction takes place, the insects produce epicuticular metabolites, proteins, and lipids to kill microbes. Moreover, the biochemical adaptations like induced fever and environmental adaptations like burrowing and grooming also keep pathogens away. In this way, insects stop pathogens from breaching the cuticle and infecting the organism (Sinha et al. 2016). Our knowledge on the interaction between ticks and EPFs, especially regarding immune responses is very limited. Nevertheless, more studies will help in selection of EPF isolates and their effective formulations for use in biological control (Fernandes et al. 2012). The species, *B. bassiana* and *M. anisopliae* are pathogenic to several species of ticks but exhibit different results for larvae and engorged females in terms of susceptibility to infection (Fernandes et al. 2011). The genetic factors and physiological characteristics of ticks might be the reason for their susceptibility to different fungal species (Fernandes et al. 2012). For ticks, EPFs only attain high mortality levels with high conidial concentrations, that too under laboratory conditions as no natural fungal epizootics are reported in ticks yet (Fernandes et al. 2012). While under lab conditions, the hemolymph of engorged females of *R. microplus*, when infected with *M. anisopliae* s.l. or *B. bassiana*, exhibits a reduced number of hemocytes and increased number of degranulated cells showing signs of an immediate and severe cellular response which activates prophenoloxidase cascade (Harrison and Bonning 2010). Within 24 h of inoculation, the engorged females displayed high levels of esterified cholesterol, hemocyte lipids, and phosphatidic acid/phosphatidylethanolamine indicating cellular immune response (Angelo et al. 2010). The prophenoloxidase cascade is a characteristic mechanism for triggering defense reactions in arthropods for limiting the infections (Harrison and Bonning 2010).

## 12.6 Efficacy of Entomopathogenic Fungi Against Ticks

The virulence of EPF strains against target pests and the cost-effective mass production are highly desirable traits for their employment against the pests (Sinha et al. 2016). The use of EPFs as biological control agents requires isolation of fungal strains in a pure culture and assessing their effectiveness through in vitro bioassays. Subsequently, pilot tests are conducted under field conditions to evaluate their efficacy (Cafarchia et al. 2022). Almost 58 fungal species have been observed to infect at least 73 species of Acari, either in natural settings or in laboratory experiments (Fernandes et al. 2012). Table 12.1 provides a thorough review on studies related to testing efficacy of EPFs against different tick species.

The most tested EPF formulation involves aqueous suspension of conidia, typically suspended in water with Tween 80), that targets different life stages of ticks (Fernandes et al. 2012; Cafarchia et al. 2022). The field or semi-field trials with aqueous suspensions have not yielded very promising results, unless applied repeatedly, most probably due to the environmental conditions where high temperature, UV radiation, and desiccation severely reduce the persistence of conidia thereby affecting viability of EPFs (Fernandes et al. 2012). Among the in vitro contact and immersion tests, water and oil-based formulations have yielded positive outcomes for adult ticks (Perinotto et al. 2012; Bernardo et al. 2018; Zhendong et al. 2019; Marciano et al. 2021). On the other hand, the spray technique seems to be more effective on larval instars (Murigu et al. 2016; Sullivan et al. 2020). The most common mode of application in the field trials is, however, the spray method with varying but encouraging outcomes (Samish et al. 2014; Tofiño Rivera et al. 2018; Lee et al. 2019). As high inoculum levels are required to control ticks, conidial concentrations higher than $1–5 \times 10^6$ are appropriate for killing them. The lethal time is also higher, more than 10 days for the adult ticks and is estimated to be more than 7 days for the unfed larvae (Cafarchia et al. 2015, 2022).

The EPF conidia, when placed on animal hosts, can effectively manage tick populations in field or semi-field settings, particularly when applied in areas protected from environmental factors that are harmful to fungi, however, the effectiveness of this method is greatly influenced by the behavior of tick species (Fernandes et al. 2012). The tick, *Anocenter nitens* (synonym *Dermacentor nitens*) primarily infests the outer ears of equines and, during severe infestations, can also be found in the perianal area and upper leg. These areas provide microclimates that protect the fungi from harsh environmental conditions like direct sunlight, excessive heat, UV exposure, and drying out, enhancing the persistence of fungal conidia. For instance, applying *B. bassiana* conidia in a polymerized cellulose gel on the ears of horses infested with *A. nitens* resulted in control rates exceeding 50% from the fourth to the 25th day after treatment (Souza et al. 2009). Similar results were seen in cattle with artificially infested ears treated with a water-based *B. bassiana* conidia solution,

**Table 12.1** A review of literature reporting the employment of entomopathogenic fungi on various life stages of tick species since year 2000

| EPF species | EPF formulation | Mode of administration | Tick species | Applied to the tick stage: egg/nymph/adult | Mortality (%) Lethal concentration (LC)/lethal time (LT) | Conclusions | References |
|---|---|---|---|---|---|---|---|
| *Beauveria bassiana*<br>*Metarizium anisopliae* | Aqueous formulation: Suspension of $10^9$ conidia per mL + water<br>Oil-based formulations: Fungal conidia+15% peanut oil+1% Tween-80 as emulsifier +84% water | Sprayed on ticks<br>Immersed on ticks sealed in nylon tetra packs | *Rhipicephalus appendiculatus*<br>*Amblyomma variegatum* | Adults<br>Nymph<br>Larvae | Ticks sealed in tetra pack:<br>100% mortality in larvae<br>80–95% mortality in nymphs and 78–80% in adults<br>Mortality with tick's life stage:<br>Larvae: 100% mortality with both formulations<br>Nymph: 80% mortality with aqueous formulation<br>100% with oil formulation<br>Adults: 20–40% with aqueous<br>65–100% with oil formulation<br>Ticks on potted grass with oil emulsion:<br>65–75% mortality in *A. variegatum* and 75–80% mortality in *R. appenduculatus* | High mortality with oil formulations<br>Egg viability of surviving ticks reduced to 30% in *B. bassiana* and 50% in *M. anisopliae* | Kaaya and Hassan (2000) |

(continued)

**Table 12.1** (continued)

| EPF species | EPF formulation | Mode of administration | Tick species | Applied to the tick stage: egg/nymph/adult | Mortality (%) Lethal concentration (LC)/lethal time (LT) | Conclusions | References |
|---|---|---|---|---|---|---|---|
| *Beauveria bassiana* *Metarhizium anisopliæ* | Aqueous formulation: Suspension of $10^9$ conidia per mL + water Oil-based formulations: Fungal conidia+15% peanut oil+1% Tween-80 as emulsifier +84% water | Sprayed on ticks and paddocks Immersed on ticks sealed in nylon tetra packs | *Amblyomma variegatum* *Rhipicephalus apendiculatus* *Boophilus decoloratus* | Larvae Nymph Adults | Higher mortalities with oil emulsion treatment. Mortality in larvae: 100% Mortality in nymphs: 80–95% Mortality in adults: 78–80% in *A. variegatum* and *R. appenduculatus* | The number of ticks on cattle is reduced due to the spraying of vegetation in paddocks. Considering both egg viability reduction and ticks' mortality, these entomogenous fungi's impact was far higher on *B. decoloratus*. The acaricide effect will be less efficient than these fungi for *B. decoloratus* | Kaaya (2000) |
| *Metarhizium flavoviride* (CG-291, MF-3) *Metarhizium anisopliae* (CG-30, CG-46) | | Inoculation of eggs with conidial suspension. Immersion of engorged females in different concentrations of conidial suspensions. | *Boophilus microplus* | Adults Eggs | $LD_{50}$ of each strain for engorged female CG-30: $2.3 \times 10^7$ Y CG-46: $1.4 \times 10^7$ Y CG-291: $3.4 \times 10^5$ Y MF-3: $4.3 \times 10^5$ Y | Mean percentage control (C%) in terms of dead females increases as the conidial concentration increases. The mean percentage of eclosion and mean reproductive efficiency decreases with increasing conidial concentration | Onofre et al. (2001) |

| | | | | | | | |
|---|---|---|---|---|---|---|---|
| *Beauveria bassiana* *Metarhizium anisopliae*, *Metarhizium avoviride* *Paecilomyces fumosoroseus* *Verticillium lecanii* | | 0.5 mL suspension of fungal spores impregnated on the filter paper over which eggs and larvae are placed<br>Immersion of engorged females in fungal spores suspension | *Boophilus annulatus* | Adults<br>Eggs<br>Larvae | *M. anisopliae* and *B. bassiana* caused 80–100% mortality of ticks engorged females.<br>70–98% mortality of eggs due to *M. anisopliae* and *B. bassiana* strains.<br>*M. anisopliae* strain (Ma-7) at a concentration of $1 \times 10^7$ spores $mL^{-1}$ cause 80.4% mortality of larvae. When concentration increased upto $1 \times 10^8$ spores $mL^{-1}$ the mortality of larvae becomes 100%.<br>$LT_{50}$ of *B. bassiana:* 7–8 days<br>$LT_{50}$ of *M. anisopliae*:<br>6–7 days<br>*M. avoviride, P. fumosoroseus*,<br>and *V. lecanii* causes 25–60% mortality of females. | Reduction of tick egg laying capacity by fungi.<br>*M. anisopliae* limit the egg laying capacity to only 7–8% of females<br>35.4%–80.8% reduction in egg weight | Gindin et al. (2001) |

(continued)

**Table 12.1** (continued)

| EPF species | EPF formulation | Mode of administration | Tick species | Applied to the tick stage: egg/nymph/adult | Mortality (%) Lethal concentration (LC)/lethal time (LT) | Conclusions | References |
|---|---|---|---|---|---|---|---|
| *Metarhizium anisopliae* *Beauveria bassiana* | $10^7$ spores/mL containing 5 mL conidia suspension+4% sunflower oil +100 mL of 0.01% Tween-80 + sterilized water for desired concentration | Adult and nymph both immersed in fungal spores suspension | *Argas (persicargas) persicus* | Adults Nymph | Mortality and $LC_{50}$ of *M. anisopliae:*<br>Unfed female: 35% with $LC_{50}$ of $2.4 \times 10^8$<br>Engorged females: 81% with $LC_{50}$ of $6.6 \times 10^3$<br>$LC_{50}$ for first nymphal instar: $3.2 \times 10^3$<br>$LC_{50}$ for 2nd nymphal instar: $>1 \times 10^{10}$<br>Mortality and $LC_{50}$ of *B. bassiana:*<br>Unfed female: 73% with $LC_{50}$ of $2.6 \times 10^7$<br>Engorged female: 74% with $LC_{50}$ of $6.9 \times 10^4$<br>$LC_{50}$ for first nymphal instar: $1.1 \times 10^4$<br>$LC_{50}$ for 2nd nymphal instar: $>1 \times 10^{10}$ | First nymphal instar and engorged female were more susceptible to fungal infection than the nymph of 2nd instar and unfed females, respectively | Sewify and Habib (2001) |

| | | | | | | | |
|---|---|---|---|---|---|---|---|
| *Beauveria bassiana* | Conidia+20 mL of 0.01% Tween-80 | Immersion of eggs, larvae, and engorged females in 1, 2, and 20 mL of suspension respectively | *Boophilus microplus* | Engorged females<br>Larvae<br>Eggs | Larvae:<br>Hatching rate reduction: 1.36–65.58%<br>Mortality increased by 0.8–70.49%<br>Engorged females:<br>Reduction of<br>1. Ovisposition period 9.69–47.80%<br>2. Egg mass weight 4.71–53.87%<br>3. Reproduction 8.3–60.62%<br>4. Egg production index 5.03–54.20%<br>5. Larval hatching 0.27–13.96%<br>Mortality rate increased by 96.60–100% | AM 09, JAB 07, and CB7 isolates were more effective against tick species | de Cássia Vieira Paião et al. (2001) |
| *Beauveria bassiana*<br>*Metarhizium anisopliae*<br>*Metarhizium flavoviride*<br>*Paecilomyces fumosoroseus* | Conidia+ aqueous solution of 0.005% Triton X-100 | Filter paper impregnated with 0.5 mL of suspension for unfed and engorged larvae. Adults submerged in 1 × $10^7$ conidia/mL for 3–5 s | *Rhipicephalus sanguineus* | Adults<br>Nymphs<br>Larvae | *M. anisopliae*-108<br>Unfed larvae/nymphs: 92–96%/7 days<br>Engorged larvae and nymphs: 82.6% and 60%<br>Unfed adults and engorged females: 100%/21 days<br>Egg laying capacity: 11.3–60.8% | *B. bassiana*, *M. flavoviride*, and *P. fumosoroseus* were less virulent to almost not virulent for most of the stages of tick | Samish et al. (2001) |

(continued)

**Table 12.1** (continued)

| EPF species | EPF formulation | Mode of administration | Tick species | Applied to the tick stage: egg/nymph/adult | Mortality (%) Lethal concentration (LC)/lethal time (LT) | Conclusions | References |
|---|---|---|---|---|---|---|---|
| *Metarhizium anisopliae*<br>*Metarhizium Flavoviride*<br>*Beauveria bassiana*<br>*Paecilomyces fumosoroseus*<br>*Verticillium lecanii* | Fungal spores+ aqueous solution of 0.0005% Triton-X 100 | Immersion of adult ticks in suspension (1 × $10^7$ spores/mL)<br>Eggs placed on 0.5 mL spore suspension (2.5 × $10^3$ spores/$mm^3$) impregnated filter paper | *Boophilus annulatus*<br>*Hyalomma excavatum*<br>*Rhipicephalus sanguineus* | Adults<br>Eggs<br>Larvae | $LT_{50}$ for eggs: 2–6 days<br>$LT_{50}$ for engorged female of *B. annulatus*: 5–6 days<br>Mortality of unfed larvae<br>*M. anisopliae*: 70–100% killed in 4–7 days<br>*M. flavoviride*: 97% and 82% of *B. annulatus* and *H. excavatum*, respectively, and 8% mortality of *R. sanguineus*<br>*B. bassiana*, *P. fumosoroseus*, and *V. lecanii*: 2–22% of all three tick species' larvae<br>Mortality of engorged females:<br>*M. annisopliae* and *B. bassiana*: 80–100% of *B. annulatus* and *R. sanguineus* | *M. anisopliae* was found to be more virulent against tick survival, engorged females' fecundity, and viability of eggs. *H. excavatum* engorged female highly resistant to fungal spores of *M. anisopliae* and *B. bassiana* | Gindin et al. (2002) |

| | | | | | | | |
|---|---|---|---|---|---|---|---|
| *Metarhizium anisopliae*<br>*Beauveria bassiana* | 2 types of formulations, (i) conidial spores harvested from liquid medium (SDY)<br>(ii) Conidial spores harvested from agar plates (SDAY) | Ticks immersed for 30 seconds in fungal suspension | *Ambylomma americanum*<br>*Ambylomma maculatum* | Adults<br>Nymphs | *A. maculatum* ticks with *B. bassiana*<br>Blastospore/mL:<br>Adult:<br>86%/28 days/$10^6$ conidia $mL^{-1}$<br>100%/$10^8$ conidia $mL^{-1}$<br>With conidia/mL:<br>95%/28 days<br>Nymph: nearly 98%/28 days<br>Conidia/mL: 95%/28 days<br>With *M. anisopliae:*<br>Adults: 61%/28 days<br>Nymphs: 99%/28 days<br>*A. americanum* with *B. bassiana:*<br>Blastospore/mL adult:<br>18%/28 days<br>Conidia/mL: 6%/28 days<br>Nymph: 20–35%/28 days<br>Conidia/mL: 26%/28 days<br>With *M. anisopliae*:<br>Adults: 13%/28 days<br>Nymph: 21%/28 days<br>From liquid medium:<br>7% mortality/$10^6$ cells $mL^{-1}$ of maculatum | Nymphs of both ticks found to be more affected by the fungal infection.<br>Both tick species had different level of resistance and susceptibility towards entomopathogenic fungus species | Kirkland et al. (2004a) |

(continued)

**Table 12.1** (continued)

| EPF species | EPF formulation | Mode of administration | Tick species | Applied to the tick stage: egg/nymph/adult | Mortality (%)<br>Lethal concentration (LC)/lethal time (LT) | Conclusions | References |
|---|---|---|---|---|---|---|---|
| *Beauveria bassiana*<br>*Metarhizium anisopliae* | Water conidial suspension+0.01% Tween-20 | Sprayed and submerged | *Dermacentor variabilis*<br>*Ixodes scapularis,*<br>*Rhipicephalus sanguineus* | Adults<br>Nymphs | 50–70%/28 days of adults of *I. scapularis* and *R. sanguineus*<br><20% of *D. variabilis* ticks<br>Nymphs:<br>*R. sanguineus:*<br>>90%/21–28 days<br>*D. variabilis*:<br>20–40%/28 days<br>*I. scapularis*:<br>45%/28 days | Addition of nutrients in fungal suspension didn't have any significant effect on mortality.<br>$10^8$/mL threshold dose for mortality of *R. sanguineus* and *I. scapularis* | Kirkland et al. (2004b) |
| *Beauveria bassiana* | – | Eggs immersed in 1 mL conidial suspension | *Boophilus. microplus* | Engorged females<br>Eggs | Eclosion percentage:<br>20–86.6%<br>Larval mortality: 10–96%<br>Highest mortality at a concentration of $10^8$/mL | – | Fernandes et al. (2003) |
| *Metarhizium anisopliae* | 50 mL of conidia in sterile distilled water with 0.2% Tween-80, coconut oil and paraffin wax separately | Immersion of engorged female in fungal inoculum for 10 s | *Boophilus microplus* | Engorged females | Average survival time (AST):<br>4.4 ± 0.15 days<br>4.6 ± 0.28 days<br>8.4 ± 0.42 days<br>With 10% liquid paraffin, coconut oil and water respectively | 10% liquid paraffin EAO and coconut oil enhanced the pathogenicity of *M. Anisopliae* to cause mortality when compared to water | Polar et al. (2005) |

| | | | | | | | |
|---|---|---|---|---|---|---|---|
| *Metarhizium anisopliae* | Conidial suspension in 0.1% Tween-80 and distilled water for controlling concentration | $1.8 \times 10^8$ conidia per mL suspension sprayed on the fields infested with engorged females | *Boophilus. microplus* | Engorged females | 87% to 94% efficacy of fungus for the control of larvae at different time such as exactly after | *B. brizantha* has higher larval count than the Tifton 85 | Basso et al. (2005) |
| *Metarhizium anisopliae* | Conidial suspension in 100 mL distilled water and 0.1% Tween-80 | Immersion of all three stages in conidial suspension after that incubated | *Boophilus. microplus* | Eggs<br>Larvae<br>Engorged females | – | Oviposition period decreased by 2.6 ± 1.4 to 2.7 ± 3.1 days.<br>Egg production decreased and became 0.013 g at $10^8$ conidia $mL^{-1}$<br>Egg hatchability reduced to 20.0 ± 8.9% at 108 conidia $mL^{-1}$<br>Reproductive efficiency reduced to 11.0 ± 6.6 and 5.6 ± 3.9% at $10^8$ conidia per mL | de Melo et al. (2006) |

(continued)

**Table 12.1** (continued)

| EPF species | EPF formulation | Mode of administration | Tick species | Applied to the tick stage: egg/nymph/adult | Mortality (%)<br>Lethal concentration (LC)/lethal time (LT) | Conclusions | References |
|---|---|---|---|---|---|---|---|
| *Metarhizium anisopliae* | Oil-based formulation: 0.074 g fungal spores in 1 mL of vegetable oil (sterilized) and 9 mL of distilled water = $3 \times 10^8$ spores/mL<br>Aqueous formulation: 0.074 g fungal spores in 10 mL of sterilized water with 0.1% of Tween-80 | Engorged females were submerged in the high dose of suspension from $8.5 \times 10^6$ to $9.5 \times 10^8$ conidia/mL for 1 min | *Boophilus microplus* | Engorged females | Aqueous suspension: 0–100% mortality based on concentration of solution. 100% mortality for oil-based and aqueous solution at $1 \times 10^8$ conidia/mL after day 2 and 5, respectively | Growth of all isolates occured at temperature of 20 °C, 25 °C and 30 °C | Leemon and Jonsson (2008) |
| *Metarhizium anisopliae* | Conidia in distilled water with 0.1% Tween-80 solution. Diluted till concentration of $1 \times 10^8$ conidia/mL | Spraying of $1 \times 10^8$ conidia/mL solution on tick infested animals after every 15 days (four treatments) | *Boophilus microplus* | Engorged females | Percentage efficacy:<br>After day 7 (second application treatment) the efficacy was 9.6%, 52.9%, 80%, and 88.1%, calculated after every dip | – | Alonso-Díaz et al. (2007) |
| *Metarhizium anisopliae* | *M. anisopliae* $1 \times 10^8$ conidia/mL solution<br>Deltamethrin 25 ppm | Spraying of *M. anisopliae* suspension and deltamethrin solution on ticks | *Boophilus microplus* (pyrethroid-resistant strain) | Engorged females | Mortality:<br>With *M. anisopliae* suspension: 32.57%<br>With deltamethrin: 38.58%<br>With both: 30.92% | Entomopathogenic fungi, i.e., *M. anisopliae* and deltamethrin both can be used as integrated management for tick control | Bahiense et al. (2008) |

| | | | | | | | |
|---|---|---|---|---|---|---|---|
| *Metarhizium anisopliae*<br>*Beauveria bassiana* | Conidial suspension formulation in:<br>i) Emulsifiable concentrate (EC)<br>ii) Polymerized cellulose gel (PCG)<br>iii) EC + PCG | Immersion in conidial solution for 3 min | *Rhipicephalus sanguineus* | Engorged females | Control percentage: 1.PCG+ *M. anisopliae*: 41.75%<br>2.PCG + *B. bassiana*: 64.34%<br>3.EC+ *M. anisopliae*: 65.25%<br>4.EC+ *B. bassiana*: 70.22%<br>5.EC + PCG + *M. anisopliae*: 80.13%<br>6.EC + PCG+ *B. bassiana*: 86.79% | Highest mortality by EC + PCG+ *B. bassiana* | Reis et al. (2008) |
| *Metarhizium anisopliae*<br>*Beauveria bassiana*<br>*Paecilomyces fumosoroseus* | Conidia in 0.85% NaCl solution and 0.1% Tween-80 | Larvae and nymph placed on petri dish having conidial suspension containing filter paper with $2.4 \times 10^3$ to $9.6 \times 10^6$ per cm$^2$ | *Ixodes ricinus* | Larvae<br>Nymphs | $LT_{50}$<br>*M. anisopliae* 97 ($1.4 \times 10^6$ per cm$^2$)<br>Unfed larvae: 14 days<br>Unfed nymphs: 21 days<br>80% mortality in unfed nymphs after 30 days | – | Hartelt et al. (2008) |
| *Beauveria bassiana* (Bb1764 and Bb2157)<br>*Lecanicillium lecanii* (Ll586, Ll618, and Ll3047)<br>*Tolypocladium cylindrosporum* (Tc3398) | Conidia in 5 mL distilled water with 0.01% Tween-80 | Immersion in 2 mL of conidial solution | *Ornithodoros erraticus*<br>*Ornithodoros moubata* | Unfed males<br>Females<br>Nymphs-4,3,2 | 34.4–62% mortality of *O. erraticus* by strains Bb1764, Bb2157, and Tc3398. Bb2157 induced 31.9% mortality of *O. moubata* | All the strains such as Ll586, Ll618, and Ll3047 did not cause any mortality in ticks | Zabalgogeazcoa et al. (2008) |

(continued)

**Table 12.1** (continued)

| EPF species | EPF formulation | Mode of administration | Tick species | Applied to the tick stage: egg/nymph/adult | Mortality (%) Lethal concentration (LC)/lethal time (LT) | Conclusions | References |
|---|---|---|---|---|---|---|---|
| *Metarhizium anisopliae* (689 and 685 strains) | Conidia suspension prepared by using Tween-80 | Immersion of larvae in the suspension for about 3 s | *H. anatolicum anatolicum*<br>*Haemaphysalis punctata* | Larvae | 50–88.2% mortality of *H. anatolicum anatolicum*<br>74.7–100% of *H. punctata* at $10^3$ and $10^4$ conidia/mL concentrations | Virulence of *M. anisopliae* 689 was higher for *H. punctata* and of 685 for *H. anatolicum anatolicum* | Tavasoli et al. (2009) |
| *Beauveria bassiana* | – | i) Both ticks submerged in various spore concentrations for 1 min<br>ii) *H. marginatum* engorged females dipped for 2 min in $1 \times 10^3$ spores/mL<br>iii) Unfed adults of *H. marginatum* suspended in concentrations of $1 \times 10^6$ and $2 \times 10^6$ spores/mL<br>Engorged nymphs of *H. marginatum* also suspended<br>iv). Suspended in spore suspension for 15 min | *H. marginatum*<br>*H. anatolicum anatolicum* | Engorged females<br>Larvae<br>Eggs | No mortality difference among experimented groups, but a decreased hatchability was observed.<br>No mortality difference, no oviposition rate difference but hatchability decreased<br>No difference of mortality rate among groups<br>Immediate tremors and paralysis were observed | The treated ticks died after 4 months of experiment | Abdigoudarzi et al. (2009) |

| | | | | | | | |
|---|---|---|---|---|---|---|---|
| *Lecanicilium lecanii* | Oil-based formulation: Conidial suspension in 15 mL of mineral oil (sterilized), 1 mL of Tween-80 solution, and 84 mL of distilled water<br>Water-based formulation: Conidial suspension in 0.1% Tween-80 in distilled water | Immersion in both conidial solutions, i.e., oil based, and water based with concentration $1 \times 10^8$ conidial $mL^{-1}$ for oil-based to several concentrations of water-based. Females were immersed for 5 min and larvae were immersed for 3 min | *Rhipicephalus microplus* | Eggs<br>Larvae<br>Engorged females | Oil suspension: Engorged females: 97.6% mortality<br>Larval mortality: 100% after 5 days<br>Water-based: 41.02% at $10^8$ concentrations<br>$LC_{50}$ range from day 5–20 is $1.16 \times 10^{14}$ -$1.16 \times 10^6$ conidia $mL^{-1}$<br>$LC_{90}$ range from $7.4 \times 10^{19}$–$1.35 \times 10^7$ conidia $mL^{-1}$ | Egg hatchability was not much affected. Only highest concentration of water suspension caused significant mortality | Angelo et al. (2010) |
| *Beauveria bassiana Beauveria amorpha, Beauveria brongniartii Beauveria velata Beauveria vermiconia* | Conidia are suspended in Polyoxyethylene Sorbitene monooleate and $1 \times 10^8$ condia/mL suspension is obtained | Immersion of larvae for 5 min | *Rhipicephalus microplus* | Larvae | $LC_{50}$ for five *Beauveria bassiana* isolates: $10^7$ to $10^8$ conidia/mL | Five isolates of *Beauveria bassiana* from 53 CG 481, CG 484, CG 206, CG 235, and CG 487 were found to be affected for biological control of ticks | Fernandes et al. (2011) |

(continued)

**Table 12.1** (continued)

| EPF species | EPF formulation | Mode of administration | Tick species | Applied to the tick stage: egg/nymph/adult | Mortality (%) Lethal concentration (LC)/ lethal time (LT) | Conclusions | References |
|---|---|---|---|---|---|---|---|
| *Metarhizium anisopliae* | Both water and oil formulations were made | Eggs and larval instars placed in petri dish with filter paper soaked in 1 mL of conidial suspension | *Amblyomma. variegatum, Rhipicephalus appendiculatus, Rhipicephalus evertsi evertsi* | Eggs<br>Larval instar | Eggs:<br>50–77% in water<br>65–87% in oil formulation<br>Unfed larvae: 55–95% in water<br>73–<br>100% in oil formulation<br>Fed larvae:<br>51–84% in water<br>59–<br>90% in oil formulation.<br>Unfed nymph:<br>52–59% in water<br>71–98% in<br>Oil formulations.<br>Fed nymph:<br>63–80% in water<br>72–92% in oil formulation.<br>Unfed adults:<br>56–83% in water<br>73–91% in oil formulation.<br>Fed adults: 71–90% in water<br>88–97% in oil | Unfed adults with *R. e. evertsi* had the highest mortality.<br>High mortality in *A. variegatum* than *R. appendiculatus* and *R. e. evertsi.*<br>In fed and unfed larvae, high mortality in *R. appendiculatus* for water suspension and *A. variegatum* for oil formulation of fed larvae,<br>For unfed larvae with oil formulation, high mortality in *R. e. evertsi* observed,<br>Mortality and infection of eggs with both water and oil suspension found high in *R. e. evertsi* | Hedimbi et al. (2011) |

| | | | | | | | |
|---|---|---|---|---|---|---|---|
| *Beauveria bassiana*<br>*Metarhizium anisopliae* | Water formulation:<br>Conidia in sterile distilled water and 0.05% Triton-X 100.<br>Oil formulation:<br>Conidia in oil emulsion which have 20% sunflower oil and distilled water containing 0.05% of Trition-X 100 | Engorged female and nymphs are submerged in conidial suspension | *Rhipicephalus (Boophilus) appendiculatus*<br>*Amblyomma variegatum*<br>*Rhipicephalus evertsi evertsi*<br>*Boophilus decoloratus* | Nymphs<br>Adults | Mortality:<br>By both fungi<br>36–64% in *R. appendiculatus*<br>40–50% in *B. decoloratus*<br>100% larval mortality with oil, 80% with aqueous, and in adults of 65–100% (oil) and 20–40% with water in *R. appendiculatus* and *A. variegatum*<br>$LC_{50}$ for Engorged nymphs and adults: $1 \times 10^8$ conidia/mL in oil<br>$1 \times 10^6$ in water | Oil formulation gave the best results compared to aqueous formulations.<br>*R. e. evertsi* was infected by *M. anisopliae* and *R appendiculatus* and *B. decoloratus* by both fungal suspensions | Kaaya and Hedimbi (2012) |
| *Metarhizium anisopliae*<br>*Beauveria bassiana* | Conidia in 0.1% Tween-80 solution of distilled water | Eggs and engorged females immersed in 1 mL of conidial solution | *Rhipicephalus microplus* | Engorged females<br>Larvae<br>Eggs | Hatching percentage of egg:<br>Population 1:3.1–49.5%<br>Population 2: 3.4–42.7%<br>Unfed larvae:<br>Population 1: 91.8–98.7%<br>Population 2: 71%–94%<br>$LT_{90}$:<br>Population 1: 19.52 to 27.51 days<br>Population 2: 22.89 to 37.31 days | Pre-oviposition period along with hatchability period and egg production index were different in both populations.<br>*B. bassiana* isolate Bb 986 was more virulent than the isolate 959 of *M. anisopliae* with 49% mortality of engorged females. | Perinotto et al. (2012) |
| *Metarhizium anisopliae* | Conidia in 30 mL of 0.1% polyoxyethylene sorbitan monooleate solution | Immersion of larvae in 3 mL of conidial suspension | *Rhipicephalus microplus* | Larvae | After 10 days, mortality was less than 10%.<br>After 20 days, mortality was between 5.8% to 100%<br>After 30 days, mortality was 37.9% to 100%<br>$LC_{50}$ :$5.861 \times 10^6$ to $5.361 \times 10^8$ conidia/mL | Difference of infection and mortality rates among different isolates | Quinelato et al. (2012) |

(continued)

**Table 12.1** (continued)

| EPF species | EPF formulation | Mode of administration | Tick species | Applied to the tick stage: egg/nymph/adult | Mortality (%) Lethal concentration (LC)/lethal time (LT) | Conclusions | References |
|---|---|---|---|---|---|---|---|
| *Metarhizium brunneum* | Water suspension: Conidia from wheat suspension in distilled water and 0.1% Triton-X 100<br>Oil suspension: Conidia in 0.01% Triton-X containing water and oils. 10% (v/v) emulsion of various oils formed | Saprying of water and oil based suspensions on engorged female ticks or sand over which females were scattered | *Rhipicephalus (Boophilus) annulatus* | Engorged females<br>Eggs | Maximum mortality: 62.2 ± 10.9% mortality of females in sprayed buckets.<br>90% females died within one week in summer<br>With oil:<br>62.5–80% of females died before laying complete full-size egg masses | Full size egg masses laid by only 30% females.<br>Hatching success of larvae was zero.<br>Egg mass reduction by suspension with mineral and paraffin oil.<br>Conidial suspension spray on different grounds affected the hatchability of eggs | Samish et al. (2014) |
| *Beauveria bassiana* | Conidia in distilled water containing 0.1% Tween-80 | Immersion in $1 \times 10^7$ conidia/mL having suspension for 3 min | *Rhipicephalus sanguineus* | Larvae<br>Nymphs<br>Adult | Engorged and unfed mortality:<br>Larvae: 98.7% and 100% after 15 days<br>Adults: 100% after 15 days 85% after 20 days<br>Nymphs: 85 and 87.5% after 20 days | Water suspension was found to be more effective on unfed larvae, engorged females and unfed nymphs | Cafarchia et al. (2015) |
| *Metarhizium anisopliae* | Blastospore of fungi in liquid medium for suspension creation | Placement of larvae on the petri dishes containing equally distributed fungal blastospore filter paper for 7 days | *Ixodes recinus* | Larvae<br>Nymph | The mortality of 96.8% of engorged larvae after a week | The reduction in the successful molt rate occurs by 3.5% | Wassermann et al. (2016) |

| | | | | | | | |
|---|---|---|---|---|---|---|---|
| *Metarhzium anisopliae* | Aqueous suspension in distilled water with 0.1% Tween-80.<br>Oil-based formulation by using 10% vegetable oil.<br>Dilution of it occurred for the desired concentration level | Spraying of formulations on the larvae and eggs<br>Eggs are placed in and on the filter paper, then 50 microliter suspension is sprayed on and poured over them | *Rhipicephalus sanguineus* | Larvae<br>Eggs | $LT_{50}$ for:<br>Water based was 9–10.2 days and<br>oil-based was 14.9–19.5 days | Oil-based emulsion proved to be more effective than the water-based ones.<br>Indirect application of water-based suspension shows the least successful results | Luz et al. (2016) |
| *Beauveria bassiana*<br>*Metarhizium anisopliae*<br>*Metarhizium robertsii* | Conidia in distilled water with 0.01–0.1% Tween-80 | Immersion of both larvae and engorged female for about 1 min | *Rhipicephalus. microplus* | Larvae<br>Engorged females | 70–100% mortality of larvae by *Metarhizium* species conidia<br>*B. bassiana* conidia caused 17–99% mortality of larvae<br>>40% mortality by blastopore of *B. bassiana*<br>All results were obtained after 14 days | Engorged females showed a reduction of egg production indices and low nutritional content when the treatment of blastopores was given.<br>But the overall conidia gave the high pathogenicity for larvae.<br>Short oviposition period | Bernardo et al. (2018) |
| *Beauveria bassiana*<br>*Metarhizium anisopliae* | Conidia in distilled water having 0.05% Triton-X 100 with the concentration of $1 \times 10^9$ conidia/mL | 10 mL fungal suspension was sprayed on the larvae of the tick | *Rhipicephalus. decoloratus* | Larvae | Percentage mortality: Amitraz susceptible strain: 10 and 100%<br>Amitraz-resistant strain: 12.1% and 100%<br>69.2% mortality with *M. anisopliae*<br>$LT_{50:}$ 3.0–4.1 days | Fungal treatment was more virulent for the amitraz-susceptible larval strain of *R. decoloratus* | Murigu et al. (2016) |

(continued)

**Table 12.1** (continued)

| EPF species | EPF formulation | Mode of administration | Tick species | Applied to the tick stage: egg/nymph/adult | Mortality (%)<br>Lethal concentration (LC)/lethal time (LT) | Conclusions | References |
|---|---|---|---|---|---|---|---|
| *Beauveria bassiana*<br>*Metarhizium anisopliae* | Conidial suspension preparation using distilled water and 0.05% Tween-80 | Nymphs were immersed in fungal suspension for 30 s | *Haemaphysalis qinghaiensis* | Nymphs | The mortality of nymphs was 52–100% after infecting tick nymphs with EPF.<br>$LC_{50}$<br>$5.88056 \times 10^4$<br>*B. bassiana*<br>$2.64973 \times 10^4$<br>*M. anisopliae*<br>$2.84857 \times 10^4$<br>*B. bassiana* and *M. anisopliae* | – | Ren et al. (2016) |
| *Metarhizium ansiopliae* | Water-based formulation by using distilled water with 0.1% Tween-80<br>Oil based suspension | Engorged females come in contact with suspension of fungus | *Rhipicephalus sanguineous* | Adults (engorged females) | – | Oil-based suspension gave greater efficacy than water-based suspension. | Alves et al. (2017) |
| *Metarhizium anisopliae* | Oil-based conidial suspension was formed and terpene D-limonene solution was used.<br>Water based formulation of conidia was also obtained | Immersion of tape stick larvae for 5 s | *Rhipicephalus sanguineous* | Larvae | Mortality/time<br>98.8% in 7 days for aqueous solutions<br>Mortality reaches 100% for oil suspension in 7 days | D-limonene caused highest mortality of 82.6%.<br>Cypermethrin mortalities varied in all groups.<br>Oil suspension surpassed water suspension in terms of effectiveness | Prado-Rebolledo et al. (2017) |

| | | | | | | | |
|---|---|---|---|---|---|---|---|
| *Beauveria bassiana* | Conidia in distilled water with 0.1% Tween-80 | Eggs were placed on filter paper submerged with conidial suspension in a petri dish.<br>Larvae nymphs and engorged female were immersed in fungal suspension for 3 min | *Haemaphysalis longicornis* | Eggs<br>Larvae<br>Nymphs<br>Engorged females | Hatching rate: 0–>10%<br>Mortality of unfed larvae: 100% in 15 days<br>For nymphs and engorged females, 100% mortality was observed after 20 days | High mortality in nymph and larvae which were unfed.<br>Hatchability of larvae decreased along with oviposition rate and egg weight | Zhendong et al. (2019) |
| *Metarhizium anisopliae* | Conidia in distilled water with 0.1% Tween-80 | Immersion of adults in suspension | *Amblyomma parvum* | Adults | Mortality on the third day was 80%, on the fourth day was 90%, and on the seventh day, 100% mortality was observed | Appropriate suspension having suspended conidia would be the best choice and protect fungi from UV radiation | Garcia et al. (2018) |
| *Metarhizium anisopliae* | Conidia in distilled water with 0.02% Triton-X 100.<br>$10^6$,$10^7$,$10^8$ conidia/mL are obtained | i) Filter paper impregnated with the suspension of fungi and then placed in a petri dish with larvae<br>ii) Larvae immersed for 5 min in the suspension | *Rhipicephalus microplus* | Larvae | $LT_{50}$ for filter paper case: 24.8 days<br>With 38% mortality after 21 days<br>$LT_{50}$ for immersion: 9.2 days with 98% mortality after 21 days<br>Both are at $10^8$ conidia/mL | The immersion test showed a high mortality in less time compared to filter paper | Webster et al. (2018) |

(continued)

**Table 12.1** (continued)

| EPF species | EPF formulation | Mode of administration | Tick species | Applied to the tick stage: egg/nymph/adult | Mortality (%)<br>Lethal concentration (LC)/<br>lethal time (LT) | Conclusions | References |
|---|---|---|---|---|---|---|---|
| *Beauveria bassiana*<br>*Purpureocilium lilacinum*<br>*Metarhizium anisopliae* | Conidia harvested and suspension was made in distilled water and 0.1% Tween-80 for the required conidial concentration | Larvae immersed in conidial suspension for 1 min | *Rhipicephalus microplus* | Larvae | In both populations of larvae about nine strains of *M. anisopliae* outperformed with mortality rate of 79.8–100%. 53.2% mortality in susceptible larvae and 41.8% in resistant larvae by *B. bassiana*. By *P. lilacinum* mortality was 92.3% and 94.9% in resistant and susceptible strains respectively.<br>$LC_{50}$ (conidia/mL):<br>*M. anisopliae*: $1.3 \times 10^6$ to $3.2 \times 10^7$<br>*P. lilacinum:*<br>$1.1 \times 10^6$ | *P. lilacinum* was identified as more effective strain. Acaricidal susceptible larvae were more prone towards the fungal infection | Fernández-Salas et al. (2019) |
| *Metarhizium anisopliae*, *Metarhizium brunneum*, *Beauveria bassiana* | Conidial suspension was prepared in sterilized distilled water and then 0.02% organosilicon surfactant was added | Tick larvae were sprayed with the conidial suspension | *Dermacentor albopictus* | Larvae | Mb-F52 isolate caused 82–99% mortality and 74–86% by Ma-ERL1582. 30–41% mortality for Bb-GHA.<br>52–64% mortality or Bb-ERL836.<br>Overall mortality by *B. bassiana* was 41–64% in 21 days.<br>By *M. anisopliae*, 100% mortality of tick larvae after 6 days | With higher mortality, granular *B. bassiana* (ERL836) were found to be more virulent than Bb-GHA | Sullivan et al. (2020) |

| | | | | | | | |
|---|---|---|---|---|---|---|---|
| *Metarhizium anisopliae* | Conidia in 500 mL of 1% polyoxyethylene sorbitane monooleate solution and one with 10% vegetable oil in water emulsion | Spraying on the engorged females | *Rhipicephalus microplus* | Larvae | 75.78–100% mortality was observed after 21 days | Vegetable oil was not as effective as mineral oil emulsion | Marciano et al. (2020) |
| *Aspergillus oryzae* | Aqueous suspension of fungi | Immersion of larvae and adult ticks in different concentrations of the prepared bio-acaricide. 500 mL of bioacaricide was sprayed on the cattle | *Rhipicephalus, Boophilus,* and *Amblyomma* spp. | Larvae<br>Adults | $LC_{50}$, $LC_{99}$ (conidia/mL), and larval mortality (%):<br>*Boophilus:* 99.691,<br>$9.8 \times 10^5$<br>95.5 ± 3.25%<br>*Rhipicephalus:*<br>$5.0 \times 10^3$<br>$3.0 \times 10^6$<br>84.95 ± 10.71%<br>*Amblyomma:*<br>$3.9 \times 10^3$<br>$1.6 \times 10^6$<br>87.90 ± 9.89%<br>$LC_{50}$, $LC_{99}$ (conidia/mL) and adult tick mortality (%):<br>*Boophilus:*<br>$5.3 \times 10^4$<br>$7.9 \times 10^6$<br>62.86 ± 23.90%<br>*Rhipicephalus*:<br>$5.7 \times 10^5$<br>$1.0 \times 10^7$<br>21.90 ± 24.42%<br>*Amblyomma*:<br>$5.3 \times 10^5$<br>$1.2 \times 10^7$<br>23.81 ± 24.99% | Reduction of egg viability and egg production ability. Concentration related increase in mortality for both larvae and adults | Msangi et al. (2022) |

(continued)

**Table 12.1** (continued)

| EPF species | EPF formulation | Mode of administration | Tick species | Applied to the tick stage: egg/nymph/adult | Mortality (%) Lethal concentration (LC)/lethal time (LT) | Conclusions | References |
|---|---|---|---|---|---|---|---|
| *Beauveria bassiana* | Conidia suspension in 15% avocado oil for the formulation | Spraying of suspension of larvae.<br>Immersion of engorged females | *Rhipicephalus microplus* | Larvae<br>Engorged female | 28–62% mortality by different strains | Reduction of egg weight, hatching ability of egg (38%), and egg production index (12.6%).<br>81% reduction in reproductive efficiency occurs | Zeina and Laing (2022) |

*EPF* entomopathogenic fungi

especially when their ears were covered (Russo et al. 2019). However, for tick species that infest more extensive areas of their hosts, using a formulated product is essential to maintain the conidia's persistence and effectiveness. Vegetation protects conidia from exposure to the direct sunlight, hence applications on pasture have yielded better results. Application of EPF to pastures is particularly important for tick species which spend a part of their life cycle off the host during ecdysis and while searching for a new host (Fernandes et al. 2012).

## 12.7 Challenges to Use Myco-Insecticides

The formulations of microbial biological control agents refer to the process of combining these with inert materials to enhance their properties (Hernandez-Tenorio et al. 2022). The goal is to produce products that are of high quality and effectiveness while being safe. In addition to enhancing their storage, application and the effectiveness of the active ingredients or the biological control agent are also important (Lacey et al. 2015). Typically, the EPF formulations include fungal spores and propagules, a delivery medium made up of inert materials and additives that enhance the protection, persistence, and functionality of the fungal agent (Fernandes et al. 2012). A variety of compounds with distinct characteristics are being used in formulation development to improve either efficacy or spore survival. Additives are included to protect spores from UV light, improve their adhesion to foliage (preventing wash-off), and elevate humidity around the spore, which aid in germination under challenging environmental conditions (Cafarchia et al. 2022). While many efforts to enhance the field longevity of microbial agents have involved incorporating UV protectants into conidia formulations, the field effectiveness of these treated fungi often remains insufficient for reliable pest management (Fernandes et al. 2015). Wettable powder formulations of EPF are the most commonly produced formulations which typically consist of 50–80% technical powder, 15–45% filler, 1–10% dispersant, and 3–5% surfactant (Sinha et al. 2016). These formulations are sprayed using standard insecticidal techniques such as ultra-low volume or hydraulic applications whereas, these can also be applied as a soil drench (Sinha et al. 2016).

A variety of oils are now being added in the formulations for improving their shelf life and performance in dry climate (Sinha et al. 2016). Conidial survival and viability are enhanced by simple addition of oil to spore powder (Lei et al. 2022). It has been observed that oil-based formulations have greater infectivity potential than aqueous suspensions (Bateman and Alves 2000). Oil-based liquid formulations, primarily made from natural substances used in food additives or cosmetics, do not cause environmental harm or toxic effects on treated plants or their products. Furthermore, the fungal species used in these emulsions are readily isolated from nature, simple to grow on culture mediums, inexpensive to maintain, and more resistant to the damaging effects of UV irradiation than those in open fields (Batta 2016). Oil formulations (paraffin, mineral, cottonseed oil, and vegetable oils) assist in disrupting and penetrating the waxy cuticle layer by enhanced spore adhesion and germination (Kim et al. 2011; Mascarin and Jaronski 2016). Another strategy to retain moisture for spore germination is using an invert emulsion in which homogenization of water is done in oil at high speed. The process results in water droplets being encapsulated by oil droplets, which helps prevent the water from evaporating at high temperature or during storage (Batta 2016).

Granular formulations of EPFs have also been highlighted for their effectiveness in managing pests in soil and on plants (Marciano et al. 2021). While they are relatively simple to produce and apply, their efficacy is heavily dependent on both biotic and abiotic factors. Once applied, factors such as wind and rain can displace the granules, preventing uniform distribution in the soil (Cafarchia et al. 2022). These EPFs are cultivated on solid substrates such as grains (e.g., corn, rice, and millet), dried and then combined with inert materials like clay minerals and ground plant residues to produce granules with a controlled and consistent size, with the active ingredient either firmly attached or embedded within (de Faria and Wraight 2007). These granules are typically distributed dry across the soil (Cafarchia et al. 2022).

Application of fungi in pastures has proven effective, targeting cattle directly appears to be a more economically viable method for controlling cattle ticks (e.g., *R. microplus*), especially given the extensive range that free-range cattle cover in most tropical and subtropical countries (Fernandes et al. 2012). Using fungi in the field remains crucial for managing certain tick species, such as those with a heteroxenous life cycle (e.g., *Amblyomma* spp. or *Rhipicephalus appendiculatus*), ticks that parasitize birds, ticks on penned animals, or ticks in wild habitats (Fernandes et al. 2012). Additionally, using fungus-treated traps baited with semi chemicals could reduce the need to treat large areas of pasture with EPF, thereby aiding in field-level tick control (Nchu et al. 2010). Despite the significant potential for a fungal product designed for topical application on cattle, the micro-environmental conditions of cattle skin could adversely impact the effectiveness of the fungi. However, advancements in formulating suitable fungal strains could potentially address these skin condition challenges (Polar et al. 2008).

Although many commercial products based on EPFs are available, they are generally costlier than chemical alternatives. The associated costs are due to the inert materials and additives used in these antimicrobial products. The mass production of EPFs still remains challenging as it requires production of conidia or propagules which should be tolerant to environmental stresses (Baker et al. 2020). The biological activity of these fungal agents can be boosted by employing nanotechnology in formulating fungal propagules, for example, encapsulation of conidia can lead to their protection to enhance their effectiveness (Fernandes et al. 2012; Cafarchia et al. 2022). Additionally, development of an effective biocontrol agent requires selection of fungal isolates with better genetic and phenotypic traits which improve their resilience in the environment. Suitable management strategies must be considered according to the environmental microclimates to make these biocontrol agents more effective (Ekesi and Maniania 2007).

## 12.8 Conclusions and Recommendations

Environmental and food safety concerns call for application of EPFs as biocontrol agents. Two common EPFs such as *B. bassiana* and *M. anisopliae* are widely used in pest management programs due to their easy delivery and infection potential for wide range of arthropod species including ticks: soft and hard. As EPFs, being natural agents, do not induce resistance among arthropods, their utilization for managing pesticide-resistant populations could be a viable option in integrated pest management programs to reduce usage of chemically formulated pesticides. Despite promising laboratory results in controlling ticks, a significant limitation in employment of these EPFs is requirement of longer duration of action compared to chemical pesticides/acaricides. Even though there is benefit of self-regeneration and dissemination, numerous hurdles exist technically for proving their effectiveness like short shelf life, slow action rate (usually taking 15–21 days to kill the ticks), dependence on favorable environmental factors like high humidity, and expensive production of commercial formulations. Moreover, risk of contamination from mycotoxins is another considerable issue. Therefore, to enhance the efficacy of EPFs, new methods of delivery and production are required. Modification of traits to improve their performance through advanced molecular techniques and a better and deeper understanding of their ecology can improve the field efficacy of entomopathogens. More research is needed as studies till date have not fully explored that how EPFs might affect the vector competence of ticks. Development of long-lasting formulations with better infective potential, at least lasting for more than 5 months after application with improved delivery methods must be undertaken. Use of biopolymers could be better approach in given circumstances when sprayable wettable powders or oil formulations face challenges related to the viability and virulence due to abiotic factors. For more cost-effective, safe, and environmentally friendly pest control, advancement in current technologies are needed to maximize the exposure of target species with minimal inoculum concentrations.

## References

Abdigoudarzi M, Esmaeilnia K, Shariat N (2009) Laboratory study on biological control of ticks (Acari: Ixodidae) by entomopathogenic indigenous fungi (*Beauveria bassiana*). Iran J Arthrop Borne Dis 3(2):36

Alonso-Díaz MA, García L, Galindo-Velasco E, Lezama-Gutierrez R, Angel-Sahagún CA, Rodríguez-Vivas RI, Fragoso-Sánchez H (2007) Evaluation of *Metarhizium anisopliae* (Hyphomycetes) for the control of Boophilus microplus (Acari: Ixodidae) on naturally infested cattle in the Mexican tropics. Vet Parasitol 147(3–4):336–340

Alves FM, Bernardo CC, Paixão FR, Barreto LP, Luz C, Humber RA, Fernandes ÉK (2017) Heat-stressed *Metarhizium anisopliae*: viability (in vitro) and virulence (in vivo) assessments against the tick *Rhipicephalus sanguineus*. Parasitol Res 116:111–121

Amiri-Besheli B, Khambay B, Cameron S, Deadman ML, Butt TM (2000) Inter-and intra-specific variation in destruxin production by insect pathogenic *Metarhizium* spp., and its significance to pathogenesis. Mycol Res 104(4):447–452

Angelo IC, Gôlo PS, Camargo MG, Kluck GEG, Folly E, Bittencourt V (2010) Haemolymph protein and lipid profile of *Rhipicephalus* (*Boophilus*) *microplus* infected by fungi. Transbound Emerg Dis 57(1–2):79–83

Bahiense TC, Fernandes ÉK, Angelo IDC, Perinotto WM, Bittencourt VR (2008) Performance of *Metarhizium anisopliae* and its combination with Deltamethrin against a Pyrethroid-resistant strain of *Boophilus microplus* in a stall test. Ann N Y Acad Sci 1149(1):242–245

Baker D, Rice S, Leemon D, Godwin R, James P (2020) Development of a mycoinsecticide bait formulation for the control of house flies, *Musca domestica* L. Insects 11(1):47

Basso LMDS, Monteiro AC, Belo MADA, Soares VE, Garcia MV, Mochi DA (2005) Controle de larvas de *Boophilus microplus* por *Metarhizium anisopliae* em pastagens infestadas artificialmente. Pesq Agrop Brasileira 40:595–600

Bateman RP, Alves RT (2000) Delivery systems for mycoinsecticides using oil-based formulations. Asp Appl Biol 57:163–170

Batta YA (2016) Recent advances in formulation and application of entomopathogenic fungi for biocontrol of stored-grain insects. Biocontrol Sci Tech 26(9):1171–1183

Benelli G, Jeffries CL, Walker T (2016) Biological control of mosquito vectors: past, present, and future. Insects 7(4):52

Bernardo CC, Barreto LP, e Silva CDS, Luz C, Arruda W, Fernandes ÉK (2018) Conidia and blastospores of *Metarhizium* spp. and *Beauveria bassiana* sl: their development during the infection process and virulence against the tick *Rhipicephalus microplus*. Ticks Tick Borne Dis 9(5):1334–1342

Beys-da-Silva WO, Rosa RL, Berger M, Coutinho-Rodrigues CJ, Vainstein MH, Schrank A, Bittencourt VREP, Santi L (2020) Updating the application of *Metarhizium anisopliae* to control cattle tick *Rhipicephalus microplus* (Acari: Ixodidae). Exp Parasitol 208:107812

Cafarchia C, Immediato D, Iatta R, Ramos RAN, Lia RP, Porretta D, Figuredo LA, Dantas-Torres F, Otranto D (2015) Native strains of *Beauveria bassiana* for the control of *Rhipicephalus sanguineus* sensu lato. Parasit Vectors 8:1–7

Cafarchia C, Pellegrino R, Romano V, Friuli M, Demitri C, Pombi M, Benelli G, Otranto D (2022) Delivery and effectiveness of entomopathogenic fungi for mosquito and tick control: current knowledge and research challenges. Acta Trop 234:106627

Castellanos-Moguel J, González-Barajas M, Mier T, del Rocío Reyes-Montes M, Aranda E, Toriello C (2007) Virulence testing and extracellular subtilisin-like (Pr1) and trypsin-like (Pr2) activity during propagule production of *Paecilomyces fumosoroseus* isolates from whiteflies (Homoptera: Aleyrodidae). Rev Iberoam Micol 24(1):62

Dannon HF, Dannon AE, Douro-Kpindou OK, Zinsou AV, Houndete AT, Toffa-Mehinto J, Elegbede IATM, Olou BD, Tamò M (2020) Toward the efficient use of *Beauveria bassiana* in integrated cotton insect pest management. J Cotton Res 3:1–21

de Cássia Vieira Paião J, Monteiro AC, do Nascimento Kronka S (2001) Susceptibility of the cattle tick *Boophilus microplus* (Acari: Ixodidae) to isolates of the fungus Beauveria bassiana. World J Microbiol Biotechnol 17:245–251

de Faria MR, Wraight SP (2007) Mycoinsecticides and mycoacaricides: a comprehensive list with worldwide coverage and international classification of formulation types. Biol Control 43(3):237–256

de Lima JDA, Vilela VO, Battisti L, Potrich M, Lozano ER (2022) Entomopathogenic fungi and plant natural products against cattle tick *Rhipicephalus microplus* (Acarina: Ixodidae). Int J Trop Insect Sci 42(5):3593–3600

de Melo DR, Reis RC, Bittencourt VRE (2006) Patogenicidade in vitro do fungo *Metarhizium anisopliae* (Metschnikoff, 1879) Sorokin, 1883, sobre o carrapato *Boophilus microplus* (Canestrini, 1887). Rev Bras Parasitol Vet 15(4):157–162

Ekesi S, Maniania NK (2007) Use of entomopathogenic fungi in biological pest management. Research Signpost, Nairobi, p 333

Fang W, Leng B, Xiao Y, Jin K, Ma J, Fan Y, Feng J, Yang X, Zhang Y, Pei Y (2005) Cloning of *Beauveria bassiana* chitinase gene Bbchit1 and its application to improve fungal strain virulence. Appl Environ Microbiol 71(1):363–370

Fernandes ÉKK, da Costa GL, de Souza EJ, de Moraes AML, Bittencourt VREP (2003) *Beauveria bassiana* isolated from engorged females and tested against eggs and larvae of *Boophilus microplus* (Acari: Ixodidae). J Basic Microbiol 43(5):393–398

Fernandes EK, Rangel DE, Moraes AM, Bittencourt VR, Roberts DW (2007) Variability in tolerance to UV-B radiation among *Beauveria* spp. isolates. J Invertebr Pathol 96(3):237–243

Fernandes EK, Rangel DE, Moraes AM, Bittencourt VR, Roberts DW (2008) Cold activity of *Beauveria* and *Metarhizium*, and thermotolerance of *Beauveria*. J Invertebr Pathol 98(1):69–78

Fernandes ÉK, Angelo IC, Rangel DE, Bahiense TC, Moraes ÁM, Roberts DW, Bittencourt VR (2011) An intensive search for promising fungal biological control agents of ticks, particularly *Rhipicephalus microplus*. Vet Parasitol 182(2–4):307–318

Fernandes ÉK, Bittencourt VR, Roberts DW (2012) Perspectives on the potential of entomopathogenic fungi in biological control of ticks. Exp Parasitol 130(3):300–305

Fernandes ÉK, Rangel DE, Braga GU, Roberts DW (2015) Tolerance of entomopathogenic fungi to ultraviolet radiation: a review on screening of strains and their formulation. Curr Genet 61:427–440

Fernández-Salas A, Alonso-Díaz MA, Alonso-Morales RA (2019) Effect of entomopathogenic native fungi from paddock soils against *Rhipicephalus microplus* larvae with different toxicological behaviors to acaricides. Exp Parasitol 204:107729

Fiorotti J, Urbanová V, Gôlo PS, Bittencourt VREP, Kopáček P (2022) The role of complement in the tick cellular immune defense against the entomopathogenic fungus *Metarhizium robertsii*. Dev Comp Immunol 126:104234

Garcia MV, da Silva Rodrigues V, Monteiro AC, Simi LD, de Oliveira Souza Higa L, Martins MM, Pretty N, Mochi DA, Andreotti R, Szabó MPJ (2018) In vitro efficacy of *Metarhizium anisopliae* sensu lato against unfed *Amblyomma parvum* (Acari: Ixodidae). Exp Appl Acarol 76:507–512

Ghosh S, Nagar G (2014) Problem of ticks and tick-borne diseases in India with special emphasis on progress in tick control research: a review. J Vector Borne Dis 51(4):259–270

Gindin G, Samish M, Alekseev E, Glazer I (2001) The susceptibility of *Boophilus annulatus* (Ixodidae) ticks to entomopathogenic fungi. Biocontrol Sci Tech 11(1):111–118

Gindin G, Samish M, Zangi G, Mishoutchenko A, Glazer I (2002) The susceptibility of different species and stages of ticks to entomopathogenic fungi. Exp Appl Acarol 28:283–288

Harrison RL, Bonning BC (2010) Proteases as insecticidal agents. Toxins 2(5):935–953

Hartelt K, Wurst E, Collatz J, Zimmermann G, Kleespies RG, Oehme RM, Kimmig P, Steidle JLM, Mackenstedt U (2008) Biological control of the tick *Ixodes ricinus* with entomopathogenic fungi and nematodes: preliminary results from laboratory experiments. Int J Med Microbiol 298:314–320

Hedimbi M, Kaaya GP, Chinsembu KC (2011) Mortalities induced by entomopathogenic fungus *Metarhizium anisopliae* to different ticks of economic importance using two formulations. Int Res J Microbiol 2(4):141–145

Herlinda S (2010) Spore density and viability of entomopathogenic fungal isolates from Indonesia, and their virulence against *Aphis gossypii* glover (Homoptera: Aphididae). Trop Life Sci Res 21(1):11

Hernandez-Tenorio F, Miranda AM, Rodríguez CA, Giraldo-Estrada C, Sáez AA (2022) Potential strategies in the biopesticide formulations: a bibliometric analysis. Agronomy 12(11):2665

Islam W, Adnan M, Shabbir A, Naveed H, Abubakar YS, Qasim M, Tayyab M, Noman A, Nisar MS, Khan KA, Ali H (2021) Insect-fungal-interactions: a detailed review on entomopathogenic fungi pathogenicity to combat insect pests. Microb Pathog 159:105122

Jarrold SL, Moore D, Potter U, Charnley AK (2007) The contribution of surface waxes to pre-penetration growth of an entomopathogenic fungus on host cuticle. Mycol Res 111(2):240–249

Kaaya GP (2000) Laboratory and field evaluation of entomogenous fungi for tick control. Ann N Y Acad Sci 916(1):559–564

Kaaya GP, Hassan S (2000) Entomogenous fungi as promising biopesticides for tick control. Exp Appl Acarol 24:913–926

Kaaya GP, Hedimbi M (2012) The use of entomopathogenic fungi, *Beauveria bassiana* and *Metarhizium anisopliae*, as bio-pesticides for tick control. Int J Agric Sci 2(6):245–250

Kim JS, Je YH, Woo EO, Park JS (2011) Persistence of *Isaria fumosorosea* (Hypocreales: Cordycipitaceae) SFP-198 conidia in corn oil-based suspension. Mycopathologia 171:67–75

Kirkland BH, Cho EM, Keyhani NO (2004a) Differential susceptibility of *Amblyomma maculatum* and *Amblyomma americanum* (Acari: Ixodidea) to the entomopathogenic fungi *Beauveria bassiana* and *Metarhizium anisopliae*. Biol Control 31(3):414–421

Kirkland BH, Westwood GS, Keyhani NO (2004b) Pathogenicity of entomopathogenic fungi *Beauveria bassiana* and *Metarhizium anisopliae* to Ixodidae tick species *Dermacentor variabilis*, *Rhipicephalus sanguineus*, and *Ixodes scapularis*. J Med Entomol 41(4):705–711

Kirkland BH, Eisa A, Keyhani NO (2005) Oxalic acid as a fungal acaracidal virulence factor. J Med Entomol 42(3):346–351

Lacey LA, Grzywacz D, Shapiro-Ilan DI, Frutos R, Brownbridge M, Goettel MS (2015) Insect pathogens as biological control agents: Back to the future. J Invertebr Pathol 132:1–41

Lee MR, Li D, Lee SJ, Kim JC, Kim S, Park SE, Baek S, Shin TY, Lee DH, Kim JS (2019) Use of *Metarhizum aniopliae* sl to control soil-dwelling longhorned tick, *Haemaphysalis longicornis*. J Invertebr Pathol 166:e107230

Leemon DM, Jonsson NN (2008) Laboratory studies on Australian isolates of *Metarhizium anisopliae* as a biopesticide for the cattle tick *Boophilus microplus*. J Invertebr Pathol 97(1):40–49

Lei CJ, Halim NA, Asib N, Zakaria A, Azmi WA (2022) Conidial emulsion formulation and thermal storability of *Metarhizium anisopliae* against red palm weevil, *Rhynchophorus ferrugineus Olivier* (Coleoptera: Dryophthoridae). Microorganisms 10(7):1460

Lorenz SC, Humbert P, Patel AV (2020) Chitin increases drying survival of encapsulated *Metarhizium pemphigi* blastospores for Ixodes ricinus control. Ticks Tick Borne Dis 11(6):101537

Luz C, D'Alessandro WB, Rodrigues J, Fernandes ÉKK (2016) Efficacy of water-and oil-in-water-formulated *Metarhizium anisopliae* in *Rhipicephalus sanguineus* eggs and eclosing larvae. Parasitol Res 115:143–149

Madison-Antenucci S, Kramer LD, Gebhardt LL, Kauffman E (2020) Emerging tick-borne diseases. Clin Microbiol Rev 33(2):10–1128

Marciano AF, Golo PS, Coutinho-Rodrigues CJB, Camargo MG, Fiorotti J, Mesquita E, Corrêa TA, Perinotto WMS, Bittencourt VREP (2020) *Metarhizium anisopliae* sensu lato (sl) oil-in-water emulsions drastically reduced *Rhipicephalus microplus* larvae outbreak population on artificially infested grass. Med Vet Entomol 34(4):488–492

Marciano AF, Mascarin GM, Franco RFF, Golo PS, Jaronski ST, Fernandes ÉKK, Bittencourt VREP (2021) Innovative granular formulation of *Metarhizium robertsii* microsclerotia and blastospores for cattle tick control. Sci Rep 11(1):4972

Mascarin GM, Jaronski ST (2016) The production and uses of *Beauveria bassiana* as a microbial insecticide. World J Microbiol Biotechnol 32:1–26

Mesquita ES, Marciano AF, Corval AR, Fiorotti J, Corrêa TA, Quinelato S, Bittencourt VREP, Golo PS (2020) Efficacy of a native isolate of the entomopathogenic fungus *Metarhizium anisopliae* against larval tick outbreaks under semifield conditions. BioControl 65:353–362

Msangi S, Zekeya N, Kimaro E, Kusiluka L, Shirima G (2022) Entomopathogenic fungi (*aspergillus oryzae*) as biological control agent of cattle ticks in Tanzania. J Vet Med Anim Health 14(3):52–61

Murigu MM, Nana P, Waruiru RM, Nga'nga CJ, Ekesi S, Maniania NK (2016) Laboratory and field evaluation of entomopathogenic fungi for the control of amitraz-resistant and susceptible strains of *Rhipicephalus decoloratus*. Vet Parasitol 225:12–18

Narladkar BW (2018) Projected economic losses due to vector and vector-borne parasitic diseases in livestock of India and its significance in implementing the concept of integrated practices for vector management. Vet World 11(2):151

Nchu F, Maniania NK, Hassanali A, Eloff JN (2010) Performance of a *Metarhizium anisopliae*-treated semiochemical-baited trap in reducing *Amblyomma variegatum* populations in the field. Vet Parasitol 169(3–4):367–372

Onofre SB, Miniuk CM, de Barros NM, Azevedo JL (2001) Pathogenicity of four strains of entomopathogenic fungi against the bovine tick *Boophilus microplus*. Am J Vet Res 62(9):1478–1480

Ortiz-Urquiza A, Keyhani NO (2013) Action on the surface: entomopathogenic fungi versus the insect cuticle. Insects 4(3):357–374

Pacheco R, Ortiz S, Haddad M, Vansteelandt M (2022) Fungal endophytes: a source of antibacterial and antiparasitic compounds. In: Chassagne, F(Ed.), medicinal plants as anti-infectives, current knowledge and new perspectives. Academic Press, New York, pp 383–437

Pedrini N, Crespo R, Juárez MP (2007) Biochemistry of insect epicuticle degradation by entomopathogenic fungi. Comparat Biochem Physiol C Toxicol Pharmacol 146(1–2):124–137

Pedrini N, Zhang S, Juarez MP, Keyhani NO (2010) Molecular characterization and expression analysis of a suite of cytochrome P450 enzymes implicated in insect hydrocarbon degradation in the entomopathogenic fungus *Beauveria bassiana*. Microbiology 156(8):2549–2557

Perinotto WMS, Angelo IC, Golo PS, Quinelato S, Camargo MG, Sá FA, Bittencourt VREP (2012) Susceptibility of different populations of ticks to entomopathogenic fungi. Exp Parasitol 130(3):257–260

Perveen N, bin Muzaffar S, Al-Deeb MA (2021) Ticks and tick-borne diseases of livestock in the middle east and noricinuica: a review. Insects 12:1–35

Polar P, Kairo MT, Moore D, Pegram R, John SA (2005) Comparison of water, oils and emulsifiable adjuvant oils as formulating agents for *Metarhizium anisopliae* for use in control of *Boophilus microplus*. Mycopathologia 160:151–157

Polar P, Moore D, Kairo MT, Ramsubhag A (2008) Topically applied myco-acaricides for the control of cattle ticks: overcoming the challenges. Exp Appl Acarol 46:119–148

Prado-Rebolledo OF, Molina-Ochoa J, Lezama-Gutiérrez R, García-Márquez LJ, Minchaca-Llerenas YB, Morales-Barrera E, Tellez G, Hargis B, Skoda SR, Foster JE (2017) Effect of *Metarhizium anisopliae* (ascomycete), cypermethrin, and D-limonene, alone and combined, on larval mortality of *Rhipicephalus sanguineus* (Acari: Ixodidae). J Med Entomol 54(5):1323–1327

Prakash BGVS, Padmaja V, Jami SK, Kirti PB (2012) Expression of chitinase genes of *Metarhizium anisopliae* isolates in lepidopteran pests and on synthetic media. J Basic Microbiol 52(6):628–635

Qayyum AM, Bilal H, Ali H, Raza H, Wajid M (2021) Factors affecting the epizootics of entomopathogenic fungi—a review. J Bioresour Manag 8(4):78–85

Quesada-Moraga E, Navas-Cortés JA, Maranhao EA, Ortiz-Urquiza A, Santiago-Álvarez C (2007) Factors affecting the occurrence and distribution of entomopathogenic fungi in natural and cultivated soils. Mycol Res 111(8):947–966

Quinelato S, Golo PS, Perinotto WM, Sá FA, Camargo MG, Angelo IC, Moraes AML, Bittencourt VREP (2012) Virulence potential of *Metarhizium anisopliae* sl isolates on *Rhipicephalus (Boophilus) microplus* larvae. Vet Parasitol 190(3–4):556–565

Rangel DE, Braga GU, Fernandes ÉK, Keyser CA, Hallsworth JE, Roberts DW (2015) Stress tolerance and virulence of insect-pathogenic fungi are determined by environmental conditions during conidial formation. Curr Genet 61:383–404

Reis RCS, Fernandes EKK, Bittencourt VREP (2008) Fungal formulations to control *Rhipicephalus sanguineus* engorged females. Ann N Y Acad Sci 1149(1):239–241

Ren Q, Chen Z, Luo J, Liu G, Guan G, Liu Z, Liu A, Li Y, Niu Q, Liu J, Yang J, Han X, Yin H, Luo J (2016) Laboratory evaluation of *Beauveria bassiana* and *Metarhizium anisopliae* in the control of *Haemaphysalis qinghaiensis* in China. Exp Appl Acarol 69:233–238

Rohrlich C, Merle I, Mze Hassani I, Verger M, Zuin M, Besse S, Robène I, Nibouche S, Costet L (2018) Variation in physiological host range in three strains of two species of the entomopathogenic fungus *Beauveria*. PLoS One 13(7):e0199199

Russo ML, Scorsetti AC, Vianna MF, Cabello M, Ferreri N, Pelizza S (2019) Endophytic effects of *Beauveria bassiana* on corn (*Zea mays*) and its herbivore, *Rachiplusia nu* (Lepidoptera: Noctuidae). Insects 10(4):110

Samish M, Gindin G, Alekseev E, Glazer I (2001) Pathogenicity of entomopathogenic fungi to different developmental stages of *Rhipicephalus sanguineus* (Acari: Ixodidae). J Parasitol 87(6):1355–1359
Samish M, Rot A, Ment D, Barel S, Glazer I, Gindin G (2014) Efficacy of the entomopathogenic fungus *Metarhizium brunneum* in controlling the tick *Rhipicephalus annulatus* under field conditions. Vet Parasitol 206(3–4):258–266
Sewify GH, Habib SM (2001) Biological control of the tick fowl Argas persicargas persicus by the entomopathogenic fungi *Beauveria bassiana* and *Metarhizium anisopliae*. J Pestic Sci 74:121–123
Sinha KK, Choudhary AK, Kumari P (2016) Entomopathogenic fungi. In: Omkar BT (ed) Ecofriendly pest management for food security. Academic Press, Cambridge, MA, pp 475–505
Souza EJ, Costa GL, Bittencourt VREP, Fagundes AS (2009) Action of the fungus *Beauveria bassiana* associated with cellulose polymerized gel in the control of the tick *Anocentor nitens* in a field test. Arquivo Brasileiro de Medicina Veterinária e Zootecnia 61:163–169
Sullivan CF, Parker BL, Davari A, Lee MR, Kim JS, Skinner M (2020) Evaluation of spray applications of *Metarhizium anisopliae*, *Metarhizium brunneum* and *Beauveria bassiana* against larval winter ticks, *Dermacentor albipictus*. Exp Appl Acarol 82:559–570
Tavasoli M, Ounagh AG, Memari R, Rahmani S, Mardani K, Butt T (2009) Laboratory evaluation of three strains of the entomopathogenic fungus *Metarhizium anisopliae* for controlling *Hyalomma anatolicum anatolicum* and *Haemaphysalis punctata*. Iran J Vet Med 3(1):11–15
Tofiño Rivera AP, Ortega Cuadros M, Pedraza Claros B, Perdomo Ayola SC, Moya Romero DC (2018) Effectiveness of *Beauveria bassiana* (Baubassil®) on the common cattle tick *Rhipicephalus microplus* in the Department of Guajira, Colombia. Rev Argent Microbiol 50(4):426–430
Wassermann M, Selzer P, Steidle JL, Mackenstedt U (2016) Biological control *of Ixodes ricinus* larvae and nymphs with *Metarhizium anisopliae* blastospores. Ticks Tick Borne Dis 7(5):768–771
Webster A, Souza UA, Martins JR, Klafke G, Reck J, Schrank A (2018) Comparative study between larval packet test and larval immersion test to assess the effect of *Metarhizium anisopliae* on *Rhipicephalus microplus* tick larvae. Exp Appl Acarol 74(4):455–461
World Health Organization (2020) Vector borne diseases. https://www.who.int/news-room/fact-sheets/detail/vector-borne-diseases
Xiao G, Ying SH, Zheng P, Wang ZL, Zhang S, Xie XQ, Shang Y, St Leger RJ, Zhao GP, Wang C, Feng MG (2012) Genomic perspectives on the evolution of fungal entomopathogenicity in *Beauveria bassiana*. Sci Rep 2(1):483
Zabalgogeazcoa I, Oleaga A, Pérez-Sánchez R (2008) Pathogenicity of endophytic entomopathogenic fungi to *Ornithodoros erraticus* and *Ornithodoros moubata* (Acari: Argasidae). Vet Parasitol 158(4):336–343
Zeina G, Laing M (2022) Isolation and evaluation of south African isolates of *Beauveria bassiana* (Hypocreales: Cordycipitaceae) on *Rhipicephalus microplus* (Acari: Ixodidae). Exp Appl Acarol 86:157–171
Zhendong H, Guangfu Y, Zhong Z, Ruiling Z (2019) Phylogenetic relationships and effectiveness of four *Beauveria bassiana* sensu lato strains for control of *Haemaphysalis longicornis* (Acari: Ixodidae). Exp Appl Acarol 77:83–92
Zheng P, Xia Y, Xiao G, Xiong C, Hu X, Zhang S, Zheng H, Huang Y, Zhou Y, Wang S, Zhao GP, Liu X, St Leger RJ, Wang C (2012) Genome sequence of the insect pathogenic fungus *Cordyceps militaris*, a valued traditional Chinese medicine. Genome Biol 12:1–22
Zibaee A, Malagoli D (2014) Immune response of *Chilo suppressalis* Walker (Lepidoptera: Crambidae) larvae to different entomopathogenic fungi. Bull Entomol Res 104(2):155–163
Zibaee A, Ramzi S (2018) Cuticle-degrading proteases of entomopathogenic fungi: from biochemistry to biological performance. Arch Phytopathol Plant Protect 51(13–14):779–794.

The manufacturer's authorised representative in the EU is Springer Nature Customer Service Centre GmbH, Europaplatz 3, 69115 Heidelberg, Germany. If you have any concerns regarding our products, please contact ProductSafety@springernature.com

Printed and bound by CPI Group (UK) Ltd, Croydon, CR0 4YY
01/10/2026
02225949-0012